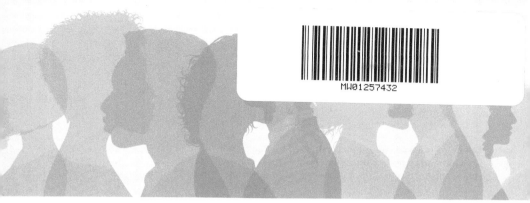

THE NEW LEADERSHIP CHALLENGE

Creating the Future of Nursing

SEVENTH EDITION

Abby E. Garlock, DNP, RN, CNE, LCCE
Professor
Hunt School of Nursing
Gardner-Webb University
Boiling Springs, North Carolina

Nicole P. Waters, DNP, RN, CNE
Professor
Hunt School of Nursing
Gardner-Webb University
Boiling Springs, North Carolina

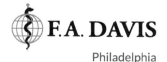

Philadelphia

F.A. Davis Company
1915 Arch Street
Philadelphia, PA 19103
www.fadavis.com

Printed in the United States of America

Last digit indicates print number: 10 9 8 7 6 5 4 3 2 1
Sponsoring Editor, Nursing: Haleahy Craven
Content Project Manager: Veronica Neff
Design and Illustration Manager: Carolyn O'Brien

As new scientific information becomes available through basic and clinical research, recommended treatments and drug therapies undergo changes. The author(s) and publisher have done everything possible to make this book accurate, up to date, and in accord with accepted standards at the time of publication. The author(s), editors, and publisher are not responsible for errors or omissions or for consequences from application of the book, and make no warranty, expressed or implied, in regard to the contents of the book. Any practice described in this book should be applied by the reader in accordance with professional standards of care used in regard to the unique circumstances that may apply in each situation. The reader is advised always to check product information (package inserts) for changes and new information regarding dose and contraindications before administering any drug. Caution is especially urged when using new or infrequently ordered drugs.

Library of Congress Cataloging-in-Publication Data

Names: Garlock, Abby E., author. | Waters, Nicole P., author. | Grossman, Sheila. New leadership challenge.
Title: The new leadership challenge : creating the future of nursing / Abby E. Garlock, Nicole P. Waters.
Description: Seventh edition. | Philadelphia : F.A. Davis, [2025] | Preceded by The new leadership challenge / Sheila C. Grossman, Theresa M. "Terry" Valiga. Sixth edition. 2020. | Includes bibliographical references and index.
Identifiers: LCCN 2024045885 (print) | LCCN 2024045886 (ebook) | ISBN 9781719650601 (paperback) | ISBN 9781719654302 (epub) | ISBN 9781719654319 (pdf)
Subjects: MESH: Nursing, Supervisory | Leadership | Nurse Administrators
Classification: LCC RT89 (print) | LCC RT89 (ebook) | NLM WY 105 | DDC 610.73068--dc23/eng/20241204
LC record available at https://lccn.loc.gov/2024045885
LC ebook record available at https://lccn.loc.gov/2024045886

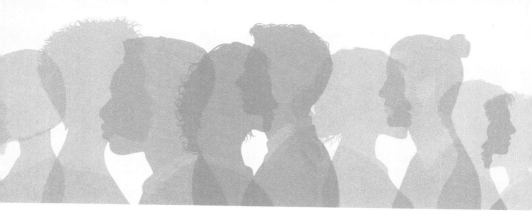

This book is dedicated to each nurse who still believes in the ability to make a difference for those we serve, and all my students and colleagues who helped me understand what it truly means to be a leader and a good follower. I also dedicate this book to my husband, Brandon, and children, Phineas and Penelope. Thank you for your love, support, and encouragement.

AEG

This book is dedicated to those who believed in me and empowered me to be my authentic self. I have experienced a life of supportive family, friends, colleagues, and students who have inspired me to lead and follow others; this book is dedicated to all of you. I dedicate this book to my husband, Nathan, for his constant support and unconditional love. To my children, Makayla, Abby, and Ethan, I dedicate this book as a lifelong example of overcoming challenges and following your dreams. This book also is dedicated in memory of my high school health sciences teacher and later a colleague, Mrs. Phyllis B. Elmore, a nurse, a mentor, and a friend. Finally, I dedicate this book to my grandmother and mother, for their unwavering love and support throughout my personal and professional pursuits. To all of you I am forever grateful.

NPW

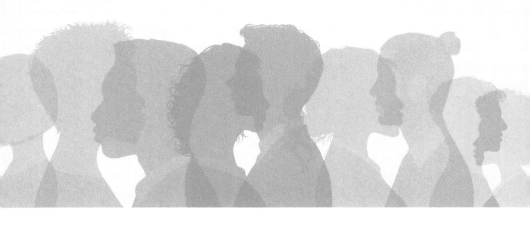

About the Authors

Dr. Abby E. Garlock, DNP, RN, CNE, LCCE, Professor, previously Chair of Doctoral Nursing Programs, and Chair of Pre-licensure Programs at the Gardner-Webb University Hunt School of Nursing, is recognized as a scholar and expert in leadership and mentoring. She has been a registered nurse since 2003 with experience in medical–surgical, pediatrics, newborn, and obstetrics. Dr. Garlock is a certified nurse educator and Lamaze-certified childbirth educator who has been engaging nursing students to foster intellect, excellence, and creativity since 2008.

Dr. Garlock has strengths in executing, strategic thinking, and relationship building. She uses these strengths, and values of integrity and learning, to create a vision for leadership and scholarship. Her primary research interests, publications, and presentations relate to learner empowerment. She also enjoys curriculum development, creative teaching strategies, and various professional issues.

Dr. Garlock earned her associate degree from Cleveland Community College, her baccalaureate degree from Winston-Salem State University, and her master's and doctoral degrees from the Gardner-Webb University.

Dr. Nicole P. Waters, DNP, RN, CNE, Professor of Hunt School of Nursing at Gardner-Webb University, has served in various leadership roles, RN-BSN Program Chair, Associate Dean and Dean of Nursing, University Faculty Chair-Elect, and currently as the Dean for the College of Health Sciences. These roles have allowed her to accumulate 10 years of collaborative leadership experience, resulting in strategic program revisions, expansion, and new program development. She is a 2015 National Lead for Nursing LEAD Alum and acknowledges the year-long formal leadership program as a pivotal point in her professional development and career trajectory.

Dr. Waters started her nursing career in 1998 as a Licensed Practical Nurse and became a Registered Nurse in 2001. She has experience in geriatrics, medical–surgical, orthopedics, and pediatrics. She is a certified nurse educator, actively engaging students since 2006. She has strengths in strategic thinking, investments in relationship building, and development. She encompasses the leadership skills to lead, influence, and co-create change within a student-focused community.

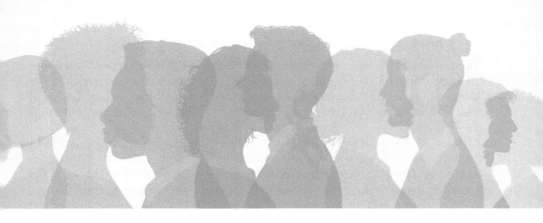

Preface

The New Leadership Challenge: Creating the Future of Nursing has been written as a reference book and textbook for undergraduate students in nursing, as well as for nurses in any practice role. The book also is helpful for nurses pursuing graduate study, including those preparing as clinical nurse leaders, nurse educators, or those pursuing Doctor of Nursing Practice (DNP) degrees. It provides an overview of significant ideas related to the multidimensional concept of "leadership" and explores the relevance of those ideas at various points throughout one's career development: beginning, intermediate, and advanced.

Each chapter includes learning objectives, a synthesis of extensive readings (from nursing and non-nursing literature) on the specific topic, a case study (except Chapter 1), and a variety of critical thinking exercises that are designed to help the reader better understand the topic and its relation to leadership and the development of individuals as leaders. In this updated edition, suggested answers to the chapter case studies have been included as a valuable resource for instructors. These answers are designed to assist instructors in facilitating both formative and summative feedback for students. Examples from clinical practice, education, and administration that relate to the specific topic and enhance learning about it are provided. Many critical thinking exercises are linked with a TED Talk, a YouTube video, or an interactive Web site. Resources from the arts and humanities that relate to the specific topic and enhance learning about it are provided, and examples from clinical practice, education, and administration are included.

Unlike many other textbooks and resource books that address leadership, this book takes that charge seriously. In many other books, particularly those written by nurses for nursing students and clinicians, the authors confuse leadership with management and, as a result, focus more on management than on leadership. Perhaps that is because the phenomenon of leadership is more elusive than that of management and because one cannot outline "steps" of leadership as one can do to some extent with management (e.g., planning, delegating, budgeting).

This book takes on the challenge of exploring the elements of authentic leadership, particularly in the "new world" context we face continually. It explores various definitions and conceptualizations of leadership, examines extant theories of leadership, analyzes the notion of vision and visionary leadership, tackles the intricacies of leader–follower relationships, and explains contemporary models of leadership that have evolved regarding the leader, follower, and context of healthcare situations.

The importance of followership, the facilitation of change, the management of conflict, the use and abuse of power, and the development of oneself and of others as leaders all are discussed. In essence, then, this book takes a broad look at the complex phenomenon of leadership and examines multiple dimensions of it.

The major points made throughout this book and its unifying elements are as follows: (1) although leadership and management are related, they are not one and the same; (2) leadership is not an innate ability, but one that can be learned and developed through conscious and purposeful effort; (3) one does not need to be in a position of authority to be a leader; (4) each of us can be, and perhaps needs to be, a leader if nursing is to advance as a profession and have a significant impact now and in the future; and (5) there are ways in which each of us can develop as a leader throughout our careers. These points are made and the goals of the book achieved through a balance of theoretical exploration; the extensive use of real-world examples from clinical practice, education, and administration; self-assessment exercises; and the integration of creative learning activities.

This seventh edition of *The New Leadership Challenge: Creating the Future of Nursing* continues to focus on nurses and nursing. It does not confuse leadership and management. It also explores the multifaceted concept of leadership in depth. As such, it is of value to several audiences.

Most undergraduate programs include a course in nursing leadership. However, although many courses carry the title "Nursing Leadership," most actually deal with management and delegation. In a world where experts recognize clearly that true leadership is needed for the future, *The New Leadership Challenge: Creating the Future of Nursing* meets a need, particularly for undergraduate programs that already have or will soon have a course that addresses true leadership.

Most graduate programs (both master's and doctoral) focus on the preparation of graduates for leadership roles in the profession; thus, a focus on leadership is appropriate. Students preparing as advanced practice nurses, clinical nurse leaders, nurse administrators, or nurse educators do not want to use a text that "advertises" leadership but "delivers" management; if they wanted management, they would have pursued an MBA or a graduate degree in healthcare administration. Instead, they want a text that helps them understand what leadership is and how it relates to the roles for which they are preparing. This book meets that need.

Finally, this book serves as a valuable resource for nurses in clinical practice, nurse researchers, nurse educators, and nurse administrators who see the need to learn more about the phenomenon of leadership and how to develop those abilities in themselves and in others (e.g., fellow clinicians, students, one's staff). One's ongoing education in an ever-changing world cannot be limited to clinical, teaching, or administrative knowledge and skills alone. It also must address broader knowledge and skills—such as those related to leadership—that are integral to one's practice.

One of the most important features of this book is the exposure to and integration of the extensive writings about leadership done by experts in that field; thus, the literature base for this book is not limited to nursing. This is purposeful and intended to broaden readers' perspectives and expose them to a much wider range of resources that can be tapped for ongoing personal development. However, many of the classic and primary sources on leadership have not been revised, so they have older publication dates. Whenever there is a revision and updated version, it has been provided. The annotated summaries of "must-read" books and articles on leadership included in this seventh edition are intended to help readers expand their horizons about leadership resources.

The New Leadership Challenge: Creating the Future of Nursing, as the title implies, also presents a clear orientation to the future. The book focused on the future—what organizations are expected to look like in the future, the skills that people associated with those organizations will need to survive and thrive, and the need to plan for a blending of professional and personal commitments. The old-model, hierarchic organization that characterizes so many healthcare agencies is no longer viable, and people in those organizations will need to be able to function and provide leadership in a contemporary environment. This book is designed to help professional nurses make this transition.

In addition to these important features, *The New Leadership Challenge: Creating the Future of Nursing* offers several other unique features. First, it includes the Grossman & Valiga Leadership Characteristics and Skills Assessment and the Creativity Ability Scale, which can be completed by the reader, who receives immediate feedback by using the answer sheets provided. Or if the reader is interested in using the tools for research studies, permission can be requested. Second, there are chapter PowerPoints and test banks available online from the F. A. Davis Web site. Third, an electronic instructor's guide is available; this resource offers numerous teaching approaches that might be used with undergraduate or graduate students and with nurses in practice. Overall, this book—conceptualized in its broadest sense—is designed to be interactive, stimulating, creative, challenging, and thought provoking.

Along with expanding on more findings from research, the seventh edition was updated, and relevant changes such as the National Academy of Medicine's (formerly the Institute of Medicine) 2020–2030 recommendations for how nurses can lead in improving healthcare are discussed. Several more contemporary perspectives on leadership, such as servant leadership, interactive leadership, and foresight leadership, are explored. Examined in greater depth are key elements of effective leadership such as trust and courage, personal power sources, organizational power sources, and willpower. Resources to support one's development as a leader; ideas for becoming a more transformational and authentic leader; strategies for becoming more innovative, creative, and resilient; hints for leading virtual teams; suggestions for becoming a board member; ideas for articulating one's message in a succinct yet comprehensive format; suggestions for using storytelling to lead change; communication strategies for dealing with difficult people and work challenges; and ideas for preparing one's legacy also are discussed.

Finally, this seventh edition provides a more in-depth exploration of concepts such as excellence; myths about mentoring; and the benefits of mentoring to the protégé, mentor, organization, and profession. Also addressed more deeply are chaos and complexity theory, adaptation to change, value-based care, creative cultures, workplace engagement, innovative intelligence, generation diversity, networking on social media in healthcare, creative leadership, artificial intelligence, the ways nurses contribute to the healthcare system reputation, and strategic foresight. All these additions/enhancements ensure that the book is relevant in today's context and the context anticipated in at least the relatively near future.

The intent of this book is to help nurses and nursing students explore the many facets of leadership and examine strategies that will aid them in (1) seeing themselves as leaders, (2) developing skills needed to function as leaders, and (3) taking on the challenges of a leadership role in the current and future healthcare, academic, or community setting. It challenges the reader's thinking, presents new ways to conceptualize leadership, and prepares nurses for their role as leaders in creating a preferred future for nursing. Readers are invited to open their minds to new perspectives; entertain the notion that the chaotic, uncertain world of today and tomorrow presents tremendous opportunities for nurse leaders to influence the future of our profession; and think of themselves as leaders who can develop in that role throughout their careers. We welcome you to the world of *The New Leadership Challenge: Creating the Future of Nursing*.

Abby E. Garlock
Nicole P. Waters

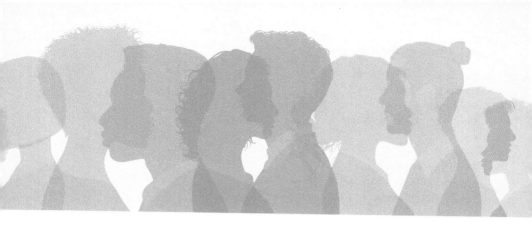

Reviewers from Previous Editions

Kay Cook, MSN, RN-BC, CNOR
Adjunct Instructor, Nursing Professional Development Specialist II, Clinical Instructor
Wilmington University, Christiana Care Health System, Neumann University
New Castle/Newark, Delaware

Lisa Drews, EdD, MSN, RN, CNE
Chair, MSN Leadership Program/Associate Professor
Wilmington University
New Castle, Delaware

Trudy Kuehn, RN, MSN, BN
Associate Professor Nursing, Lead Instructor ADN
Paul D. Camp Community College
Franklin, Virginia

Kelli Kusisto, MSN, RN
Associate Professor/Pre-Licensure Program Coordinator
Siena Heights University
Adrian, Michigan

Jan Meiers, RN, MN
BSN Faculty
North Island College
Courtenay, British Columbia

Jennifer Robinson, RN, MSN, CCRN
Instructor, Nursing
Washington Health System School of Nursing
Washington, Pennsylvania

Melody Sharp, DNP, RN-BC
Dean/Professor
Centra College of Nursing
Lynchburg, Virginia

Julie Slade, DNP, RN
Assistant Professor of Nursing/RN-BSN Program Coordinator
Chatham University
Pittsburgh, Pennsylvania

Jean Truman, DNP, RN, CNE
Assistant Dean of Academic Affairs & Associate Professor of Nursing
University of Pittsburgh at Bradford
Bradford, Pennsylvania

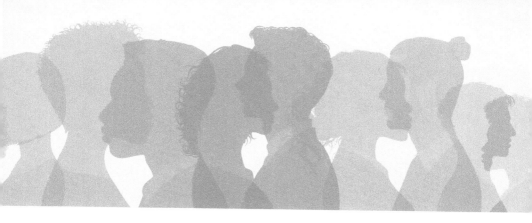

Acknowledgments

The authors wish to thank Haleahy Craven, sponsoring editor, for her expertise in guiding this seventh edition to publication. We also acknowledge Veronica Neff and Christine Abshire for all their assistance in the editing and publishing process of this book. Additionally, we express our deep gratitude to Dr. Valiga and Dr. Grossman for the foundation of this text in the previous six editions and for trusting us to carry forward their legacy in the seventh edition. Finally, we thank our families and friends for their love and support throughout the process of developing and writing this book.

AEG
NPW

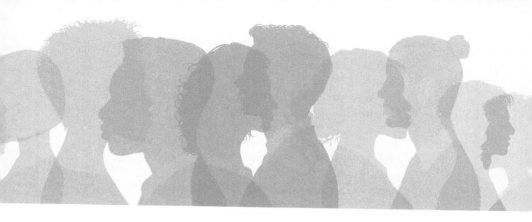

Contents

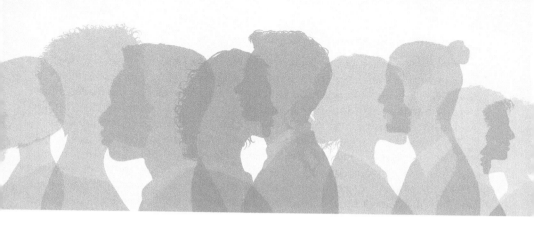

CHAPTER 1

The Phenomenon
of Leadership
Classic/Historical and Contemporary
Perspectives on Leadership

LEARNING OBJECTIVES
- Examine the multiple aspects of the phenomenon of leadership.
- Describe how leadership ability is a vital component of success for an individual; a unit, a department, or practice; and an organization, particularly in nursing.
- Compare and contrast major theoretical ideas about leadership from classic/historical and contemporary perspectives.
- Analyze how nurses can use a combination of classic and contemporary perspectives on leadership to strengthen their success as leaders of the healthcare team, within institutions, and for the profession.

INTRODUCTION

Chaos. Uncertainty. Unpredictability. Constant change. These are all characteristics of the world we live in, and all indications are that our future world will be even more chaotic, more uncertain, more unpredictable, and in even greater states of constant and unprecedented change. Such circumstances desperately call for new leaders, even though "being an effective leader in today's tumultuous world is almost impossible" (Tetenbaum & Laurence, 2011, p. 48).

Defining what leadership is, who leaders are, what leaders do, and how leadership is different from management—a phenomenon with which it is often confused—is no easy task. This chapter is intended to address these questions and help the reader understand the complex, multidimensional concept we refer to as *leadership*. It is also intended to challenge readers to consider the leadership we need in nursing today, to think about themselves as leaders, and to reflect on how leadership responsibilities can be integrated into their roles as professional nurses.

For almost a century, writers have attempted to describe leadership, and researchers have attempted to identify the defining characteristics of leaders. The outcome has been one obvious conclusion: "Leadership is one of the most observed and least understood phenomena on earth" (Burns, 1978, p. 2). It is multidimensional and multifaceted—a universal human phenomenon that many know when they see it, but few can define clearly.

In fact, there are almost as many different definitions of leadership as there are people who write about it. According to Bennis and Nanus (2003):

> Decades of academic analysis have given us more than 850 definitions of leadership. Literally thousands of empirical investigations of leaders have been conducted in the last seventy-five years alone, but no clear and unequivocal understanding exists as to what distinguishes leaders from nonleaders, and perhaps more important, what distinguishes *effective* leaders from *ineffective* leaders. (p. 4)

The lack of a "clear and unequivocal understanding" of leadership has led these experts on the subject to assert that "never have so many labored so long to say so little" (Bennis & Nanus, 2003, p. 4). Since 2003, when these authors noted more than 850 definitions in existence, even more definitions of and perspectives on the phenomenon of leadership have been proposed. Although no universally accepted definition has yet to be proposed, there is increasing clarity about what true leadership is and how it differs from the related concept of management.

The key to successful leadership today is influence, not authority. —Ken Blanchard

CLASSIC THEORIES OF LEADERSHIP

Great Man Theory

Leadership theories have evolved tremendously over the years (Bass, 2008). Among the earliest was the "great man theory," which asserted that one was a leader if one was born into the "right" family—usually a family of nobility—and possessed unique characteristics, most of which were inherited. Although some individuals who were born into the "right" family did accomplish extraordinary things and did, in fact, change the course of history, the notion that "leaders are born, not made" did not capture the imagination of the masses, and it failed to recognize that there was more to leadership than having royal blood. This conclusion has been substantiated through ample empirical research that illustrates that leadership can be learned (Dugan, 2017). In light of these limitations and insights, a search was begun for the traits or cluster of traits that would determine whether a person would be a leader.

Trait Theories

Personal trait theories of leadership attempted to distinguish leaders from other people and identify the universal characteristics of leadership. Not surprisingly, no qualities were found that were universal to all leaders, although several traits did seem to correlate with leadership: an abundant reserve of energy, an ability to maintain a high level of activity, better education, superior judgment, decisiveness, a breadth of knowledge, a high degree of verbal facility, good interpersonal skills, self-confidence, and creativity (Bass, 2008). In addition to the fact that these theories revealed no universal traits among leaders, they also failed to acknowledge the importance of the situation in which leadership occurred.

Situational Theories

Situational theories, in comparison, gave clear recognition to the significance of the environment and the particular situation as factors in the effectiveness of a leader. They asserted that the leader was the individual in a position to institute change when a situation was ready for it. In other words, the leader did not plan for a change, nor was the leader chosen by a group of followers; they just happened to be in the right place at the right time and took the action that was needed to resolve a crisis or manage a problem. Although this view of leadership was broader than merely looking at one's heritage or specific traits, it still did not capture the complexity of the phenomenon and failed to acknowledge one critical element in a leadership "event"—the followers.

As noted by Allen (2018), the study of the phenomenon of leadership "includes paradoxes and inconsistencies and is messy, hazy, and inconsistent" (p. 154). The development of new theories or new perspectives on the phenomenon are attempts, he says, to eliminate these issues.

CONTEMPORARY LEADERSHIP PERSPECTIVES

More contemporary leadership theories recognize that effective leadership depends partly on the personality of the leader, partly on the situation at hand or context of the situation, partly on the qualities and maturity of the followers, and partly on the culture of the organization or setting. In fact, multiple experts on leadership and followership (including Bennis & Nanus, 2003; Chaleff, 2009; Kellerman, 2008; Stech, 2004)—cited in *The Art of Followership* (Riggio et al., 2008)—continue to assert that without followers, there is no leadership; followers, therefore, are a most significant element in the leadership equation. Their needs, goals, abilities, sense of responsibility, degree of involvement, potential, and so forth are all important in determining the effectiveness of a leader.

The importance of followers is acknowledged by Northouse (2021) in the ninth edition of *Leadership: Theory & Practice*. In this comprehensive book, Northouse explains several leadership theories, gives examples of how each theory plays out in practice, and expands on the concept of followership—describing why this concept can be thought of as a leadership theory itself.

In addition to acknowledging the significance of followers, more modern theories recognize that leadership is not a random occurrence. Instead, it very much involves having a vision, co-creating and communicating that vision to others, planning with followers on how to make the vision a reality, effecting change, navigating conflict, empowering followers, serving as a symbol for the group, being a source of energy and renewal for the group, and taking responsibility for facilitating the ongoing development of followers. Additionally, contemporary leadership theories suggest that individuals can develop and improve their leadership ability.

Relational and Social Models

More and more, contemporary leadership theories are focused more on dyadic, relational, and complex social models than on an individual leader (Avolio, 2007; Yukl, 2006).

In her TED Talk, Torres (2013) advises people in healthcare to follow great leaders who are not "head-down but see around corners" and to surround themselves with people who think differently than they do. Tetenbaum and Laurence (2011) concur, stating that "homogenous groups tend to produce homogenous ideas. To achieve a high level of creative thought, it is necessary to bring together groups of people with different levels of expertise" (p. 44).

Leaders, therefore, must seek input from diverse groups and individuals with unique perspectives so that they will be less apt to succumb to "just going along with the group" or engaging in "groupthink," a psychological phenomenon by which the desire for conformity and harmony in a group result in dysfunctional decision making (Janus, 1982).

Despite the value of and need for leaders to work collaboratively with others, current trends suggest that leaders also need focused alone time; in other words, collaborating with a team should be balanced with having some individual alone time. Leaders need to spend time thinking about their role and responsibilities within an organization (Albert et al., 2022). Indeed, leaders and followers alike may feel more productive and creative when they have time to reflect on past and present situations and to think about future directions. The focus is on the leader and that individual's own challenges, priorities, and growth (Albert et al., 2022).

Transformational Leadership

This theory was first introduced by Burns (1978), who described it as being context based, a process for motivating followers believing in similar internal values directed toward the greater good, and having an emphasis for leaders and followers to enjoy a close bond. Bass (1985) expanded the work of Burns to explain how transformational leadership could be measured in terms of the leader's *influence* on followers and how followers could be motivated via transformational leadership to include four processes: (1) idealized influence, (2) inspirational motivation, (3) individualized consideration, and (4) intellectual stimulation. By *idealized influence*, the leader assists the follower to increase confidence, respect, and trust.

Inspirational motivation involves teaching the follower to be empowering, goal oriented, and responsible. *Individualized consideration* includes assisting the follower to increase self-esteem, continue working hard, and self-actualize. Last, *intellectual stimulation* involves assisting the follower to be creative, expand on ideas, and find new approaches to solve problems.

Transformational leaders inspire followers to "achieve extraordinary outcomes and, in the process, develop their own leadership capacity" (Clavelle & Prado-Inzerillo, 2018, p. 39). In other words, they motivate people to act and work diligently to accomplish the goal or attain the solution.

Sinek (2016) says one also has to think about the service or product in which the leader is involved. For example, people do not buy a product or service because of what it does—they buy it because of *why* it does what it does. He explains his golden circle theory of why Apple is so successful. The theory has three concentric circles: what the product or service is on the outside circle, how the product or service works in the middle circle, and why the product or service does what it does in the inside circle. This model can explain why patients need nurses—they perform an action but can also explain why it is so important to do the action and can also teach the patient this rationale, which could lead to increased patient adherence and better patient health. This is very transformational!

Certainly, transformational leaders can create adaptable, innovative teams that thrive amid change if they practice the above transformational leadership methods. Through real-life experiences, Carrig and Snell (2019) offer hints for executing excellence or, in other words, leading the transformational change so it is sustainable—for as long as it is successful. With continuous change and chaos in the healthcare system, many of our transformational solutions should not be forever. Another idea to consider is not to focus just on the product's being successful. For example, nurses and other healthcare providers obsess about attaining the highest quality care for our patients (look at how many measurements are being performed to document quality patient care!) rather than looking more at the processes that occur to obtain the highest quality of care. Christenson et al. (2016) suggest looking at what you hoped that product would do and not just at the product itself. They use the example of Uber—the product is stellar but what about the people who drive the vehicle? Once again, using transformational leadership involves the leader being aware of all aspects of new changes and leading through negative as well as positive times.

Transformational leadership involves "open communications, inspiration, enthusiasm, supporting positive change, and empowering others through shared decision-making" (Clavelle & Prado-Inzerillo, 2018, p. 39), characteristics that were highlighted in a recent comparison between transformational and disruptive leaders (Love, 2017). Love asserts that disruptive leaders are authoritarian and unrestrained, and tend to destabilize organizations and cultures because they charge forward—often as individuals—with wanting to make change and "be first" rather than being guided by a clear vision for moving forward; such individuals often create products that had been unimaginable, but they do so at a significant cost to the organizations and the individuals within them, and the sustainability of the change is likely to be low and tenuous. On the other hand, transformational leaders are inclusive, intentional, guided by clear goals, "nurture a culture that embraces change, engage with ambiguity, and relinquish the fear that naturally accompanies change" (Love, 2017, p. 2). As a result, they more fully engage followers and transform cultures, and the likelihood of success is high, as is continuous growth of the organization and of individuals.

Servant Leadership

Robert Greenleaf (1977) wrote *Servant Leadership: A Journey Into the Nature of Legitimate Power and Greatness*, which introduced the notion of servant leadership, a concept described briefly by the book's subtitle. In this seminal work—and in many subsequent writings by Greenleaf and others—the assertion is made that not only can a single individual be both a leader and a servant, but also fulfilling both of those responsibilities is essential if the essence and effectiveness of leadership is to be realized.

Greenleaf (1977) asserted that "*the great leader is seen as a servant first*, and that simple fact is the key to his greatness" (p. 7). Thus, an individual begins with a desire to serve, and that conscious choice brings him or her to aspire to lead. One can liken this "desire to serve" as having a vision of a "better" environment, organizational culture, or world, and then enacting the qualities that define a leader to work collaboratively with others to realize that vision.

Rockwell (2018) offers some signs that one is a servant leader. He says such leaders turn conversations toward others, stand behind others, and provide feedback to others that focuses on their strengths, aspirations, and capabilities. Additionally, Rockwell asserts that servant leaders take responsible risks, revel in the success of others, and concern themselves with how others feel about them, not what others think about them.

A systematic review of 39 empirical studies published between 2004 and 2011 in a variety of peer-reviewed journals regarding the servant leadership theory (Parris & Peachey, 2013) led the authors to conclude that although there is no consensus on the definition of servant leadership and researchers are using multiple measures to explore it, the theory is being investigated across a variety of contexts, disciplines, cultures, and themes. Perhaps one of the most significant conclusions from this analysis is that servant leadership is a viable leadership theory that helps organizations and improves the well-being of followers. The review identified the following 10 characteristics of servant leaders: listening, empathy, healing, awareness, persuasion, conceptualization, foresight, stewardship, commitment to the growth of people, and building community. It also noted that such leadership serves to develop followers into people who "can build a better tomorrow" (p. 378). They might also be thought of as authentic, a concept that is key to another leadership theory.

Authentic Leadership

This theory often is associated with the perception of morality and may be confused with ethical leadership, but it differs in that authentic leaders also have a strong component of effective communication skills and self-awareness. According to Gardner et al. (2005), this leadership model's underpinnings include (1) *self-awareness*, an understanding of each individual's strengths and weaknesses; (2) *relational transparency*, which encompasses honest two-way communication; (3) *balanced information processing*, which is defined as taking the time to explore other options before making a decision; and (4) *internalized moral perspective*, or the individual's moral compass. Kernis (2003) further expands on the first component of authentic leadership by emphasizing the importance of self-reflection, a concept that may be particularly important for nurses who, in many instances, do not engage in reflection because of work environment demands and the many immediate issues with which they must deal.

For 22 years, Gallup polling of Americans on the ethics of professional groups has consistently shown nurses to be rated the most honest (Brenan, 2023). This finding positions nurses well for leadership roles, as honesty is considered an essential characteristic of leadership. To become better authentic leaders, George (2015) says we need to work on developing our character, substance, and honesty, and offers suggestions that may be helpful to enhance our self-awareness. He shares several leaders' life stories and discusses how these leaders learned from their experiences, both good and bad, to find their "true north," or authenticity. All nurses need to find their "true north" and self-confidence to improve their leadership, especially when their profession is held in such high esteem. Patients respect nurses because they trust them, so it seems they can all work on being even stronger authentic leaders. Additionally, nurses must lead themselves, their followers (e.g., colleagues, students, and patients), and their organizations. We often need to be reminded of the excellent work nurses do. Such recognition will impact their self-respect and confidence, and will ultimately increase their leadership ability (Hougaard & Carter, 2018).

Interactive Leadership

Rosener (2011) identified "interactive leadership"; this theory asserts that interactive leaders "believe that people perform best when they feel good about themselves and their work" (p. 21), and they try to create environments that contribute to such a feeling. Inclusion, therefore, is "at the core of interactive leadership" (p. 21).

Interactive leaders encourage participation, use a conversational style of communication, and enhance the self-worth of others, in part by consistently letting team members know that their contributions are valued. They also ask team members, "What would you do if you were me?" and then act on the input they receive. Finally, they energize others by spreading their enthusiasm and passion, almost in an evangelistic way.

Clearly, this type of leadership takes time, requires giving up some control, opens the door to criticism, and can be interpreted as the leader not having answers (Rosener, 2011, p. 22). It also is important for interactive leaders to appreciate that not everyone wants to participate, but they still are inclusive, inviting others to participate in shaping and realizing a vision and to "willingly share power and information rather than guard it" (p. 22).

Adaptive Leadership

Heifetz et al. (2009) created the adaptation leadership model in 1994, defining it as "the practice of mobilizing people to tackle tough challenges and thrive" (p. 13). At the same time that these authors proposed this model, Schore (1994), a prestigious neuropsychologist, suggested that the evolution of any system generates greater complexity, stability, and adaptability. Just as any living system evolves, so does the healthcare delivery system, and those who are part of that system must be able to relate to the context of what is happening in it and adapt to the continuous changes that occur. In other words, nurses need to be agile leaders in today's demanding environment and be flexible, adaptive in knowing what leadership style to use, and aware of the consequences of one's leadership style (Meyer & Meijers, 2018).

Northouse (2021) further explains that adaptive leadership is about helping people change and adjust to new situations. Adaptive leadership focuses on the adaptations in response to chaos, disequilibrium, and change in organizational structures. Heifetz et al. (2009) outline the role of the leader as one who disturbs equilibrium and engages followers in solving an organization's problems, a theory, they assert, that is useful in the face of chaos, ambiguity, and rapid change.

Successful adaptable leaders, therefore, must do the following:

- Demonstrate integrity in all circumstances
- Surround themselves with people who possess different opinions
- Be flexible but not always willing to compromise
- Be able to defend their vision(s)
- Learn from the past and enjoy the present
- Remain aware of having a stake in one's future by continuously gathering data from all sources (Galuska, 2014)

The notion of leaders disturbing equilibrium also is advanced by Gryskiewicz (2005), who notes that "probably the most important challenge a leader faces today is building an organization that continually renews itself—an organization in which creativity . . . and innovation . . . are ongoing" (p. 8). Thus, engendering "positive turbulence" is a critical factor in contemporary theories of leadership.

Innovative Leadership

Johnson (2014) describes how innovation over the years has generated historical consequences and how unexpected connections have yielded successes in far-reaching ways. Reading *How We Got to Now: Six Innovations That Made the Modern World* can help nurses to follow previous entrepreneurs by being more innovative regarding how we provide, document, and evaluate care. Examples of healthcare inventions, best practices of care delivery, and employee engagement techniques are emerging at some Magnet-recognized hospitals and healthcare delivery centers, both serendipitously and as a result of planned initiatives.

Canton (2015) asserts that future leaders must be more innovative than they are now, and the paradigm of having one individual leader must change to having a leader force. The leaders must "inspire greatness in others and evangelize the future vision" as well as develop "a new set of values that embrace purpose, sustainability and innovation" (p. 47). Perhaps Mckeown's definition (2014) will serve to better explain innovation leadership: it is about practical creativity and making new ideas useful to solve problems and make something better plus creating new opportunities. He recommends that *innovation + strategy about shaping the future = adaptability.*

If nurses aspire to become more innovative leaders, they will need to engage in formal leadership training and mentoring. Engaging in more formal leadership activities, participating in leadership courses or workshops, and identifying one's strengths should assist leaders to practice more effective innovative leadership. During our professional learning we learn how knowledge and our experiences (i.e., analytic intelligence) would assist us in succeeding with our careers. During our professional career learning it is important to learn that knowledge and experiences will help us solve some work challenges, but not all of them. Weiss and Legrand (2011) call this innovative intelligence—being able to answer or at least try some solution—"ambiguities of work." Innovative leaders introduce new ideas that challenge the status quo and recommend new operating systems (Northouse, 2021).

Denning and Dunham (2010, pp. 381–383) offer eight practices leaders can follow to generate an innovative leadership model: sensing, envisioning, offering, adopting, sustaining, executing, leading, and embodying. They also have an innovation assessment tool that can be used to describe an individual's or organization's innovative strengths. By engaging in these eight practices, nurse leaders may be more prepared to implement innovative leadership. It is of significance that everyone has innovative ideas, but many individuals often need assistance to launch, implement, and sustain them (Krippendorf, 2019). Also, we can learn from reading biographies of respected leaders. For example, Goodwin (2018) wrote about past presidents and describes how we can learn to communicate better, be more resilient, and be inspirational, all of which can serve to enhance our leadership skills.

Foresight Leadership

One of nursing's prominent leaders and scholars, Dan Pesut, extended the notion of innovative leadership through the conceptualization of a perspective he applies directly to nursing and names *foresight leadership*. This type of leadership "is the ability and act of forecasting what will be needed in the future" (Pesut, 2019, p. 198), in light of changing healthcare needs and the evolving role of the nurse. Such leadership requires one to have a future time orientation, anticipatory planning skills, constant environmental scanning of signals and trends that are "likely to become movements" (p. 198), partnerships that bring diverse perspectives to our thinking, and envisioning possible, probable, and preferred scenarios. Such a perspective clearly aligns with having a vision of a preferred future and collaborating with others to shape that future, rather than merely waiting for something to happen and then passively accepting it when it does. Clearly, nurses engaged daily in caring for diverse, vulnerable populations are in an excellent position to be aware of trends, envision a preferred future, and work collaboratively to create such a future; thus, they are excellent candidates to enact foresight leadership.

Appreciative Inquiry

Although appreciative inquiry (AI) is promoted as a theory related to change, the concepts inherent in it have relevance to leadership. As noted in Whitney and Trosten-Bloom's preface (2010), "appreciative inquiry transforms organizations into places that are free and alive, where people are eager and filled with positive power, and where the creativity of the whole never ceases to amaze, surprise, and innovate" (p. xi). It would seem that leaders have the responsibility for creating environments where all participants are respected and valued, all share a common vision, and all are excited about the journey to achieve that vision.

Such environments are characterized by the six freedoms outlined by Whitney and Trosten-Bloom (2010, p. 1): freedom to be known in relationship, freedom to be heard, freedom to dream in community, freedom to choose to contribute, freedom to act with support, and freedom to be positive.

Current conceptualizations of leadership center on a clear purpose where any and all individuals in the group may fill the role of leader or follower, and internalizing an AI perspective when serving in the role of leader would encourage all participants to be heard, to recognize the unique gifts of all participants, to support collective action, and to contribute in a positive way to the group's goal.

Using an AI approach in organizations has been shown to improve communication and collaboration, increase involvement in decision making, and "get employees engaged in shared governance" (Therady, 2022, p. 71). Perhaps if more leaders adopted the "4-D" cycle of AI—*discover* (appreciating what is), *dream* (imagining what might be), *design* (determining what should be), and *deliver* or *destiny* (creating what will be)—as described by these nurse researchers, there would be greater engagement of followers and greater success in achieving articulated visions.

Complexity Theory

Complexity science acknowledges the "messiness" and complexity of social processes and the growing realization that effective leadership does not necessarily reside within the actions of the individual designated as "leader" but instead is "an emergent event, an outcome of relational interactions . . . [that] emerges through dynamic interactions" (Lichtenstein et al., 2006, p. 2). This complex, dynamic process emerges in the interactive spaces between people and ideas.

In this contemporary view, leadership is a complex dynamic that is more than the capabilities of any single individual. In essence, it is a product of interaction, tension, and exchange, making it a system phenomenon. Such a view of leadership (Uhl-Bien & Marion, 2008) supports the notion that all participants learn; grow; constantly interact; can be innovative; can develop their capabilities; and can "step up" to articulate the group's vision, facilitate change, or inspire others. Indeed, it reflects web-type structures, rather than hierarchical ones, and a distributed leadership approach.

Humanbecoming Leading-Following Model

In our own field of nursing, Parse (2008) proposed the humanbecoming leading-following model that challenges traditional notions of leadership. The author asserts that "power resides with the constituents of a situation and . . . there are at least three essentials inherent in leading: commitment to a vision, willingness to risk, and reverence for others" (p. 369). This model, therefore, places high value on all those who interact together (i.e., what we typically think of as "leaders" and "followers") to create change, innovate, and "co-create infinite possibilities" (p. 375).

PERSPECTIVES ON LEADERSHIP AND QUALITY HEALTHCARE

We often think that the various perspectives on leadership discussed here apply only in the corporate world or the world of politics. However, the healthcare system also is in desperate need of leaders who reflect all the contemporary theories just discussed—relational and social, transformational, servant leader, authentic, adaptive, innovative, positive (i.e., AI), dynamic (i.e., complexity theory), values-based (i.e., humanbecoming leading-following), and culturally relevant. Such leaders are essential if healthcare systems and the care provided to those in such systems are to be effective and advance the health of our nation.

As noted in the 1999 Institute of Medicine (IOM, 1999) report *To Err Is Human: Building a Safer Health System*, approximately 44,000 to 98,000 people die annually from a preventable adverse event during their hospitalization, and recent approximations of the number of patients harmed in primary and ambulatory settings because of unsafe care is approximately 4 in every 10 patients, while up to 80% of this harm can be avoided (World Health Organization, 2023). This number increases when individuals in nonhospital settings who experience a preventable medical error are included, but no estimates of these numbers have been published. Numbers such as these are startling and challenge all healthcare workers to design and implement practices to reduce them.

Recommendations to lead the healthcare industry to safer and higher quality systems were given in the 1999 IOM report, and the 2001 IOM report, *Crossing the Quality Chasm*, also made recommendations to the healthcare industry to improve care. Such leadership is expected of nurses and others. Indeed, the IOM made specific recommendations in 2004 regarding nurses, indicating that nurse managers, directors, and administrators should use transformational leadership to increase patient safety and decrease healthcare errors. The IOM's 2010 report, *The Future of Nursing: Leading Change, Advancing Health*, recommended that all nurses be prepared to assume leadership positions, and the National Academy of Medicine's current work recommends that nurses must be prepared to assume responsibility to "serve as change agents in creating systems that bridge the delivery of healthcare and social needs care in the community" (n.d.).

It is clear that all nurses, regardless of setting, must use their knowledge and experience to lead in making changes that will improve the quality of care, ensure patient safety, and decrease patient deaths from preventable errors. Many nursing groups are responding to this call, the most widely known of which is the Quality and Safety Education for Nurses (QSEN) Institute.

The QSEN (2014) project began in 2005 with funding from the Robert Wood Johnson Foundation to augment the IOM in improving nurses' leadership and education with the goal of improving safe healthcare. There have been four phases of education implemented since 2005, with the last, phase IV, beginning in 2012 with a specific goal of having 80% of all registered nurses hold a bachelor's degree or higher (QSEN, 2014).

CONCLUSION

The phenomenon of leadership has been the focus of study for many years, and over time, a number of theories about and perspectives on this phenomenon have emerged. Such theories evolved (1) from beliefs that one is born to be a leader because of noble heritage, (2) to attempts to define leaders by a list of characteristics or traits, and (3) to then exploring the interactions among the person of leader, the persons of followers, and the situation at hand. More recently, leadership has been viewed as a relation or social dynamic, the ability to influence followers and transform individuals and systems, self-awareness and transparency, inspiring others to greatness, innovating and creating new opportunities, focusing the group on appreciating group members, and the co-creation of infinite possibilities. Current discussions of leadership also acknowledge the influence of culture on how the phenomenon is conceptualized, and some suggest that we need a more holistic understanding of and global perspective on leadership (Allen, 2018, p. 155). Additionally, contemporary views of leadership describe it as an emergent event that results from the interaction of all those involved in a situation, group, or organization rather than as activities that reside in an individual.

Nurses who will influence today's practice environments and shape those of tomorrow will be strengthened in their ability to achieve such goals if they have an understanding of a variety of leadership theories, evaluate each theory for its relevance and applicability in their setting and situation, be aware that they may apply different leadership theories when dealing with a single challenging situation, and enact a leadership role in ways that have already been shown to be effective. This is, indeed, quite a challenge, but we must take responsibility for serving our patients, our colleagues, and our profession in this way because if we do not, we will be able only to react to the future rather than help create it.

 CRITICAL THINKING 1-1

1. Compare and contrast one classic/historical and one contemporary leadership theory and propose how using parts of each may facilitate successful leadership as a nurse with any level of preparation and in any setting. How can knowing a variety of leadership theories help you lead in different ways? For example, what leadership framework(s) would you use to deliver the highest quality healthcare to more patients but at a lower cost?

2. Describe the leadership practices you have observed or participated in that were designed to implement an organizational change to help nurses engage in evidence-based practice. What contemporary leadership theories were evident in the actions of the organization's senior leadership team, governance groups, and human and financial resource facilitators, and how effective were those actions?

3. An authentic leader is genuine, honest, trustworthy, humble, knowledgeable, and passionate, and is one who does things right. Identify specific examples from journal articles that highlight the impact of authentic leadership on employee engagement and job satisfaction.

4. Do you believe leadership is an inherent trait or do you think it can be developed through experience and learning? Research some ideas on developing your leadership skills and improving your leadership ability.

References

Albert, N., Pappas, S., O'Grady, T., & Malloch, K. (2022). *Quantum leadership: Creating sustainable value in healthcare* (6th ed.). Jones & Bartlett Learning.

Allen, W. E. (2018). Leadership theory: A different conceptual approach. *Journal of Leadership Education, 17,* 149–160.

Avolio, B. J. (2007). Promoting more integrative strategies for leadership theory-building. *American Psychology, 62,* 25–33.

Bass, B. M. (1985). *Leadership and performance beyond expectations.* Free Press.

Bass, B. M. (2008). *The Bass handbook of leadership: Theory, research, and managerial applications* (4th ed.). Free Press.

Bennis, W., & Nanus, B. (2003). *Leaders: The strategies for taking charge* (3rd ed.). HarperCollins.

Brenan, M. (2023). Nurses retain top ethics rating in U.S., but below 2020 high. *Gallup News.* https://news.gallup.com/poll/467804/nurses-retain-top-ethics-rating-below-2020-high.aspx

Burns, J. M. (1978). *Leadership.* Harper Torchbooks.

Canton, J. (2015). *Future smart: Managing the game changing trends that will transform your world.* DaCapo Press.

Carrig, K., & Snell, S. (2019). *Strategic execution: Driving breakthrough performance in business.* Stanford University Press.

Chaleff, I. (2009). *The courageous follower: Standing up to and for our leaders* (3rd ed.). Harvard Business Press.

Christenson, C., Dillon, K., Hall, T., & Duncan, D. (2016). *Competing against luck: The story of innovation and customer choice.* HarperCollins.

Clavelle, J. T., & Prado-Inzerillo, M. (2018). Inspire others through transformational leadership. *American Nurse Today, 13*(11), 39–41.

Denning, P., & Dunham, R. (2010). *The innovator's way: Essential practices for successful innovation.* MIT Press.

Dugan, J. P. (2017). *Leadership theory—Cultivating critical perspectives.* Jossey-Bass.

Galuska, L. (2014). Enabling leadership: Unleashing creativity, adaptation, and learning in an organization. *Nurse Leader, 12*(2), 34–38.

Gardner, W. L., Avolio, B. J., Luthans, F., May, D. R., & Walumbwa, F. (2005). Can you see the real me? A self-based model of authentic leaders and follower development. *Leadership Quarterly, 19,* 343–372.

George, B. (2015). *Discover your TRUE NORTH.* John Wiley & Sons.

Goodwin, D. (2018). *Leadership: In turbulent times.* Simon & Schuster.

Greenleaf, R. K. (1977). *Servant leadership: A journey into the nature of legitimate power and greatness.* Paulist Press.

Gryskiewicz, S. S. (2005). Leading renewal: The value of positive turbulence. *Leadership in Action, 25*(1), 8–12.

Heifetz, R., Grashow, A., & Linsky, M. (2009). *The practice of adaptive leadership: Tools and tactics for changing your organization and the world.* Harvard Business Press.

Hougaard, R., & Carter, J. (2018). *The mind of the leader: How to lead yourself, your people, and your organization for extraordinary results.* Harvard Business Review Press.

Institute of Medicine. (1999). *To err is human: Building a safe health system.* National Academy Press.

Institute of Medicine. (2001). *Crossing the quality chasm: A new health system for the 21st century.* National Academy Press.

Institute of Medicine. (2010). *The future of nursing: Leading change and advancing health.* National Academies Press.

Janus, I. (1982). *Groupthink: Psychological studies of policy decisions and fiascoes.* Houghton Mifflin.

Johnson, S. (2014). *How we got to now: Six innovations that made the modern world.* Penguin Books.

Kellerman, B. (2008). *Followership: How followers are creating change and changing leaders.* Harvard Business Press.

Kernis, M. H. (2003). Toward a conceptualization of optimal self-esteem. *Psychological Inquiry, 14*(1), 1–26.

Krippendorf, K. (2019). *Driving innovation from within: A guide for internal entrepreneurs.* Columbia Business School Publishing.

Lichtenstein, B. B., Uhl-Bien, M., Marion, R., Seers, A., Orton, J. D., & Schreiber, C. (2006). Complexity leadership theory: An interactive perspective on leading in complex adaptive systems. *Emergence: Complexity and Organization, 8*(4), 2–12.

Love, A. (2017, January). Are you a disruptive or transformational leader? *SmartBrief.* https://www.smartbrief.com/original/2017/01/are-you-disruptive-or-transformational-leader

Mckeown, M. (2014). *The innovative book: How to manage ideas and execution for outstanding results.* Maverick & Strong.

Meyer, R., & Meijers, R. (2018). *Leadership agility: Developing your repertoire of leadership styles.* Routledge.

National Academy of Medicine. (n.d.) *The future of nursing: 2020–2030.* https://nam.edu/publications/the-future-of-nursing-2020-2030/

Northouse, P. (2021). *Leadership: Theory & practice* (9th ed.). SAGE.

Parris, D. L., & Peachey, J. W. (2013). A systematic literature review of servant leadership theory in organizational contexts. *Journal of Business Ethics, 113*(3), 377–393.

Parse, R. R. (2008). The humanbecoming leading-following model. *Nursing Science Quarterly, 21*(4), 369–375.

Pesut, D. J. (2019). Anticipating disruptive innovations with foresight leadership. *Nursing Administration Quarterly, 43*(3), 196–204.

Quality and Safety Education in Nursing Institute. (2014). *About QSEN: Project overview.* http://qsen.org/about-qsen

Riggio, R. E., Chaleff, I., & Lippman-Blumen, J. (Eds.). (2008). *The art of followership.* Jossey Bass.

Rockwell, D. (2018, September 6). The top signs you're a servant-leader. *Leadership Freak.* https://leadershipfreak.blog/2018/09/06/the-top-signs-youre-a-servant-leader/

Rosener, J. B. (2011). Ways women lead. In P. H. Werhane & M. Painter-Moreland (Eds.), *Leadership, gender, and organization.* Springer.

Schore, A. (1994). *Affect regulation and the origin of the self: The neurobiology of emotional development.* Psychology Press.

Sinek, S. (2016, April 8). *Start with why to inspire action [Video].* YouTube. https://www.youtube.com/watch?v=HjriwYrGL28

Stech, E. L. (2004). *The transformed leader.* Trafford Publishing.

Tetenbaum, T., & Laurence, H. (2011). Leading in the chaos of the 21st century. *Journal of Leadership Studies, 4*(4), 41–49.

Therady, A. (2022). A leadership lesson learned: Employees come first. *Journal of Healthcare Management, 67*(2), 71–74.

Torres, R. (2013, October). *What it takes to be a great leader* [Video]. TED Conferences. http://www.ted .com/talks/roselinde_torres_what_it_takes_to_be_a_great_leader?language=en

Uhl-Bien, M., & Marion, R. (Eds.). (2008). *Complexity leadership, part 1: Conceptual foundations.* Information Age.

Weiss, D., & Legrand, C. (2011). *Innovative intelligence: The art and practice.* John Wiley & Sons, Canada, Ltd.

Whitney, D. D., & Trosten-Bloom, A. (2010). *The power of appreciative inquiry: A practical guide to positive change* (2nd ed.). Berrett-Kohler.

World Health Organization. (2023, September 11). *Patient safety.* https://www.who.int/news-room/ fact-sheets/detail/patient-safety#:~:text=Above%2050%25%20of%20harm%20(1,can%20be%20 avoided%20(4)

Yukl, G. A. (2006). *Leadership in organizations.* Pearson/Prentice Hall.

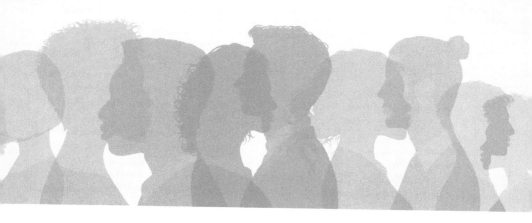

CHAPTER 2

The Nature of Leadership
Distinguishing Leadership From Management

LEARNING OBJECTIVES
• Discuss the essential elements of leadership.
• Describe the tasks of leadership.
• Distinguish leadership from management.
• Create a personal definition of leadership that reflects its essential elements.

INTRODUCTION

Leadership is a complex, multifaceted phenomenon that does not "just happen" and is not limited to an elite few. It can be learned. It is deliberative. And it is not necessarily tied to a position of authority. In other words, a leadership role is something each of us has the potential to fulfill. To be most effective in taking on that role, one must understand the dimensions of leadership and be able to distinguish it from the related, but different, concept of management. This chapter is designed to provide an in-depth analysis of the phenomenon of leadership, clarify the distinctions between that role and others, and challenge the reader to create a personal conceptualization of leadership that can be used throughout a lifetime career in nursing.

Leadership is action, not position. —Donald H. McGannon

Consider this case study on the nature of leadership as you continue reading this chapter.

Case Study

Georgia, Sarah, and Ron worked the evening shift in the psychiatric emergency department (ED) at a large acute care urban healthcare organization. They all began employment three years ago, immediately after graduating from their baccalaureate nursing programs, and have been working together ever since. Each of these nurses was getting discouraged and experiencing the same problem—there was no clear triage process to follow for individuals who came to the ED with suspected mental health problems, although a clear triage process for patients with no suspected psychiatric issues was in place.

Georgia, Sarah, and Ron decided to talk with their psychiatric emergency department (PED) nurse colleagues about the lack of a protocol, and were affirmed when all agreed that it was an issue. However, these colleagues also said, "You are right, but using a triage protocol for psychiatric patients will never happen here. Don't waste your time." The three nurses decided to talk with their nurse manager about developing a triage checklist. The nurse manager did not support their suggestion, saying, "It is not necessary, and will be a waste of time. We have to accept everyone; it is different with psychiatric patients."

REFLECTION QUESTIONS

1. As "new" nurses, should Georgia, Sarah, and Ron challenge their colleagues' response to the concern?
2. How could Georgia, Sarah, and Ron use the Clinical Judgment Measurement Model to respond to their manager's statement?

LEADERSHIP AND MANAGEMENT

The vast array of textbooks on leadership—particularly in nursing—often have the words "leadership" and "management" in their titles. A careful analysis of the content of those textbooks frequently reveals, however, that a great deal of attention is given to management and very little to leadership. In fact, although the authors of many such textbooks make a point at the outset to say that leadership and management are not the same thing, they often go on to use the terms interchangeably and imply that the only person who is providing leadership to a group is the person who is in the management position. Kotter (2013) asserts this is common in many discussions and writings about leadership. Despite the tendency to suggest that only chief executive officers (CEOs) and others in upper-management positions are leaders, nothing can be further from the truth.

It is true that leadership and management are related and that many managers are also leaders. However, these phenomena are not the same and should not be confused. Most important, one must remember that **leadership is not necessarily tied to a position of authority** and that each of us has the potential, and perhaps the responsibility, to provide leadership in our specific area of practice, our institution, our professional organizations, our community, and our profession as a whole. Leadership, therefore, should be thought of as a role, rather than as a position.

TASKS OF LEADERSHIP

One of the most noted experts in the field of leadership, John Gardner, outlined nine tasks of leadership that help distinguish it from management. These tasks of leadership, which still have relevance today, are as follows (Gardner, 1989):

1. **Envisioning goals:** Pointing others in the right direction and helping the group members balance and deal with any tension between long- and short-term goals
2. **Affirming values:** Regenerating and revitalizing the beliefs, values, purposes, and vision shared by members of the group and challenging the values held by some
3. **Motivating:** Unlocking or channeling motives that exist within members of the group, having and promoting positive attitudes, being creative, and encouraging others to be excited about the future and about how they can be part of it and part of shaping it
4. **Managing:** Planning, setting priorities, making decisions, facilitating change, and keeping the system functioning, all in an effort to move the group toward achieving the goals and realizing the vision
5. **Achieving a workable unity:** Establishing trust, striving toward cohesion and mutual tolerance, managing conflict, and "creating loyalty to the larger venture" (p. 29)
6. **Explaining:** Helping others understand what the vision is, why they are being asked to do certain things, and how their contributions relate to the larger picture
7. **Serving as a symbol:** Serving as a risk-taker and acting as the group's source of unity, voice of anger, collective identity, and continuity, as well as its source of hope
8. **Representing the group:** Speaking and acting for or on behalf of the group and being an advocate for the group
9. **Renewing:** Blending continuity and change and breaking routines, habits, fixed attitudes, perceptions, assumptions, and unwritten rules . . . and keeping hope alive

Gardner (1989) asserted that the *"sine qua non* of leadership" (p. 29) is the ability to achieve a workable unity in the group and build community, a perspective supported by Schweitzer (2006), who talked about the leader moving from being a soloist to being an orchestrator.

In essence, "leadership is not tidy" (Gardner, 1989, p. 33); it is more of an art than a science. It also is an ongoing learning process. Management, in comparison, often is thought of as a science in which a series of steps can be followed to implement the role. McCarthy (2012) summed this up nicely when he said, "You can *do* management to manage, but you have to *be* a leader to lead." Elements of the tasks of leadership will be explored in greater depth, but a careful look now at how leadership differs from management can facilitate a more thorough understanding of leadership.

DISTINCTIONS BETWEEN LEADERSHIP AND MANAGEMENT

"If you believe that management and leadership are identical then you are wrong. You're about as wrong as wrong can be. . . . All organizations need both management and leadership [and] the same person can and frequently does possess both skill sets. But many times, they do not. When they don't it is usually the leadership skills that are missing." So Keating (2018) contends in his discussion of when leadership is lacking. He also notes that we manage things, but human beings resist being managed and insist on being led instead.

One of the first to explore the differences between leadership and management in depth was Abraham Zaleznik. In his classic work, Zaleznik (1981) asserted that leaders and managers are very different kinds of people:

- They differ in their motivation, their personal history, and how they think and act.
- They differ in their orientation toward goals, work, human relationships, and themselves.
- They differ in their worldviews.

Goals

Leaders are proactive in formulating goals, primarily because they typically arise out of some passion for a better world. The goals are developed through dialogue and collaboration with others, engagement with the literature, and self-reflection. Leaders shape ideas instead of merely responding to the ideas of others. They act to change the way people think about what is desirable, possible, and necessary. *Managers*, by comparison, adopt impersonal attitudes toward goals because someone higher in the organizational hierarchy often formulates those goals, which are deeply embedded in the history and culture of the organization and arise out of necessity rather than passion and desire.

Conceptions of Work

Regarding their conceptions of work, *leaders* act to develop fresh approaches to long-standing problems and to open issues for new options. Leaders provide a direction and impetus for others to see what lies ahead by creating a group vision of what might be achieved (Gutterman, 2023). Their instinct is to take risks, challenge norms, question existing assumptions, and ask, "Why not?" True leaders do not merely engage in routine activities of work, but instead anticipate hindrances and create novel solutions to keep the group pressing forward toward the goal (Gutterman, 2023).

Managers see work as a task to be accomplished with the least amount of turmoil and the greatest amount of coordination, balance, and efficiency. They act to limit choices and rock the boat as little as possible. Their instinct, in contrast to that of leaders, is for survival. According to Gutterman (2023), management has to do with directing and coordinating the work of others, and lacks an interpersonal relationship seen with true leadership.

Relationships With Others

In their relationships with others, *leaders* are concerned with what events and decisions mean to those who are affected by them. They care about the people with whom they work, and they want to promote the development and individual creativity of their followers. They facilitate, focus on personal issues, and encourage the growth of others. Relationships with leaders may appear turbulent, intense, and at times even disorganized because of the involvement of all concerned. Despite this ability to work effectively with others, leaders also are comfortable with solitary activity because it provides time for reflection, creative thinking, and incubation of ideas.

Although *managers* are often thought of as "human engineers" (Holle & Blatchley, 1987) and like working with people, they tend to maintain a lower level of emotional involvement in their relationships with employees. They assign work or tasks, focus on personnel issues, and promote the growth of the organization. They prefer to reconcile differences, seek compromises, and not become involved with what events may mean to others. Instead, managers are concerned with how events occur, how things get done, and whether tasks are accomplished, preferably in the most efficient, cost-effective manner.

Sense of Self

Managers and leaders also have a different sense of self, according to Zaleznik (1981). Using the terms coined by William James many years ago, Zaleznik says *leaders* are "twice born" individuals—those who are separate from their environment, never "belong" to organizations, and have had many challenges in life. Put another way, leaders are made during defining moments of meaningful resonance with potential followers (Ruben & Gigliotti, 2021). They are not threatened by the ideas of others because their sense of self comes from within, not from their roles or the expectations of others.

Managers, on the other hand, often define themselves in terms of the organization and prefer not to have their ideas challenged. According to Zaleznik (1981), they are "once born" individuals, whose lives are rather harmonious and who are very much influenced by others' opinions.

Summary

The differences between leaders and managers outlined by Zaleznik (1981) were extended by Kotter in 1990, who noted that the core of modern management involves planning and budgeting, organizing and staffing, and controlling and problem-solving, while the essence of leadership involves establishing direction, aligning people, and motivating and inspiring. And the distinctions continued in a 2023 article by Cloud and Leturmy, who noted that *manager* and *leader* are two uniquely different concepts based on their underlying philosophies and functions. Although the terms *leader* and *manager,* as well as the terms *leadership* and *management,* are often confused and used interchangeably, they are not synonymous. Effective leadership is not controlled by a person's title within an organization, and not all managers display effective leadership (Cloud & Leturmy, 2023).

Table 2-1 summarizes these and other differences between leaders and managers. It is important to note that this table compares the extreme "ideal" leader with the extremely "organization-focused" manager for purposes of illustration, and does not define all managers or leaders. For example, many managers also serve as

TABLE 2-1 Differences Between Leadership and Management

	LEADERSHIP	MANAGEMENT
Position	Selected or allowed by a group of followers	Appointed by someone higher in the organizational hierarchy
Power base	Comes from knowledge, credibility, and ability to motivate followers	Arises from one's position of authority
Goals/visions	Arise from personal interests and passion that may not be synonymous with the goals of the organization	Espoused or prescribed by the organization
Innovative ideas	Developed, tested, and encouraged among all members of the group	Allowed, provided they do not interfere with task accomplishment, but not necessarily encouraged
Risk level	High risk, creativity, innovation	Low risk, balance, maintaining the status quo
Degree of order	Relative disorder seems to be generated	Rationality and control prevail
Nature of activities	Related to vision and judgment	Related to efficiency and cost-effectiveness
Focus	People	Systems and structure
Perspective	Long range, with an eye on the horizon	Short range, with an eye on the bottom line
Degree of "freedom"	Extensive since not limited to an organizational position of authority	May be limited since tied to a designated position in an organization
Actions	Does the right thing (Bennis & Nanus, 1985, p. 21).	Does things right (Bennis & Nanus, 1985, p. 21)

leaders in their organizations, and people in positions of authority often are leaders; therefore, the distinctions are not as clear-cut as Table 2-1 may imply. In fact, more recent literature (Cloud & Leturmy, 2023) suggests that today's healthcare environment requires both effective managers and effective leaders, because both unique skill sets are needed if we want to guide healthcare to the next level.

The important point to emphasize is that **one can be a leader without being in a position of authority**. It is this aspect that professional nurses need to keep in mind when they face challenges in the practice arena: each of us has the potential to provide leadership that will create new futures, and one need not be in a position of authority to do that. In fact, if one considers how leaders rock the boat, challenge existing ways of doing things, constantly ask "Why not?" questions, and are comfortable with—and indeed, thrive on—turbulence, one can see that it is sometimes easier to be a leader if one is *not* in a hierarchical position of authority.

ELEMENTS OF LEADERSHIP

Leadership is a complex, multifaceted phenomenon with numerous definitions, and a quick Google search of the term "leadership" produces over 500 million results. Clearly, this is a concept that is of great interest to researchers, corporate executives, educators, community leaders, religious organizations, and individuals, and it is a concept about which we are still learning. Despite the array of ideas, however, certain elements of leadership emerge again and again.

Ken Robinson (2009) was one of the world's leading thinkers on creativity and innovation and proposed that finding one's passion is all that is needed to change the world. Although he did not frame this discussion in the context of leadership, Robinson made a strong case for the power of passion.

In the current climate, one of the skills integral to successful leadership is being a "human expert" rather than a "strategy expert" (Hale, 2023). Leadership is understanding human behavior and how to motivate change. "Ultimately, leadership is about intentional influencing of behavioral change. Leaders don't influence outcomes; they influence humans to act in ways that drive outcomes. Behavior change is the job of a leader" (Hale, 2023).

Despite these myriad definitions, several fundamental elements of leadership recur in writings about the concept. Those elements—vision, communication skills, trust, change, courage, stewardship, and developing and renewing followers (Box 2-1)—are discussed in depth to help the reader better understand leadership.

Vision

Few would argue that having, creating, and expressing a vision are important elements of leadership. Manfredi (1995) asserted that one of the primary roles of leaders is that of creating visions—"engag[ing] in the process of traveling into the future" (p. 62). Leadership involves dreaming of possibilities, believing there can be a better world, exploring uncharted waters, and asking questions such as, "Why not?" Indeed, great leaders are idealists, dreamers, and "possibility thinkers" (Kouzes & Posner, 2017, p. 98).

The significance of vision to leadership has been identified by numerous experts in the field (Bennis, 1989, 2004; Gardner, 1990; Jackman, 2005; Kouzes & Posner, 2017; Nanus, 1992; Phillips, 1997; Thornberry, 2006). In fact, the ability to see a new world, or a different world, and mobilize others to help make it a reality are

---

BOX 2-1 **Elements of Leadership**

Vision
Communication skills
Trust
Change
Courage
Stewardship
Developing and renewing followers

two of the hallmarks of leadership. Consider the following individuals, many of whose dreams became realities as a result of their determination, persistence, and passion:

- **Florence Nightingale:** Reduced battlefield fatalities resulting from poor care and founded modern nursing.
- **Jeff Bezos:** Started Amazon, one of the largest and most successful e-commerce companies in the world.
- **Martin Luther King Jr.:** Civil rights leader who fought for racial equality.
- **Mother Teresa:** Devoted her life to providing compassionate care for the sick and poor.
- **Oprah Winfrey:** Businessperson who turned her dreams into reality with a media empire that includes television, magazines, and more.
- **Taylor Swift:** Musician and businessperson whose determination and talent propelled her to become one of the most successful artists of her generation.
- **Tim Cook:** Continued the legacy of Steve Jobs, leading Apple to new heights with innovative products and services.

Although we think of these individuals today as significant figures in our nation's or world's history, they were little-known people when their visions began to take shape, when they began talking to others about their vision, and when they initiated actions to turn those dreams into reality. As a result, we now see more scientific and nursing-oriented approaches to healthcare, the worldwide impact of the Missionaries of Charity, greater racial equality, the convenience of online shopping, the positive outcomes of nonviolence, freedom of people in various parts of the world, and a computer in nearly every home and office. It has been said that "in creating a vision, we are creating a power, not a place, an influence, not a destination" (Wheatley, 1999, p. 55). Surely, individuals like these have created a power and an influence that have touched millions.

As professional nurses in practice, each of us can envision a better world. One might think of ways to promote greater involvement of patients' families in care decisions or a more powerful role for the professional nurse on the healthcare team. Another person might see a more effective way to prepare patients for the transition from the critical care unit to a step-down unit or from the hospital to home care. And yet another may look at ways to increase hospital stays for certain patients, such as those undergoing mastectomy, or encourage greater autonomy for the nurse in making referrals to needed services.

Whatever the vision, if it is something about which one cares, as a leader, one cannot sit idly waiting for others to make it happen. Instead, one must learn to ask great questions and imagine possibilities. As leaders, nurses must talk about their vision, the imagined possibility, to other nurses, nurse managers and administrators, patients, patients' families, other health professionals, members of the media, legislators—in fact, anyone who will or should listen. Nurses must be passionate about the "little corner of the world" that needs change and take every opportunity to do something to make that change happen. They must move beyond the current policy, practice, and assumptions that are less than ideal, and share their vision, especially in areas requiring innovative change (Abbas & Ali, 2023). Nurses do not have to be in positions of authority to raise the issues, to argue the necessity for the change, to elicit support for the idea, to speak eloquently and enthusiastically about possible solutions, or to convince others that it is a vision worth working toward. But they must have the vision.

Communication Skills

Leadership involves communicating one's ideas and visions, explaining to others how that vision has relevance for them and how they can be a part of making it a reality, and inspiring others to invest their energies on behalf of the group and the goal (Gardner, 1989). In essence, excellent communication skills are essential for effective leadership.

Individuals who have great ideas but refuse to share them with others or who communicate them in a way that does not generate excitement in others are not likely to see their visions become reality. Individuals who cannot help others clearly see the vision probably will not effectively convince potential followers to join in the struggle. Likewise, individuals who are unable to listen to the ideas of others, respond to their suggestions, and convey enthusiasm for input from all group members are not likely to facilitate change, sustain an effort over time, or effectively manage the conflict that is almost certain to arise as new goals are being realized.

Interestingly, the seemingly simple act of listening may be one of the skills leaders need to develop so they can "[listen] for a higher order and perhaps a more nuanced set of [issues]," better understand how members of the group "ask questions and diagnose issues," and "[gain] insights from what one does NOT hear" (Hoban, 2018). In fact, in an interview, leadership and management guru Tom Peters claimed that "listening is the bedrock of leadership excellence" (Kinni, 2018).

Nurses excel in communication. They know how to listen and how to encourage people to keep trying when there seems to be no hope of success or when the effort is extraordinarily difficult. They know how to encourage others to respond openly and how to overcome barriers to communication. Nurses are, therefore, particularly advantaged in this element of leadership, and they should use this skill to its fullest.

The public puts a great deal of trust in nurses, and the credibility of nurses is strong in the eyes of patients, families, legislators, and the general public. Nurses who provide leadership can benefit from this favorable perception by communicating their vision at every opportunity. Such opportunities are more readily available than many nurses realize. They include serving on a committee at one's institution or professional association, speaking at a conference, writing for a professional journal or organizational newsletter, meeting with a legislator, talking with patients and their families, being interviewed for a podcast, holding office in one's professional association, campaigning for a candidate or a particular issue, confronting a healthcare team member; networking at professional meetings; forming alliances with other healthcare professionals, seeking and using a mentor, and so on. We are limited only by our imaginations and willingness to take risks.

Trust

Nursing is the most trusted profession in the United States, with 79% of respondents rating the honesty and ethical standards of nurses as high or very high (Brenan, 2023). In fact, 2022 marked the 20th consecutive year that nursing received this top rating (Brenan, 2023).

Because "trust is the engine of team performance" (Rockwell, 2019), it is essential for leaders. But what does a trustworthy leader look like? Trustworthy leaders celebrate the accomplishments of others, rather than tearing them down. They talk openly about weaknesses and how to turn them into strengths, rather than focusing on what others cannot do. They admit to their own mistakes, assume goodwill, and can be counted on to do what they say they will do. They also consistently match their actions with their words. With trust being a key element of successful leaders and nurses being seen as trustworthy, we are in an excellent position to enact change and transform the care provided to all individuals to create the world we want to see.

Change

If leadership requires trust and involves articulating and realizing visions, the process by which that happens is change. Indeed, "learning to lead is, on one level, learning to manage change" (Bennis, 1989, p. 145). Leaders, therefore, need to be effective change agents, knowing when change is needed, "stretch[ing] the imagination of followers" (Manfredi, 1995, p. 63) to appreciate the need for change, planning effectively for change to occur, involving those who will be affected by change in the process, helping others realize their role in making change and creating new worlds, maintaining a positive attitude throughout the challenges of change, and knowing when to maintain the status quo. Monehin and Diers-Lawson (2022) discuss the benefits of sustaining appropriate optimism and keeping hope alive, especially when challenges become particularly difficult for the group or in crisis situations.

As Gardner (1990) noted, "[L]eaders must understand the interweaving of continuity and change" (p. 124). They must realize that not all change is good or necessary and that changing only for the sake of changing is not always healthy. Therefore, continuity often is what a group needs, at least for a certain period. But leadership also involves a willingness to create change and manage the chaos that often is associated with change. In fact, navigating change successfully requires leaders to focus more on encouraging others to overcome uncertainty rather than focusing all attention on the change itself (Monehin & Diers-Lawson, 2022).

Professional nurses have a responsibility to create change in their work or professional arenas. Nurses who are dissatisfied with current feelings of burnout or the increased stress of nursing shortages, for example, can complain to their colleagues and blame someone else for issues. But a professional nurse who is a leader will do more than just complain. They will outline what is needed to make changes in the unit, perhaps test it out in practice (by informally creating a self-care plan or trying a new team approach to care), develop a plan for pilot testing it on a wider scale, and propose a culture of self-care for nurses in that unit. Such an approach creates change that is intended to improve the overall quality of patient care, and although it takes more effort than merely complaining about the existing problems, the outcomes are worth the effort. This closely aligns with the National Council of State Boards of Nursing's (NCSBN, 2019) Clinical Judgment Measurement Model in which nurses cycle through the process of recognizing cues, analyzing cues, prioritizing hypotheses, generating solutions, taking action, and evaluating outcomes. By being willing to generate solutions for existing problems and taking action to initiate these solutions, nurses are not only using clinical judgment to improve patient outcomes, they are exemplifying an element of leadership. Remember, leaders do not need to be in positions of authority, and they do not need to wait for guaranteed success before trying new approaches and creating change.

Case Study, continued

Georgia, Sarah, and Ron sensed that on just about every shift someone ended up in the PED who did not require psychiatric emergency care, and they were convinced this would not be happening if more specific screening were conducted. They set about collecting data informally and found that in one month's time, 10 to 12 individuals per week were ending up receiving acute psychiatric care when they really did not require that level of care.

They shared the data with the nurse manager, who realized that there was a problem, that it was large in scope, and that it needed attention. Together, the three nurses and their nurse manager spoke to the medical director of the PED, who encouraged them to develop a triage checklist for patients presenting to the PED.

The team collaborated to develop a checklist and shared it with the nursing and medical staff, who made a few simple changes and agreed that they would support the protocol. Then they submitted this draft to the medical director, who accepted it fully and suggested a trial period. Georgia, Sarah, Ron, and the nurse manager assisted with the implementation.

REFLECTION QUESTIONS

3. How did Georgia, Sarah, and Ron determine that change was needed and what helped their manager see change was needed to promote patient safety?
4. Who is acting as a leader in this situation, and how does their role contribute to moving toward a common vision of improving patient outcomes?

Courage

In a TED Talk, Tómasdóttir and Freedman (2019) asserted that our world currently faces a crisis of conformity where we continue to do things the way we've always done them despite evidence that we need to change. They say there is a crisis of trust, anger is rampant, and the world is calling for responsible leadership now. In light of these circumstances, they claim, we need courageous leaders who are humble, who are guided by a moral compass and other-focused principles, who think holistically, who are transparent, and who hold themselves accountable for improving society or some small part of it.

If one is to stimulate and guide change, support self and others throughout that process, say what needs to be said, and, in essence, provide effective leadership, one must have courage. Indeed, one must have the heart to "step up" in order to turn a vision into reality. But what are the components of courageous leadership? Brené Brown (2018) explains there are four skills of courageous leadership:

- Leaning into vulnerability (stepping into tough conversations)
- Living your values (walking the walk, not just taking the talk)
- Braving trust (and being the first one to trust another)
- Learning to rise (having a growth mindset, rather than a fixed mindset)

Clearly, serving as a leader is no easy task. It takes strength, passion, and the courage to be vulnerable. Such an individual might also be thought of as a contrarian (Begoun, 2018), someone who is "willing to speak truth to power even when doing so can put [one's] best interests at risk," someone who resists "within the tribe," and who willingly challenges the group's thinking. Begoun acknowledges that being a contrarian leader is the most difficult and rarest form of leadership, and although it may be thought of as a form of radical leadership, it is sorely needed, as "we can't disrupt and innovate by simply going along with the tribe."

Stewardship

"Stewardship is to hold something in trust for another" (Block, 1996, p. xx) and to be responsible for something more than just oneself. It has to do with serving others rather than serving one's own self-interests or attempting to control others, and it involves a balance of power. In essence, stewardship incorporates engendering partnerships, empowerment, and investing in things we care about (Block, 1996). Block's discussion of stewardship is congruent with the elements of leadership described previously: deep commitment, risk-taking, high energy, working with others, and an enormous investment of self.

If leaders are to move forward with creating new worlds and helping visions become realities, they must have a sense of stewardship. They must feel responsible for the larger picture, oversee the implementation of change, ensure that it is the overarching vision that drives decisions and actions, establish partnerships with followers or group members, and give their personal self-interests a back seat. They must, in the words of Robert Greenleaf (1977), be servant-leaders, those who "first serve others [and] whose primary motivation is a desire to help others" (Spears, 1995, p. 3).

Professional nurses at all levels need to have a sense of stewardship about their practice arenas—whether in the clinical area, education, administration, or research—and be concerned with overall excellence in those arenas. Educators, for example, who have a vision of creating positive learning experiences for students—where they are fully engaged in the learning process, work collaboratively with each other, are excited about what they are learning, use their creativity and other potentials to the fullest, and use the teacher as a guide and a resource to facilitate their own learning—cannot be concerned with doing this only in their own courses. If they are to be leaders and demonstrate the essential element of stewardship, there must be an effort to see that such positive learning experiences are provided for students throughout the curriculum and a willingness to oversee that what is being done in the name of positive learning experiences is based on theory and research.

Developing and Renewing Followers

Finally, leadership involves the continual development of followers and ongoing renewal of their commitment, understanding, and involvement. In fact, Maxwell (2022) asserted that one of the truly defining characteristics of leaders is they are "other-focused" instead of self-focused.

More than accomplishing tasks or meeting deadlines, leadership is about keeping people "thirsty" for what motivates them and developing the abilities of others (Maxwell, 2022) as well as "challenging comfort zones" (Levine, 2019, p. 50). Leaders who have a vision for the future need to ensure that there are people to carry that vision forward and continue to work to make it become a reality. Building toward a vision requires collaboration between leaders and followers, as well as a cadre of effective followers who provide leadership.

It is the leader's responsibility to build such a cadre and develop the next generation of leaders. Because "all people have untapped leadership potential" (Tichy, 1997, p. 6), part of the leader's role is to recognize that potential and capitalize on it so that an effort or change can be sustained. Developing and renewing others can occur through personal attention, role modeling, precepting, and mentoring, each of which is described briefly to show their similarities and differences.

Personal Attention

Personal attention involves the personal guidance one gives to another. It requires that the strengths, limitations, and goals of the recipients are known and are used as a basis for the challenges presented to those individuals, the opportunities made available to them, and the expectations that are set regarding their contributions to the group.

Role Modeling

Role modeling occurs when a more experienced individual performs a role in such a way that novice leaders follow the individual's actions, style, values, behaviors, and so on. Because one can be a role model for another without even knowing it, this method of developing and renewing others is considered a more passive approach.

Precepting

Precepting is a strategy often used in nursing in which an experienced individual may be assigned to teach, guide, and assist another who is learning a role. The preceptor relationship often has a specific time limitation, and specific responsibilities of the preceptor and preceptee are clearly outlined.

Mentoring

Mentoring, in comparison with precepting, is a purposeful relationship in which an experienced, accomplished individual chooses to enter a relationship with a less experienced individual (mentee) who shares certain values or goals, is seen as having potential, shares a certain chemistry with the mentor, and is willing to work with the mentor. Mentors open doors for mentees, give critical feedback and personal guidance about career goals, improve outcomes for the mentee's health and well-being, provide psychological empowerment, and can enhance job satisfaction (Rosser et al., 2023).

Commitment
It is clear that there are many approaches to developing and renewing followers. Some are conscious and purposeful (e.g., mentoring, personal attention), some are assigned (e.g., precepting), and some may occur without the leader even being aware of their occurrence (e.g., role modeling). Regardless of the strategy used, the leader is committed to the development of the followers and to their continued renewal and involvement.

CONCLUSION

Leadership is a complex, multifaceted phenomenon that is quite different from management. It is a potential that each of us has and a set of skills (Box 2-2) that can be learned, developed, and nurtured. Most important, it is not necessarily tied to a position of authority in an organization.

Based on an analysis of more than 130,000 leaders worldwide, Kitt et al. (2023) reported on the characteristics of highly-effective leaders, based on written 360-degree feedback, a process that gathers feedback from an individual's colleagues, associates, and managers, as well as a self-evaluation by the individual. Characteristics include having balance between being task focused (skills) and relationally focused (people skills). Highly effective leaders also demonstrate high creative orientation and low reactivity (being controlling, autocratic, or expecting perfection).

A review of the characteristics of leaders described by Kitt et al. (2023) reveals that none are "earth-shattering" or impossible to achieve, yet very few people see themselves as leaders. "We've made leadership something bigger than—and beyond—us. We think it means changing the world and maybe someday we'll deserve to be called a leader. If we call ourselves leaders now, we think it's cocky and arrogant" (Dudley, 2010). According to Dudley, however, the truth of the matter is that we are important to others, often without even knowing it. We often do or say something that makes another's life fundamentally better, and we are more powerful than we realize. When we harness that power and purposefully act to improve situations, we act as leaders.

Leadership is by no means easy, but it is incredibly rewarding. Opportunities to provide leadership exist in all aspects of our lives, and enacting that role can lead to significant change in the lives of individuals, the success of organizations, and the power of a profession. Leaders do not need to be appointed or even "invited" to exercise leadership; they do it because they are willing to "risk more than others think is safe. Care more than others think is wise. Dream more than others think is practical. Expect more than others think is possible" (Bissell, n.d.).

The idea also is evident in Tómasdóttir and Freedman's TED Talk (2019). They noted that "there is a leader inside every one of us, not just in those in positions of power. We must release that leader and think about how we are making a positive impact on the world." We must avoid what they called the "hubris syndrome"—leaders who think they know it all, can do it all, have all the answers, and think they do not need to surround themselves with others who can make *them* better.

BOX 2-2 **Summary of Leader Characteristics**

VISION

- Challenge long-held assumptions and traditions; question continually.
- Inspire others to act (Sinek, 2009a, 2009b).
- Have a clear and compelling vision.
- Know your WHY.
- See the bigger picture and leave an impact.

COMMUNICATION SKILLS

- Be positive in appearance as well as in attitude.
- Communicate truthfully, effectively, and often; persuade, don't coerce.
- Take risks; be willing to make "brilliant mistakes" (Bleich, 2015).
- Be willing to be unpopular when presenting new ideas.
- Model the way; be an example; be someone to look up to.

TRUST AND STEWARDSHIP

- Form personal connections; care about others.
- Be approachable and accessible.
- Ensure that followers "live in a circle of safety" (Sinek, 2014) where they feel they belong and can trust others.
- Demonstrate integrity; be reliable and trustworthy, and honest.
- Know yourself—your strengths, weaknesses, and biases; be authentic.
- Seek and respond thoughtfully to feedback or criticism.
- Show gratitude and sustain optimism.

CHANGE AND COURAGE

- Continually learn; engage in deep reflection of self and situations.
- Seek out diverse views; embrace differences; encourage dissent; see diversity as a strength.
- Be flexible and dynamic; be willing to improvise.
- Learn to be comfortable with ambiguity.

DEVELOPING AND RENEWING FOLLOWERS

- Surround yourself with strong people and call on their strengths; bring out the leader and the best in others.
- Challenge complacency and mediocrity; encourage innovation.
- Appreciate the potential of followers; challenge them to stretch and go beyond what they thought they could do (Sinek, 2017).
- Empower others to achieve things they did not believe possible.

Leadership is needed for growth and progress—of individuals, groups, organizations, and institutions. As Harry Truman once said, "In periods where there is no leadership, society stands still. Progress occurs when courageous, skillful leaders seize the opportunity to change things for the better." In this world of increasing chaos, uncertainty, unpredictability, interdependence, and constant change, leadership is desperately needed. In fact, we have a "deeply wired-in need for leaders who will guide us well and safely; who care more about the success of the enterprise than about their own comfort; who call out our best and take full advantage of who we are" (Andersen, 2012, p. 1). Nowhere is this more evident than in today's healthcare arena.

As can be seen from the discussions here, the acknowledged leader is "farsighted, passionate, courageous, wise, generous, and trustworthy" (Andersen, 2012, p. 8). This individual sees beyond the current situation, expresses a compelling vision in an inclusive way, is deeply committed, "doesn't wimp out" (p. 9), learns from mistakes, is thoughtful, and is humble. Finally, leaders are curious, a skill we may need to practice (Barton, 2019), refine, and continually improve.

Professional nurses are in an excellent position to provide leadership within their work settings, professional associations, communities, and society at large. Their communication skills, ability to work collaboratively, sense of service to others, well-established credibility, and commitment to high-quality patient care make them excellent candidates to provide this much-needed leadership. In fact, a recent analysis of the top leadership skills for nurses (Guibert-Lacasa & Vázquez-Calatayud, 2022) include many of these very assets: communication, problem-solving, working with a team, respect, empathy, emotional intelligence, critical reflexivity (the ability to be aware of themselves and their influence on others), and trust. Interestingly, this review focused on clinical nurses who influenced teams to improve patient care, even though they were not in formal leadership positions, which provides support for nurses to think about leadership in different ways.

After a systematic review and meta-analysis of the literature related to leadership effectiveness in healthcare settings, Restivo et al. (2022) determined that "healthcare systems' quality could improve with effective leadership actions" (p. 9). Healthcare workers should be motivated to apply leadership strategies in healthcare systems to improve patient outcomes (Restivo et al., 2022). Nurses can and must be such leaders.

Although *The Future of Nursing* report (Institute of Medicine, 2010) clearly called for nursing to shape its own future and have nurses be prepared as leaders to improve the nation's health, the call for nurse leaders is stronger than ever. In the *Future of Nursing 2020–2030* report (National Academies of Sciences, Engineering, and Medicine et al., 2021), the need for a "new generation of nurse leaders" to address healthcare disparities and strengthen the profession's commitment to health equity is paramount.

Broome and Marshall (2021) emphasize the need for new leadership and how the visions of leaders must be developed, acknowledging the power of followers and the importance of the leader–follower relationship in creating change. Creating a resonant team, one in which both leaders and followers are in a relationship moving toward a shared vision, is necessary to effect lasting change. The leader cannot think the vision can be accomplished alone because a "solitary vision that is not shared is only daydreaming" (Broome & Marshall, 2021, p. 191). The current healthcare climate needs more than a daydream—it needs a new generation of nurse leaders who will shape effective organizations, polices, and patient outcomes. This book presents such a challenge to readers.

Case Study, continued

Before implementing the checklist, the staff asked for a team meeting to review its use and enjoyed the 20-minute meeting so much that the nurse manager instituted weekly team meetings. (This was a bonus win since the nurse manager had always wanted to have weekly team meetings.) Additionally, the nurse manager clearly recognized Georgia, Sarah, and Ron for their leadership and excellence. After the trial period, the triage checklist was accepted as part of their admission protocol and has been in use ever since.

The nurse manager asked Georgia, Sarah, and Ron to collect outcome data related to using the checklist, and they found positive improvements in care as well as decreased cost. The three nurses presented the results at the Hospital Annual Research Day and published the triage checklist in a refereed journal under the title "Best Practice in Care Delivery: Use of a Triage Protocol in a Psychiatric Emergency Department." The nurse manager set up a Grand Rounds, *Emphasizing Safe and Best Practice in the Psychiatric ED*, that Georgia, Sarah, and Ron led for the entire healthcare organization, including senior administrators. Approximately 340 interprofessional staff members attended and evaluated the process of developing the triage protocol as well as safety outcomes of the protocol very highly; in fact, many are now implementing interprofessional changes in their units to foster safe, high-quality care and meet financial goals.

Given that Georgia, Sarah, and Ron really wanted to change the protocol of the PED to give better and safer patient care, they demonstrated strong adaptation behaviors with the nurse manager and staff, demonstrated innovative leadership skills, and used aspects of several other leadership models to make positive changes. A way to implement a big change such as this would be by using the S (strengths), O (opportunities), A (aspirations), and R (results) model, which is based in appreciative inquiry leadership theory. Leaders take what already works in the system and build on those strengths, rather than focus on problems and try to fix them (Stavros & Hinrichs, 2019).

REFLECTION QUESTIONS

5. How did Georgia, Sarah, and Ron demonstrate leadership and work with formal leaders to implement a change?
6. Who benefitted from the leadership displayed by Georgia, Sarah, and Ron; was the outcome worth the effort of embracing leadership?

CRITICAL THINKING 2-1

1. Given the opportunity to publish "the definitive definition of leadership," what would you write? How does your definition reflect the tasks of leadership and the essential elements of leadership?

2. Ask several nursing colleagues and several people outside the health professions (including children) to define leadership. What are the similarities in the definitions offered by these individuals? Are there any significant differences in their definitions? If so, what are they? How do you explain those differences?

3. If an alien came to Earth, approached you, and said, "I see you are a nurse. Take me to your leader," to whom would you take the alien? Who, in your opinion, is providing true leadership within the profession or even within your own institution? Why would you take the alien to this person?

4. Complete the following Grossman & Valiga Leadership Characteristics and Skills Assessment tool to get a sense of how you measure up as a leader. How did you score? Were your scores consistent with how you think of yourself as a leader? Where were your greatest areas of strength? How can you use this information for your future role?

APPENDIX: GROSSMAN & VALIGA LEADERSHIP CHARACTERISTICS AND SKILLS ASSESSMENT

Directions: Part 1 lists statements that are useful in determining a person's perception of what makes for a good leader. Part 2 lists skills that are useful in determining a person's ability to lead. Answer "SA" to those statements with which you Strongly Agree and "A" to those statements with which you Agree. Answer "D" to those statements with which you Disagree and "SD" to those statements with which you Strongly Disagree.

Part 1: Perception of What Makes for a Good Leader				
STATEMENT	SA	A	D	SD
1. Leaders are very creative.				
2. The most important goal of a leader is to be sure the job gets done.				
3. Leaders should focus on people, not on the system.				
4. One does not need to be in a position of authority to be a leader.				
5. Credibility is an important characteristic of a leader.				
6. Leaders tend to be people with high energy who are passionate about their work.				
7. Leaders focus more on being creative than on accomplishing their vision or goal(s).				
8. Persistence is a trademark of an effective leader.				
9. Leaders are committed to their vision and tend not to adapt to change well.				
10. Leaders are good at empowering others to grow.				
11. It is important for leaders to have a dream and to be future oriented.				
12. A person's ability to lead in a professional setting depends on their self-esteem.				
13. A leader's style of leading is determined by the situation and/or task at hand.				

Continued

Part 1: Perception of What Makes for a Good Leader—cont'd

	STATEMENT	SA	A	D	SD
14.	A good leader must have integrity.				
15.	Leaders mentor others to assist them in pursuing their dreams.				
16.	Leadership is a quality one is born with, and it cannot be acquired.				
17.	Good leaders help others to resolve conflict.				
18.	One does not need to be an excellent critical thinker in order to be a great leader.				
19.	A good leader should have excellent communication skills.				
20.	Leaders always follow the rules.				

Part 2: Perception of Your Own Ability to Lead

	STATEMENT	SA	A	D	SD
1.	I value integrity higher than power.				
2.	People tend to think I have the ability to influence others.				
3.	I feel confident about my knowledge base and skills, given my years of experience.				
4.	I have a definite dream for where I want to be in my profession.				
5.	I have mentored another person and found the experience rewarding.				
6.	Change usually makes me feel nervous, and I tend to lose my self-confidence.				
7.	I feel energized taking risks unless they are life-threatening.				
8.	I do not feel confident calling a physician about my patient's status.				
9.	When I experience conflict, I usually give in and accommodate the other person.				
10.	I feel I do make a difference as a nurse and plan to continue to do so.				

Continued

Part 2: Perception of Your Own Ability to Lead—cont'd					
	STATEMENT	SA	A	D	SD
11.	Because I am only a nurse, I am not responsible for patient care errors.				
12.	I often follow others when I am not sure what to do about something.				
13.	I notice I agree with others easily unless the issue is very dear to my heart.				
14.	I attempt to empower ancillary workers because I find the team spirit is enhanced.				
15.	Personally, I do not really have a vision as to where I plan to be in a few years.				
16.	I enjoy conflict and rarely compromise my needs.				
17.	I am an autonomous person.				
18.	I have been told I am extremely reliable and dependable.				
19.	I have great passion for my nursing career.				
20.	It is important to me to think about and plan for the future.				

Scoring. Assign the number shown in the box below to the response you gave to each question in **Part 1** and each question in **Part 2**.

Part 1: Perception of What Makes for a Good Leader					
	STATEMENT	SA	A	D	SD
1.	Leaders are very creative.	4	3	0	0
2.	The most important goal of a leader is to be sure the job gets done.	4	3	2	1
3.	Leaders should focus on people, not on the system.	4	3	2	1
4.	One does not need to be in a position of authority to be a leader.	4	3	0	0
5.	Credibility is an important characteristic of a leader.	4	3	0	0
6.	Leaders tend to be people with high energy who are passionate about their work.	4	3	0	0
7.	Leaders focus more on being creative than on accomplishing their vision or goal(s).	4	3	3	4

Continued

Part 1: Perception of What Makes for a Good Leader—cont'd				
STATEMENT	SA	A	D	SD
8. Persistence is a trademark of an effective leader.	1	2	3	4
9. Leaders are committed to their vision and tend not to adapt to change well.	0	0	3	4
10. Leaders are good at empowering others to grow.	4	3	0	0
11. It is important for leaders to have a dream and to be future oriented.	4	3	0	0
12. A person's ability to lead in a professional setting depends on their self-esteem.	4	3	0	0
13. A leader's style of leading is determined by the situation and/or task at hand.	4	3	0	4
14. A good leader must have integrity.	4	3	2	1
15. Leaders mentor others to assist them in pursuing their dreams.	4	3	0	0
16. Leadership is a quality one is born with, and it cannot be acquired.	0	0	3	4
17. Good leaders help others to resolve conflict.	4	3	2	1
18. One does not need to be an excellent critical thinker in order to be a great leader.	0	0	3	4
19. A good leader should have excellent communication skills.	4	3	0	0
20. Leaders always follow the rules.	0	0	3	4

Part 2: Perception of Your Own Ability to Lead				
STATEMENT	SA	A	D	SD
1. I value integrity higher than power.	4	3	0	0
2. People tend to think I have the ability to influence others.	4	3	0	0
3. I feel confident about my knowledge base and skills, given my years of experience.	4	3	0	0
4. I have a definite dream for where I want to be in my profession.	4	3	3	4
5. I have mentored another person and found the experience rewarding.	4	3	0	0

Continued

		SA	A	D	SD
Part 2: Perception of Your Own Ability to Lead—cont'd					
	STATEMENT	SA	A	D	SD
6.	Change usually makes me feel nervous, and I tend to lose my self-confidence.	4	3	0	0
7.	I feel energized taking risks unless they are life-threatening.	4	3	0	0
8.	I do not feel confident calling a physician about my patient's status.	0	0	3	4
9.	When I experience conflict, I usually give in and accommodate the other person.	0	0	3	4
10.	I feel I do make a difference as a nurse and plan to continue to do so.	4	3	0	0
11.	Since I am only a nurse, I am not responsible for patient care errors.	0	0	3	4
12.	I often follow others when I am not sure what to do about something.	0	0	3	4
13.	I notice I agree with others easily unless the issue is very dear to my heart.	4	3	3	4
14.	I attempt to empower ancillary workers because I find the team spirit is enhanced.	4	3	0	0
15.	Personally, I do not really have a vision as to where I plan to be in a few years.	4	3	2	2
16.	I enjoy conflict and rarely compromise my needs.	4	3	0	0
17.	I am an autonomous person.	4	3	0	0
18.	I have been told I am extremely reliable and dependable.	4	3	0	0
19.	I have great passion for my nursing career.	4	3	0	0
20.	It is important to me to think about and plan for the future.	4	3	0	0

Interpretation of Scores

Part 1: Perception of What Makes for a Good Leader

Add up your score for Part 1. Here's what the scores indicate:

70 to 80 = Excellent perception of a good leader.

60 to 69 = Good perception of a good leader.

50 to 59 = Probably mixing up the difference between management and leadership.

40 to 49 = Definitely mixing up the difference between management and leadership.

39 or less = Need to do some reading on what good leadership is.

Part 2: Perception of Your Own Ability to Lead

Add up your score for Part 2. Here's what the scores indicate:

70 to 80 = Extremely high perceived leadership ability.

60 to 69 = High perceived leadership ability.

50 to 59 = Moderate perceived leadership ability.

40 to 49 = Low perceived leadership ability.

39 or less = Extremely low perceived leadership ability.

References

Abbas, M., & Ali, R. (2023). Transformational versus transactional leadership styles and project success: A meta-analytic review. *European Management Journal, 41*(1),125–142. https://doi.org/10.1016/j.emj.2021.10.011

Andersen, E. (2012). *Leading so people will follow.* Jossey-Bass.

Barton, A. J. (2019). Practicing curiosity (Editorial). *Journal of Nursing Education, 58*(8), 439–440.

Begoun, E. (2018, August 21). Where are the contrarian leaders? *SmartBrief on Leadership.* http://smartbrief.com/original/2018/08/where-are-contrarian-leaders?utm_source=brief

Bennis, W. (1989). *On becoming a leader.* Addison-Wesley.

Bennis, W. (2004, April 20). A leadership discussion with Warren Bennis. Webcast sponsored by the American Society of Association Executives Foundation.

Bennis, W., & Nanus, B. (1985). *Leaders: The strategies for taking charge.* Harper & Row.

Bissell, C. T. (n.d.). Claude Thomas Bissell > quotes. Goodreads. https://www.goodreads.com/author/quotes/1555218.Claude_Thomas_Bissell

Bleich, M. R. (2015). Leadership and brilliant mistakes. *Journal of Continuing Education in Nursing, 46*(5), 203–204.

Block, P. (1996). *Stewardship: Choosing service over self-interest.* Berrett-Koehler.

Brenan, M. (2023, January 10). Nurses retain top ethics rating in U.S., but below 2020 high. *Gallup.* https://news.gallup.com/poll/467804/nurses-retain-top-ethics-rating-below-2020-high.aspx

Broome, M. E., & Marshall, E. S. (2021). *Transformational leadership in nursing: From expert clinician to influential leader* (3rd ed.). Springer.

Brown, B. (2018). *Dare to lead: Brave work. Tough conversations. Whole hearts.* Random House.

Cloud, K., & Leturmy, A. (2023). Management vs. leadership: Would you rather? *College and University, 98*(1), 75–80. https:// www.proquest.com/scholarly-journals/management-vs-leadership-would-you-rather/docview/2785685210/se-2?accountid=11041

Dudley, D. (2010, February). *Everyday leadership* [Video]. TED Conferences. https://www.ted.com/talks/drew_dudley_everyday_leadership?subtitle=en

Gardner, J. W. (1989). The tasks of leadership. In W. E. Rosenbach & R. L. Taylor (Eds.), *Contemporary issues in leadership* (2nd ed., pp. 24–33). Westview Press.

Gardner, J. W. (1990). *On leadership.* Free Press.

Greenleaf, R. K. (1977). *Servant leadership: A journey into the nature of legitimate power and greatness.* Paulist Press.

Guibert-Lacasa, C., & Vázquez-Calatayud, M. (2022). Nurses' clinical leadership in the hospital setting: A systematic review. *Journal of Nursing Management, 30*(4), 913–925. https://doi.org/10.1111/jonm.13570

Gutterman, A. S. (2023). Definitions and conceptions of leadership. Older Persons' Rights Project. https://www.researchgate.net/publication/371169414_Definitions_and_Conceptions_of_Leadership

Hale, J. (2023, February 17). The most important leadership skill for 2023. *Forbes.* https://www.forbes.com/sites/forbescoachescouncil/2023/02/17/the-most-important-leadership-skill-for-2023/?sh=24193e97403f

Hoban, M. (2018, November 7). Strategic leadership means learning to listen—Differently. *Leader Pulse.* https://www.ddiworld.com/blog/tmi/november-2018/strategic-leadership-means-learning-to-listen

Holle, M. L., & Blatchley, M. E. (1987). *Introduction to leadership and management in nursing* (2nd ed.). Jones & Bartlett.

Institute of Medicine. (2010). *The future of nursing: Leading change, advancing health*. National Academies Press.

Jackman, I. (Ed.). (2005). *The leader's mentor: Inspiration from the world's most effective leaders.* Random House.

Keating, S. (2018, December 28). When leadership is lacking. *LeadToday*. https://stevekeating.me/2018/12/28/when-leadership-is-lacking/

Kinni, T. (2018, September 28). A blinding flash of the obvious. *Insights by Stanford Business*. https://www.gsb.stanford.edu/insights/blinding-flash-obvious

Kitt, A., Van Dusen, L., & Athey, S. (2023). *Integrated leadership: The pathway to transforming healthcare and healing the world*. Leadership Circle. https://leadershipcircle.com/wp-content/uploads/2023/09/Integrated-Leadership-The-Pathway-to-Transforming-Healthcare-and-Healing-the-World-Unlocking-EveLC-White-Paper-2023-09.pdf

Kotter, J. P. (1990). *A force for change: How leadership differs from management*. The Free Press.

Kotter, J. P. (2013, January 9). Management is (still) not leadership. *Harvard Business Review*. https://hbr.org/2013/01/management-is-still-not-leadership

Kouzes, J. M., & Posner, B. Z. (2017). *The leadership challenge: How to make extraordinary things happen in organizations* (6th ed.). Wiley.

Levine, J. (2019). On board; Getting better all the time. *TC Today, 43*(2), 50.

Manfredi, C. (1995). The art of legendary leadership. *Nursing Leadership Forum, 1*(2), 62–64.

Maxwell, J. (2022, May 18). Motivation: How leaders inspire effort [Audio podcast episode]. In *Maxwell Leadership Podcast*. https://johnmaxwellleadershippodcast.com/episodes/john-maxwell-motivation-how-leaders-inspire-effort

McCarthy, D. (2012, July 17). 10 simple "truths" about management vs. leadership. *Great Leadership*.

Monehin, D. & Diers-Lawson, A. (2022). Pragmatic optimism, crisis leadership, and contingency theory: A view from the C-suite. *Public Relations Review, 48*(4), 102224. https://doi.org/10.1016/j.pubrev.2022.102224

Nanus, B. (1992). *Visionary leadership*. Jossey-Bass.

National Academies of Sciences, Engineering, and Medicine; National Academy of Medicine; Committee on the Future of Nursing 2020–2030; Flaubert, J. L., Le Menestrel, S., Williams, D. R., & Wakefield, M. K. (Eds.). (2021, May 11). *The future of nursing 2020–2030: Charting a path to achieve health equity*. National Academies Press (US). https://www.ncbi.nlm.nih.gov/books/NBK573919/

National Council of State Boards of Nursing. (2019, Spring). Clinical Judgment Measurement Model and Action Mode. *Next Generation NCLEX News*. https://www.ncsbn.org/public-files/NGN_Spring19_ENG_29Aug2019.pdf

Phillips, D. T. (1997). *The founding fathers on leadership*. Warner Books.

Restivo, V., Minutolo, G., Battaglini, A., Carli, A., Capraro, M., Gaeta, M., Odone, A., Trucchi, C., Favaretti, C., Vitale, F., & Casuccio, A. (2022). Leadership effectiveness in healthcare settings: A systematic review and meta-analysis of cross-sectional and before-after studies. *International Journal of Environmental Research and Public Health, 19*(17), 10995. https://doi.org/10.3390/ijerph191710995

Robinson, K. (2009). *The element: How finding your passion changes everything*. Penguin Books.

Rockwell, D. (2019, May 8). 7 faces of distrust. *Leadership Freak*. https://leadershipfreak.blog/2019/05/08/7-faces-of-distrust/

Rosser, E. A., Edwards, S., Kwan, R. Y. C., Ito, M., Potter, D. R., Hodges, K. T., & Buckner, E. (2023). The Global Leadership Mentoring Community: An evaluation of its impact on nursing leadership. *International Nursing Review, 70*(3), 279–285. https://doi.org/10.1111/inr.12860

Ruben, B. D., & Gigliotti, R. A. (2021). Explaining incongruities between leadership theory and practice: Integrating theories of resonance, communication and systems. *Leadership & Organization Development Journal, 42*(6), 942–957. https://doi.org/10.1108/LODJ-02-2021-0072

Schweitzer, C. (2006, March). From soloist to orchestrator. *Associations Now*, 33–36.

Sinek, S. (2009a). *How great leaders inspire action* [Video]. TED Conferences. https://www.ted.com/talks/simon_sinek_how_great_leaders_inspire_action

Sinek, S. (2009b). *Start with why: How great leaders inspire everyone to take action*. Penguin Group.

Sinek, S. (2014, March). *Why good leaders make you feel safe* [Video]. TED Conferences. https://www
.ted.com/talks/simon_sinek_why_good_leaders_make_you_feel_safe.

Sinek, S. (2017). *Leaders eat last: Why some teams pull together and others don't.* Penguin Group.

Spears, L. C. (Ed.). (1995). *Reflections on leadership: How Robert K. Greenleaf's theory of servant-leader-ship influenced today's top management thinkers.* John Wiley & Sons.

Stavros, J., & Hinrichs, G. (2019). *The Thin book of SOAR: Creating strategy that inspires innovation and engagement.* Thin Book Publishing.

Thornberry, N. (2006). A view about "vision." In W. E. Rosenbach & R. L. Taylor (Eds.). *Contemporary issues in leadership* (6th ed., pp. 31–43). Westview Press.

Tichy, N. M. (1997). *The leadership engine: How winning companies build leaders at every level.* HarperBusiness.

Tómasdóttir, H., & Freedman, B. (2019, February). *The crisis of leadership—and a new way forward* [Video]. TED Conferences. https://www.ted.com/talks/halla_tomasdottir_and_bryn_freedman
_the_crisis_of_leadership_and_a_new_way_forward?subtitle=en

Wheatley, M. J. (1999). *Leadership and the new science: Discovering order in a chaotic world* (2nd ed.). Berrett-Koehler.

Zaleznik, A. (1981). Managers and leaders: Are they different? *Journal of Nursing Administration, 11*(7), 25–31.

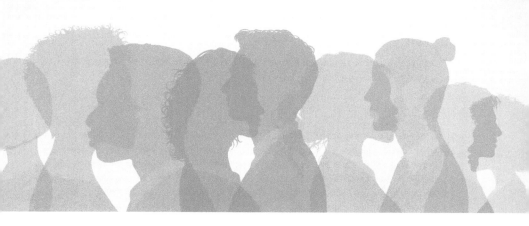

CHAPTER 3

Uncertainty and Chaos
Challenging, Invigorating, and Growth Producing

LEARNING OBJECTIVES
- Describe the process by which leaders and followers can thrive and grow despite the challenges of today's healthcare system.
- Describe how chaos and complexity science can propel individuals and organizations to accomplish goals.
- Analyze how nurse leaders can use the change process effectively in the realization of a vision.
- Formulate innovative strategies that decrease resistance to change.
- Describe how purposeful introduction of conflict can generate change.

INTRODUCTION

Surviving the tumultuous changes and problems of the current healthcare system is a tremendous challenge for nurses and other healthcare professionals, as well as for patients, families, communities, and organizations. Providers must continue to create new and effective delivery systems, partner more effectively with one another and with patients, and work cohesively to provide cost-effective quality care and achieve desired patient outcomes (Marshall & Broome, 2021).

As we move from the scientific (or Newtonian) age to the relationship (or new leadership) age, nurses must incorporate a new perspective—that chaos can be advantageous because unpredictability is what makes us evolve and grow. Nursing leaders need to be willing to make educated guesses, be more flexible and adaptable, use their intuition, and be comfortable with uncertainty and ambiguity. Nurses must take the time to develop leadership ability so that they can be part of the force that drives the profession's evolution and creates our preferred future.

Consider the following case study related to leadership during uncertainty and chaos as you continue reading this chapter.

Case Study

Susan, a registered nurse (RN), and her colleagues in a high-acuity medical unit have extremely challenging patient assignments due to an increase in patients with COVID and the growing staff shortage. Additionally, they are usually assigned new unlicensed assistive personnel (UAPs) to assist them. Despite the challenging circumstances, Susan and the other RNs feel that it would be easier to do the work themselves because they have to explain details to the UAPs, and they rarely have any consistency with the UAPs. Generally, there are different UAP assignments each day. Often, as is happening today, the RNs have to orient a new float or travel nurse who has their own separate patient assignment and who has been told by the supervisor to ask the staff RN for assistance with anything about which they feel uncomfortable. The staff RN has a new UAP to orient, another staff RN not familiar with the unit's policies and staff who are asking questions, and responsibility for an extremely challenging patient assignment.

REFLECTION QUESTIONS

1. How can Susan foster teamwork and collaboration among the RNs, UAPs, and other staff members in the face of the challenges of high-acuity and staff shortage?
2. What strategies can be implemented to communicate critical information effectively to all team members, including new staff and float nurses?

UNCERTAINTY AND AMBIGUITY: NEED FOR FLEXIBILITY AND ADAPTATION

Healthcare is complex and unpredictable, requiring flexible and adaptable professionals to deliver patient care and leadership. The global pandemic that began in 2020 heightened the need for employees to be flexible and adaptable because of the uncertainties of the disease, limited resources, workforce shortages, stress, and burnout. More than ever, nurses must become comfortable with chaos and disequilibrium and be willing to adopt a new perspective on change. In a classic example, Wheatley (2006, p. 137) remembered listening to a geologist during a radio interview regarding his perspective on a huge hurricane in the North Carolina Outer Banks. The interviewer asked what he expected to find after the hurricane. Instead of saying all the negative findings one would expect, the geologist said, "I expect to find a new beach." In organizations, nurses also have to be willing to "find a new beach" and adapt. They need to appreciate "how life is capable of so much change, so much newness," and "embrace this newness instead of trying to control it" (Wheatley, 2006, p. 139). They need to use their intuition to solve problems rather than focusing all their energy on finding the parts that are not working and trying to fix them. By taking a new view of problems, nurses can identify "images, words or patterns that surface" (Wheatley, 2005, 2006, p. 141) that will help them focus on the whole and anticipate how growth and positive outcomes can be generated from the situation.

Nurses must embrace the idea that there is no usual routine in their profession. They must develop adaptive skills to manage change and conflict daily. The ability to delegate effectively to other healthcare workers and to develop new delivery of care strategies is paramount. Nurses require maturity to recognize their lifelong learning needs, and have the astuteness to position themselves in arenas where significant decisions are being made so that they can be a part of implementing the changes that are so necessary.

In time of change and uncertainty, leaders and those they lead may become easily paralyzed by the uncertainty they are experiencing; leading during these periods requires pushing through the perceived inability to move forward or make decisions (Polson, 2020). Nurses must acclimate themselves to feelings of uneasiness, ambiguity, and the unknown. They must plan for uncertainty and remain focused to harness the positive aspects of chaos. By applying quantum theory principles (Malloch & Porter-O'Grady, 2009), we can realize that all systems work from the inside out, not from the top down or bottom up, and appreciate that relationship is as significant as control in maintaining effectiveness. Although systems cannot be predicted with certainty, we know that tension between stability and chaos creates change. The new leader, therefore, must do the following:

- Analyze current models of care delivery and be willing to create new models when necessary.
- Collaborate with and obtain information from all members of the interdisciplinary team in an effort to co-create change. Despite some of the autonomy involved in nursing practice, it is important to remember your role in the team.
- Be aware of new methods, listen to ideas that may not make sense today, and embrace a degree of uncertainty.
- Engage in continuous learning and quality improvement.

Leadership has changed from an individualized, unit-focused perspective to a more participative, collaborative focus. Essentially, successful organizations will need to have adaptive cultures if they want to succeed (Kotter, 2012). We cannot just sit back and hold on to the status quo in our individual departments and practices and "let the next generation of executives do it" (p. 179). The time is now—we need to transform our work settings and gain new skills. The Center for Creative Leadership (CCL) offers transformational and human-centered workshops and programs on leadership, which can be accessed at the CCL's Web site (http://www.ccl.org).

One of CCL's reports (2019) is especially helpful for reviewing how to successfully lead a transformational change. The report explains the seven trends that transformative leaders must be aware of when leading their constantly changing organizations: recognizing accidental leaders, improving change endurance, using digital fluency, embracing disruption, kicking glass, reimagining the review process, and developing a culture reboot. The familiar 360-degree assessment strategy or 365-day assessment (Scott, 2009) is also available as a tool for individuals to obtain data regarding their performance in a specific area, such as, adaptation to change. The assessments are designed to provide a snapshot of practical feedback on skills and behaviors. It allows an individual to view data privately from people with whom they come in contact but do not necessarily work for, while avoiding data sharing with specific people in their work organization. Upon finalizing the assessment strategy, it is crucial to participate in discussions with individuals offering feedback. While the feedback providers' perceptions may not necessarily represent the absolute truth of a situation, they serve as the basis for decision making. Otherwise, the individual receiving the feedback might not give much importance to following the feedback. Additional assessment tools are available on the Internet.

> *Use the constant change around you as your opportunity to change people's perceptions of you, and to prove your skills and ability to contribute.* —Susan Rehwaldt and Mary Lou Higgerson

DEFINING CHAOS

Chaos, or extreme, unpredictable disorganization and surprise, is most apparent today. Lorenz (1993, p. 4) defined chaos as "processes [systems] that appear to proceed according to chance, even though their behaviour is in fact determined by precise laws." Wheatley and Kellner-Rogers (1996) remind us that a "system maintains itself only if change is occurring somewhere in it all the time" (p. 33). So, one must view chaos or unrest as a means of survival. In other words, if there were no arguments or differences of opinion, the status quo would be maintained, and there would be no individual growth. In addition, organizational survival would be threatened. The following questions were posed by Wheatley (2006, p. 73) to those who tend to believe that everything has to have a place and be labeled and filed away:

- Why would we stay locked in our belief that "truth" exists in objective form?
- Why would we stay locked in our belief that there is one way to do something or one correct interpretation to a situation, when the universe welcomes diversity and seems to thrive on a plurality of meaning?
- Why would we avoid participation and worry only about its risks?
- Why would we resist the powerful visions and futures that emerge when we come together to co-create the world?
- Why would we ever choose rigidity or predictability when we have been invited to be part of the generative dance of life?

Questions such as these invite one to discard old ways and embrace new ideas. Many creative, motivated, and enthusiastic individuals thrive on chaos and are most successful in their personal and professional lives despite the incredibly confusing climate in which they function (Gribbin, 2004). Hawking (1987) viewed this uncertainty as opening the way to randomness and unpredictability, ideas many perceive as refreshing. Others may become disengaged and not flourish in the uncertain environment. For example, some nurses temporarily assigned to a different unit see that situation as an opportunity to expand their knowledge, skills, and networks. However, other nurses may become angry with having to work in a different unit and allow their anger to interfere with the assignment; barely maintain safety; and complain to anyone who will listen, including patients, their families, and nursing students. If situations such as these were to be seen as opportunities for personal and professional growth, fear of the unknown could be minimized, and individuals would learn new skills and acquire greater decision-making abilities. As a result, one would expect such individuals to increase their confidence and increase their ability to survive the "chaos" associated with having to work in different units.

How we perceive our situations in life, at work, and in our personal lives will significantly affect the outcome of our work. Fackler et al. (2015) found that staff nurses perceived they do have the power to improve patient care. So, with this perceived power, the nursing workforce can impact substantive change in healthcare delivery. For example, conducting patient rounds during which nurses share their approaches to caring for a patient allows new and experienced nurses to dialogue, learn from one another, feel empowered, and refocus the negative energy that may accompany new experiences. When everyone and everything can link together, systems form that create more possibilities for all.

This perspective helps explain why nurses need to start leading as soon as they graduate and why they need to develop their leadership skills as they grow and evolve throughout their professional careers. Likewise, hospitals and organizations must sustain ways for nurses to buy in to new initiatives, take risks, and adapt to practice changes to maintain nurse engagement and ultimately improve quality care (French-Bravo & Crow, 2015). For example, nurses can change care delivery to include the patient and family or significant others as important stakeholders in their health. These patient–provider partnerships are frequently seen in primary and specialty care, as well as close patient–nurse relationships in the hospital and community. Berger-Hoger et al. (2019) conducted a study of 64 patients with primary ductal carcinoma in situ with no other breast malignancy history and found that nurses' coaching increased patients' shared decision making regarding their treatment determination and ultimately patient satisfaction. Nurses can participate in multiple methods of encouraging patients to be a more productive part of their healthcare plan by offering group sessions on mindfulness, exercise, and nutrition tips, and creating sample diets. Additionally, by following specific policies, most of these patient educational sessions can be reimbursable to the practice. Elwyn et al. (2016) offer multiple tools that can be used to facilitate more shared decision making with patients.

In attempting to attain the most positive outcome for each patient, nurses need to manage multiple variables and be alert to the possible influence of variables we do not even know about. Nurses who are leaders attend to the realities and possibilities of chaos inherent in life and learn and grow as a result of the unanticipated occurrences in our lives every day.

CHAOS IN NURSING

From a Newtonian (scientific) perspective, a leader is expected to help organizations adapt to change by establishing goals, obtaining commitment from employees at all levels of the bureaucracy, and decreasing uncertainty (Malloch & Porter-O'Grady, 2009). Such behaviors reflect the following assumptions:

- If something works once, keep trying it.
- If employees' needs are identified, managers can manipulate the employee to improve the organization but not necessarily improve the employee.
- Large effects have large causes.
- Each employee should confine themself to their specific job description.
- Given the organizational structure, one should know that lines of authority and information flow are similar.

This view emphasizes management, planning, and controlling rather than leadership and empowering a group. The new leadership paradigm helps us realize that individuals are more effective leaders when they can keep their groups curious and open to change, because it is only then that the whole organization can grow creatively and productively.

The uncertainty of healthcare flows from the quantum and chaotic nature of the world over time. Nurses should, therefore, stop trying to plan every step and predict each happening. They must realize that they can never come close to knowing all there is to know about a topic or a patient situation, nor is it possible to plan every step. Hence, they must accept that no matter how much they know about the world, there are far more questions than answers, and uncertainty is a natural part of their lives.

For example, the COVID-19 pandemic brought about challenging circumstances and unpredictable changes. Before the world knew of COVID-19, The World Health Organization (WHO) declared 2020 to be The Year of the Nurse and the Midwife to bring awareness to the need for nurses in healthcare worldwide (WHO, 2020). "Little did the profession of nursing know at the time, that the Year of the Nurse would reveal to the world, yet again, what the role of professional nursing does to uphold the healthcare of the most vulnerable, even in the midst of great personal risk" (Zipf et al., 2021, p. 101). Nurses and healthcare professionals had to learn quickly, plan in the present, and adapt to future changes with uncertainty during the pandemic crisis. Nurses had to work collaboratively with the healthcare team to implement new protocols, issue immediate staff training for employees, and adapt to rapidly changing information. They had to plan for an influx of patients and embrace technology for virtual patient care and communication with patient families and friends. During the COVID-19 pandemic, nurses faced challenging circumstances and unpredictable changes in their profession and personal lives as the world navigated the uncertainty.

Additionally, nurses must realize they cannot go it alone when they are dealing with a changing environment. Indeed, it is paramount that nurses interconnect with members of other disciplines to make innovative changes. By using diverse skill sets, incorporating multiple perspectives for improving care for various patient populations, and seeing the patient and family as the focus of care, nurses will be more successful in accomplishing the profession's goals. Nurses must think collaboratively and innovatively, and not accept the status quo when planning and providing quality care for patients and their families.

Nurses must also realize that the lengthy to-do lists they routinely develop at the beginning of a workday can be nothing more than skeletal frameworks, because such lists cannot encompass all that nurses need to do that day. Being task oriented and using a minute-to-minute structure to organize one's work must give way to critical thinking and constantly adapting as new problems and challenges arise. Because of the exceptional complexity of the nursing role, organizational charts, time-management lists, and critical pathways have served almost as survival techniques by giving some structure in a highly chaotic environment. Unfortunately, to-do lists and predictive pathways inhibit our ability to see things globally. Instead of trying to block out the chaos and unpredictability inherent in healthcare, nurses need to learn how to embrace it. One must embrace relationships with others and be aware that the order of life is based more on principles of emergence and less on a predetermined order. Variables such as communication and collaborative relationships among individuals energize a system and help it to be effective.

However, nurses cannot simply wait and see how things evolve. Haigh (2008) reported on a strategy to use chaos theory to help an acute pain practice (with an overwhelming 20% patient growth each year) plan more effectively for providing nursing services. Although it is impossible (and perhaps contrary to chaos theory) to predict the details of each desired patient outcome, one can plan to reach specific levels of effectiveness in fulfilling the several components of a patient's plan of care. This prediction is made possible by creating various ranges of what constitutes effectiveness. The next step involves developing numerous possibilities (e.g., increasing the number of professionals needed for safe and quality care delivery in the growing pain practice) that can be used to achieve each outcome; this is accomplished using a population equation that can help with forecasting appropriate provider-to-patient care delivery. Chaos theory assisted this organization in obtaining insight into the number and types of patients who would most likely present at the pain service; as a result, reasonable staffing could be positioned with the right resources for likely success. Nurses could accomplish this by hiring a diverse staff to work with the diverse patient population, focusing on retaining current staff instead of recruiting new staff to regenerate their energy and passion, trying methods that do not require the same expensive resources that have been used in the past, and assisting staff in experimenting with new ideas that will help develop new practice models.

Many healthcare agencies and institutions have experienced change through merging or acquisition or from an internal governance model shift. For example, when a practice or clinic is bought out or merged with a different care system, several chronically ill patients may be required to transfer to a new primary care provider. When that happens, no patient–provider relationship exists, and all involved parties must begin again. In addition, it probably will take more time for the new provider to care for these complex patients, compared with the original provider, because they do not know the patient; the patient and provider will have to invest energy into starting a new relationship. The nurse can be the consistent piece in this puzzle and assume the role of coordinating patients and providers to deliver consistency with the patient, family, and healthcare system. This type of case management is needed to advocate for the maximal quality of patient care. Nurse leaders can also help avoid some of the problems that have accompanied such change and be more successful with the ultimate change if they do the following (Ponte et al., 2007):

- Obtain representation from every healthcare group that is involved, especially those who are directly engaged in patient care.
- Be sure to keep each representative accountable—by ensuring that the representative returns to their constituents to gather their ideas and share what is happening in the planning meetings for a redesign of the governance model.
- Define each leader's role (including oneself) involved in the change initiative and be sure each of these leaders is part of defining their responsibilities and that these duties are transparent to the entire staff.
- Be very cognizant of developing a governance model that promotes safe, high-quality patient- and family-centered care.
- Build in metrics that measure the model's effectiveness regarding quality, patient and staff satisfaction, cost-effectiveness, productivity, and safety.

Case Study, continued

The staff RNs are likely to expend only so much energy and accept this type of working condition with the UAPs and travel nurses only so many times before becoming angry and unwilling to follow this patient assignment model. Whether the nurses stay in this job or not depends greatly on how effectively the leader can help them manage the anger or conflict; create a new model of orienting travel nurses; and, even more important, assist in retaining nurses so that there is less need for travel nurses.

3. What proactive measures can leaders implement to address the root causes of dissatisfaction and enhance overall job satisfaction among nursing staff?

PROVIDING LEADERSHIP IN THE MIDST OF CHAOS

Tetenbaum and Laurence (2011) describe ways of dealing with volatile and chaotic organizations. Using Heifetz's adaptation theory of leadership (Heifetz, 1994), they suggest leaders do the following:

- Change the leader role to one of facilitator.
- Continue to disturb the status quo or what might seem to be the status quo.
- Delegate the hard work to the followers so that they participate.
- Guide the new ideas and initiatives.
- Encourage conflict.

Continue to negotiate the chaos until the "best adaptive solution to the problem facing you is reached" (Heifetz, 1994, p. 46).

Undoubtedly, we are being confronted with multiple challenges, such as climate change, political instability, and a pandemic, to name a few. Nurse leaders need to hone their skills in policy advocacy so the status quo does not prevail in these chaotic times. Jurns (2019) offers suggestions to nurses on how they can communicate with policymakers about their identified problem/challenge, starting with making an appointment to discuss the topic and following up after the meeting to achieve the most effective results regarding the desired change.

It is wise to realize that no matter how much energy is spent trying to lead through chaos, the stability one might long for is not really the solution, because stability will only limit the growth that occurs when some degree of chaos remains. Thus, each of us must become comfortable with constant change. Heifetz and Linsky (2017) remind us that a productive change needs to be adaptable if we are looking for sustainability and offer helpful tools for assisting us in surviving.

CONSTANT CHANGE: INCREASINGLY CHARACTERIZING OUR WORLD

One of the most pervasive and significant concepts affecting our lives is that of change—change that comes about through our own development and maturation, change that takes place as a result of our education and our interactions with others, change that is imposed on us from outside sources, and change that we impose on ourselves and others. If we are to cope effectively with change and use it to our advantage, we must be able to recognize when it occurs, when it needs to occur, how to facilitate it, how it can be blocked, and the impact various changes and change strategies have on individuals and groups.

Change is making something different from the way it was. It is an alteration; it results from differences and conflicts in a system, from information, or sometimes from unfulfilled needs. Change potentiates or allows the possibility of accomplishing goals. It can be planned or an unexpected result of a decision or other event (Nickerson, 2014). Change can be subtle, or it can be spontaneous, even revolutionary. Change in one's personal and professional life can involve a transition period, during which adjustment may be successful or not. No matter what the change is, an actual change does not affect only a single person; instead, it permeates the ambiance of a setting and triggers some type of change in anyone who comes in contact with the individual or setting that changed. Examples of changes that have profoundly affected most healthcare workers and patients include the emerging delivery of healthcare via telehealth. With the global pandemic of 2020, telehealth became a primary method of delivering care. Suddenly, nurses with very little training in telehealth were expected to use technology (Rutledge & Gustin, 2021). Nurses practiced, and continue to practice, telehealth by implementing videoconferencing to conduct remote patient assessments, provide medication management, and communicate with patients regarding self-care and education, showcasing adaptability.

Denhardt and Denhardt (2006) also speak to the dance of leadership. They assert that leadership can be perceived as being "drawn directly from the arts" (p. 6) and of being an "intense textured interplay of space, time, and energy" (p. 6).

These two authors also differentiate leadership from management by saying leadership is all about "what energizes people," and to energize others, a leader must try one thing and then another until a path reveals itself (p. 10). Additionally, whereas "leadership is a way of working within a world of openness and change," "management is a way of working within a world of order and regulation" (Denhardt & Denhardt, 2006, p. 10).

It seems that many people are dissatisfied with their lives but do not know how to change. They have, in a sense, been conditioned to accept their lot in life and do not know how to move away from their routine—no matter how uncomfortable or dissatisfying that life has become. Perhaps by better understanding some principles of change (Box 3-1), we can be more willing to engage in it and change our lives.

THE LEADER AS A CHANGE AGENT

As nurses acquire new abilities and transform into leaders, they will demonstrate courage by involving others in clarifying the vision and making decisions about how to realize it. Nurses will need to be involved and influence decisions about quality of clinical outcomes, work content, and performance effectiveness of workers and not just the managers. Nurses are responsible for their practice; thus, they should exercise leadership and direct that practice. Nurses must collectively share ownership of the workplace with others, while empowering others to make necessary changes.

Kouzes and Posner (2017) believe that leaders do not always seek the challenges and consequential ramifications of change that occur but that these challenges seek the leaders. They also believe that challenge is the motivating milieu for excellence. They have found through their research that "ordinary" individuals are able to accomplish extraordinary feats, and those who function as leaders in the group realize they have skills they never knew they had, including the ability to manage change.

An important skill for a leader to exercise when involved in change is that of mentoring and coaching. This is the ability to facilitate others' understanding of themselves and their own abilities. It is the process by which one person (the coach–leader) helps followers understand that answers to questions or solutions

---

BOX 3-1 **Principles of Change**

- A change in one part affects other parts and other systems.
- People affected by the change should participate in making the change.
- People should be informed of the reasons for the change.
- Concrete and specific feedback about the process of change will enhance its acceptance.
- People need assistance in dealing with the effects of the change.
- People's suggestions and contributions about the implementation of change should be sought and incorporated.
- A change must be reinforced, or the system will revert to its old practices.
- Conflict may occur at any step during the change process.
- The more compatible the new ideas are with one's values and needs, the more easily a change will be adopted.
- The more trust one has in the initiator of change, the more likely one is to support the change.
- One's past experience with change can profoundly affect one's willingness to support a new idea.

to problems lie within themselves. Being able to role-model behaviors that assist individuals' adaptation to change is also helpful. Leaders who can help facilitate connections among followers should be successful in orchestrating change. For example, fostering collaboration, addressing internal conflicts, and cultivating a positive work environment help boost meaningful connections among leaders and followers (Zhang et al., 2022).

The new leadership is about forming relationships and connecting with others to challenge old, bureaucratic organizational structures and old ways of doing things. The delay in committing to a decision allows followers or all those affected by the decision to discuss all issues fully and explore all possible options. Change requires discarding old behaviors and replacing them with new ones, which will undoubtedly cause conflict. However, if this conflict is addressed effectively, the new behaviors will be adopted, and the ultimate outcome will be superior. It is likely that as followers explore various options and points of view, turmoil in the group or organization will occur. Rather than being distressed by this turmoil, however, leaders are excited by it because it is exactly what the organization needs if change is to be successful. Teams of followers should be expected to cause continuous change in the group's or organization's strategy as they generate ideas for action and identify new directions. Reducing the existing hierarchy and challenging the group's or organization's belief system are necessary to prevent an organization from maintaining the status quo. When an individual, group, community, or team is able to empower itself, effective leadership has occurred, positive change is likely, and the organization can grow tremendously. With this new perspective, the importance of developing self-directed teams of effective followers in any organization is made abundantly clear (Fig. 3-1).

FACILITATING THE CHANGE PROCESS

Leaders are necessary to facilitate change. There must be a reason for the change to occur, and the players must be willing to try to change. The change must also yield growth—positive or negative. Such actions require that the leader be willing to think in new ways and try new approaches despite the barriers to change that they are likely to confront.

Often, patients do not comply with taking their medications, following a diet, stopping smoking, or engaging in other behaviors that health professionals recommend. What about nurses facilitating change in the patient arena? Change revolves around patient behavior, and essentially, much of the discouragement that nurses, staff, and advanced practice nurses experience is due to their patients not complying with their treatment protocol, both pharmacological and nonpharmacological. It is essential for nurses and healthcare professionals to assess the root cause and to be aware of any barriers preventing compliance. For example, is the patient unable to comply due to lack of resources? Suppose it is determined that patient behavior is the cause of noncompliance. In that case, the Model for Health Behavior Change (Prochaska et al., 1992) is a method for assisting patients in changing their behavior and is often used in setting up a contract between a patient and a health provider regarding the steps the patient will follow to make a change that will positively affect their health. An important aspect of this model is that the patient

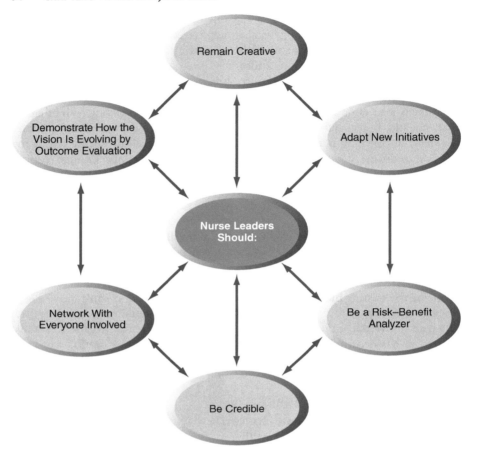

FIGURE 3-1 • Implications for nurses to be successful change agents.

and provider mutually decide the goals of the contract. For example, when working with a patient who overeats and needs to change their eating habits, the nurse and the patient mutually develop a contract with goals and target dates for measuring changes and outcome results of the change. Communication methods are set up according to what is appropriate to share between the nurse and the patient and includes a list of the consequences the patient will encounter if the change in eating habits does not occur. There has been much success with this framework with all healthcare providers and their patients. Some suggestions regarding communicating with patients who need to change a health behavior include the following (Van Servellen, 2009):

- Change can occur in minimal steps.
- An individual must be motivated to change for the change to be permanent.

- Outside reinforcement of changed behavior can be negative or positive but still be productive for the person making the changes.
- The patient must see the importance of making the change for overall health.
- The patient needs a social network for support in making the change.
- Patients must feel they are able to make the change.
- Nurses need to show confidence in the patient making the change.

Effective communication, recognition of staff welfare in addition to patient safety during a transition, and empowerment of staff to accomplish the processes necessary for the change to evolve are necessary components for a successful change similar to the above suggestions of change with patients.

There is no doubt that effective change requires leadership; however, both leaders and followers must be motivated and energized to implement positive changes and thrive in the chaos that will ensue. Having informal discussions regarding new ideas for changing care is one way to stimulate nurses' thinking about how they can shape future changes in healthcare and how open they and their organization are to change. Continuous dialogue can offer insight into nurses' and organizations' readiness for the changes confronted by healthcare today and can help leaders who want to implement a change. Readiness to Change Assessment Tools are available on the Internet to formally assess an individual's, unit's, or department's ideas about change. It is important to create a work culture supportive of change so that individuals develop an appreciation for change, adapt values that motivate them to seek change when needed, and realize that successful change yields positive incentives for both patients and staff.

PROCESS OF CHANGE

The current and predicted rate of change in society in general and in healthcare in particular is phenomenal. Such change requires professions, groups, and institutions to reassess their goals, structure, culture, and planning processes. Leaders are faced, therefore, with enormous challenges that are not only energy consuming but are also revitalizing and rewarding. Leaders must help others see the need for change, work with others to implement change, evaluate the effect of change, and participate in each stage of the change process. They also must understand what people may experience as they go through change.

Perhaps one of the most useful theories to help us understand this phenomenon is that espoused by Lewin (1951). He identified three stages of change:

1. **Unfreezing,** in which people are preparing for change
2. **Moving,** in which people have accepted the need for a change and actually engage in implementing the change
3. **Refreezing,** in which the new change is integrated into the system and becomes part of the new norm or culture

For example, a unit practicing primary nursing is experiencing turmoil related to staffing and reporting as a result of the increased acuity of patients and decreased number of nurses. It becomes obvious that old assignment methods are no longer working, and some unfreezing must occur. The staff and nurse manager engage in brainstorming activities and decide, after exploring many options, to institute a charge position for each shift. When the new charge position is started, the unit enters Lewin's moving stage and works to refine the position and its duties to make it most effective. As the unit adjusts to and incorporates the new position, refreezing, or the integration of the position into daily work, occurs. This approach to change is congruent with the new leadership style because it is a dynamic process planned or facilitated by the leader and followers but then allowed to evolve spontaneously and mesh into the system.

Whenever applying Lewin's change theory, it is important to realize that the stages of change are merely categories to help our thinking, not discrete steps that begin and end abruptly. In other words, change typically is not a clear-cut process that can be achieved by following a formula. In fact, it is often the case that a change process may advance to stage 2 and then move back to stage 1 when using Lewin's change model. Transformational change, as noted earlier, is an evolving process that tends to be the product of a group's vision over time, and, again, revolutionary change follows no clear-cut formula. Perhaps nursing is in the process of a revolution. It appears the profession has moved through the unfreezing stage and is now moving toward a more autonomous role in the healthcare arena. Advanced practice nursing is taking hold in every setting of healthcare delivery, and patient outcomes are beginning to validate the significance of nurses' contributions. Nurses and hiring institutions are realizing the need for continuing education as the staff nurse position becomes more integrated into the healthcare team structure. Nurses and physicians are collaborating more than ever before, and patient outcomes are being tracked to identify both the nursing and medical interventions responsible for outcomes. As outcomes become publicized, our profession must move toward the refreezing or integration of change stage.

Kotter (2012) developed a more specific model of change built on Lewin's framework to emphasize the importance of team collaboration and follow-through. The author offers the first four steps as Lewin's first stage of unfreezing; steps 5 through 7 are stage 2, or moving; and step 8 is Lewin's stage 3, or refreezing. The following is Kotter's Eight Step Plan for Integrating Change:

1. Identify a need and communicate the necessity for implementing a change.
2. Gather the stakeholders and create power in numbers to lead the change.
3. Develop a vision and strategies to enforce change to lead the initiative.
4. Communicate the new vision for the change to everyone in the organization.
5. Encourage risk-taking and creative troubleshooting to move the change along.
6. Move the change and offer incentives for success.

7. Evaluate the implications of the change as it takes hold and offer suggestions to improve it as it progresses.

8. Evaluate the change and offer reinforcement of the successful outcomes of the change.

BARRIERS TO CHANGE

The captain of a ship steers the vessel from one port to another using carefully plotted coordinates. Why then does the ship veer off its course, sometimes miles off track of the destination? Why does the ship end up beached on a shoal not marked on the charts? Why does an iceberg cut up the ship? The answer to all these questions is that life is unpredictable, and captains must consider many other factors beside coordinates when navigating their ships. Nurse leaders must also consider multiple factors and anticipate potential problems when instituting changes.

Many factors can serve as barriers to change, including decreased resources, lack of support, resistance, poor communication mechanisms, burnout, or pressures to get the daily work done. The more barriers there are to the change, the more effort will be needed to deal with those barriers and, consequently, the less energy will be available to institute the actual change.

DEALING WITH CONFLICT GENERATED BY CHANGE

Perhaps one of the biggest barriers to change is the conflict that it generates. Although leaders work to implement changes that will have positive outcomes, they also must realize the negative situations that are likely to occur along the way. One of the most common outcomes of change is *conflict,* which is historically viewed as negative but can be quite positive. The positive results of conflict are the following:

- Growth
- An ability to accept that what was can no longer be
- Collaboration, which builds healthy relationships

In the new science of leadership, conflict can be an outcome of change or serve as an instigator of change and ultimately growth. To deal with the conflict generated, some goals may need to be abandoned, the vision may need to be altered, and an extraordinary amount of energy may need to be invested to help the group navigate the change. The evolution of individuals, groups, and organizations experiencing the change, however, far surpasses the time and effort involved. Dreher (1996) reminds us that the Tao says one can develop better harmony by looking for it within—by decreasing one's anxiety and defensiveness in conflict. Using both the yin (patience, process, and empathy) and yang (courage and positive action), Taoism suggests leaders must balance opposites within themselves and be able to manage and grow from conflict.

Leaders must be confident, focused, proactive, and able to balance personal and professional goals to successfully orchestrate a change. This gives them the energy needed to take on the challenge of change. People must have a clear perspective and life balance. To lead in the midst of change and chaos, it is necessary to have a clear vision and support from one's followers. Ultimately, it is better to choose to change and design one's own approach to change than to have a change imposed by some external force.

It appears that many nurses use avoidance to manage conflict. Although this may seem like an ideal approach initially, avoiding a conflict ultimately causes issues to escalate. Avoidance generally does not solve the problem but perpetuates the conflict (Kennison, 2019). An example that portrays the conflict of many nurses follows.

Case Study, continued

Leaders must know how to deal with change and the conflict typically associated with it. It is important for the leader to assist the staff in developing champions for a new model of orientating and cross-training RNs. Being confident that a change can be made and that the staff RNs can be responsible for creating a new way of thinking about floating will be paramount for success (Runde & Flanagan, 2013). Some ideas to manage this case include the following:

- Create a champion among the staff who believes in the need for a change and who will guide the creation of a new orientation and cross-training policy.
- Brainstorm so that all staff nurses (those assigned to the unit and those who float to it on occasions) can participate in developing the new cross-training model.
- Obtain feedback regarding the change from other units, an objective party, and administration.
- Facilitate collaboration between representatives of the staff RN group and nursing administration to find a solution that incorporates both parties' perspectives and allows for a win-win outcome for all.
- Evaluate the effect of the change after piloting it.
- Incorporate findings from the pilot to revise the new practice policy.
- Periodically evaluate the effects of the new cross-training policy.
- Implement the new policy on a broader scale.
- Offer positive reinforcement to the nurses who succeed in orienting float staff and stress relievers such as meditation.

It is important to teach nurses how to express their feelings and ideas appropriately. Allowing frequent opportunities to both share ideas and receive feedback among multiple individuals (staff nurses, physicians, social workers, pharmacists, and all members of the healthcare team) would improve everyone's ability to contribute their two cents to solving challenges such as the staffing problem in the above case. This would aid in obtaining the best solutions and assisting all staff in gaining increased competence and capability. Because nurses are responsible for their patients' care, it stands to reason they should be part of planning how to best make patient assignments and how to most effectively orient new staff— both permanent staff and temporary staff (including travel nurses). By using the above-mentioned strategies, nurses can better manage conflict and facilitate change in their units and even in the overall organization. Another framework to follow is to facilitate more organizational and individual resilience in order to assist nurses in handling challenges more as "opportunities." Witmore and Mellinger (2016) shared how hope and optimism, transformational leadership, fiscal transparency so staff are more aware of the finances, improvisation so limited resources could be better used, commitment to the organization's mission, and community reciprocity all assisted an organization to adapt to various problems, including staffing shortages. It seems that the more creative leaders (meaning all levels of nurses) can be, the more successful adaptation to change will be in both the unit and in the overall organization. Additionally, all of us have to realize that change is not something that happens once in a while, but rather that change is normal and is constantly happening (Arussy, 2018).

CONCLUSION

There is no doubt that nurses are experiencing continuous change in their practice and the environments in which they practice. Although nurses may bemoan the fact that leaders cannot control or predict what will happen in these uncertain times, they need to rethink situations, because the chaos that exists can be used to promote extraordinary growth for the profession, the organization, and all individuals involved in it.

Leaders must have the ability to know when the strategies selected to realize a vision need to be altered, and they must surround themselves with a team of effective followers who bring diverse and innovative perspectives to the situation. Networking, partnering, and collaborating are skills that nurses have used with success, and they need to draw on those skills to coach followers and help them identify their strengths and build their self-esteem so that they can more effectively manage the many changes the profession faces.

Leaders should strive to make changes in incentives for bedside nurses that recognize their significant contributions and allow them to continue to develop their expertise in that role and changes that create more opportunities for nurses to engage in collaborative efforts with their nurse colleagues and other healthcare workers. As we experience the chaos of the 21st century, it is even more important for nurses to lead and participate in change that reshapes healthcare practices and policy and education. Groups, organizations, and professions that survive will encourage all members to think beyond what is currently possible and continuously participate in change.

CRITICAL THINKING 3-1

1. Several authors assert that resistance to change grows out of fear. Talk to your colleagues about why they have resisted change. Is the bottom-line reason that of fear? If so, what seems to be feared? If not, what is the bottom-line reason given?

2. What strategies have you used or experienced being used that have resulted in reduced resistance to and a successful outcome of change?

3. Use a personality inventory such as the Myers-Briggs (n.d.) to identify your personality style. Discuss how the results affect your ability to communicate and to resolve and grow from conflict.

References

Arussy, L. (2018). *Next is now: 5 steps for embracing change: Building a business that thrives into the future.* Simon & Schuster.

Berger-Hoger, B., Liethmann, K., Muhlhauser, I., Haastert, B., & Steckelberg, A. (2019). Nurse-led coaching of shared decision-making for women with ductal carcinoma in situ in breast care centers: A cluster randomized controlled trial. *International Journal of Nursing Studies, 93*, 141–152.

Center for Creative Leadership. (2019, February 26). *Emerging trends report: Talent reimagined (2019).* https://www.ccl.org/articles/research-reports/trends-report-talent-reimagined/

Denhardt, R., & Denhardt, J. (2006). *The dance of leadership: The art of leading in business, government, and society.* M. E. Sharpe.

Dreher, D. (1996). *The Tao of personal leadership.* Harper Business.

Elwyn, G., Edwards, A., & Thompson, R. (2016). *Shared decision making in health care: Achieving evidence-based patient choice* (3rd ed.). Oxford University Press.

Fackler, C., Chambers, A., & Bourbonniere, M. (2015). Hospital nurses' lived experience of power. *Journal of Nursing Scholarship, 47*(3), 267–274.

French-Bravo, M., & Crow, G. (2015). Shared governance: The role of buy-in in bringing about change. *Online Journal of Issues in Nursing, 20*(2), 8.

Gribbin, J. (2004). *Deep simplicity: Chaos, complexity and the emergence of life.* Allan Lane.

Haigh, C. A. (2008). Using simplified chaos theory to manage nursing services. *Journal of Nursing Management, 16*, 298–304.

Hawking, S. (1987). *A brief history of time.* Bantam Press.

Heifetz, R. (1994). *Leadership without easy answers.* Belknap Press of Harvard University Press.

Heifetz, R., & Linsky, M. (2017). *Leadership on the line with a new preface: Staying alive through the dangers of change.* Harvard Business Review Press.

Jurns, C. (2019). Policy advocacy motivators and barriers: Research results and applications. *Online Journal of Issues in Nursing, 24*(3).

Kennison, M. (2019). Overcoming workplace interpersonal conflict. *Reflections on Nursing Leadership, 45*(1), 1–6.

Kotter, J. P. (2012). *Leading change* (2nd ed.) Harvard Business School Press.

Kouzes, J., & Posner, B. (2017). *The leadership challenge: How to keep getting extraordinary things done in organizations* (6th ed.). Jossey-Bass.

Lewin, K. (1951). *Field theory in social science: Selected theoretical papers.* Harper & Row.

Lorenz, E. (1993). *The essence of chaos.* UCL Press.

Malloch, K., & Porter-O'Grady, T. (2009). *The quantum leader: Applications for the new world of work* (2nd ed.). Jones & Bartlett.

Marshall, E. S., & Broome, M. E. (2021). *Transformational leadership in nursing: From expert clinician to influential leader* (3rd ed.). Springer.

Myers & Briggs Foundation. (n.d.). *Myers-Briggs® Overview.* https://www.myersbriggs.org/my-mbti -personality-type/mbti-basics/home.htm?bhcp=1

Nickerson, J. (2014). *Leading change from the middle: A practical guide to building extraordinary capabilities.* Brookings Institution Press.

Polson, S. (2020). Exercising grit in challenging times. *Leader to Leader, 98*, 33–37. https://doi.org/ 10.1002/ltl.20532

Ponte, P. R., Gross, A. H., Winer, E., Connaughton, M. J., & Hassinger, J. (2007). Implementing an interdisciplinary governance model in a comprehensive cancer center. *Oncology Nursing Forum, 34*(3), 611–616.

Prochaska, J., DiClemente, C., & Norcross, J. (1992). In search of how people change: Applications to addictive behavior. *American Psychologist, 47*, 1102–1114.

Runde, C., & Flanagan, T. (2013). *Becoming a conflict competent leader: How you and your organization can manage conflict effectively* (2nd ed.). John Wiley & Sons.

Rutledge, C., & Gustin, T. (2021) Preparing nurses for roles in telehealth: Now is the time! *Online Journal of Issues in Nursing, 26*(1), 3.

Scott, S. (2009). *Fierce leadership: A bold alternative to the worst "best" practices of business today.* Broadway Business.

Tetenbaum, T., & Laurence, H. (2011). Leading in the chaos of the 21st century. *Journal of Leadership Studies, 4*(4), 41–49.

Van Servellen, G. (2009). *Communication skills for the health professional.* Jones & Bartlett.

Wheatley, M. (2005). *Finding our way: Leadership for an uncertain time.* Berrett-Koehler.

Wheatley, M. (2006). *Leadership and the new science: Discovering order in a chaotic world* (3rd ed.). Berrett-Koehler.

Wheatley, M., & Kellner-Rogers, M. (1996). *A simpler way.* Berrett-Koehler.

Witmore, H., & Mellinger, M. (2016). Organizational resilience: Nonprofit organization's response to change. *Work, 54*(2), 255–265.

World Health Organization. (2020). *Year of the nurse and the midwife 2020.* https://www.who.int/campaigns/annual-theme/year-of-the-nurse-and-the-midwife-2020

Zhang, F., Peng, X., Huang, L. Liu, Y., Xu, J., He, J., Guan, C., Chang, H., & Chen Y. (2022). A caring leadership model in nursing: A grounded theory approach. *Journal of Nursing Management, 30*(4), 981–992.

Zipf, A., Polifroni, E., & Beck, C. (2021). The experience of the nurse during the COVID-19 pandemic: A global meta-synthesis in the year of the nurse. *Journal of Nursing Scholarship, 54*(1), 92–103.

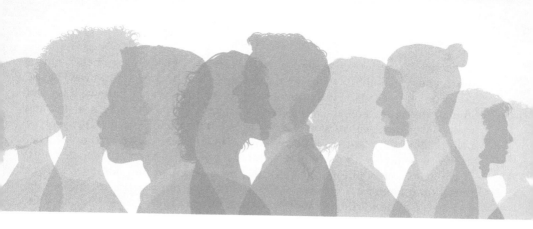

CHAPTER 4

The World and New Leadership
Changing Our Thinking About Leadership

LEARNING OBJECTIVES
- Define the new leadership that nurses must adopt in order to participate successfully in and shape our chaotic healthcare system.
- Examine how chaos in today's world creates new opportunities for nurses to function as leaders in the healthcare delivery system.
- Describe how each of the following theories is congruent with new perspectives of nursing leadership: chaos, quantum, developmental, cognitive, complexity, and perspective transformation.
- Identify how new leadership has a positive effect on the nursing profession and on individual nurses.
- Outline strategies to assist nurses' development as new leaders.

INTRODUCTION

Evidence-based practice, patient outcomes, quality and safety, accountability, information management, interprofessional collaboration, partnerships, value-based healthcare acquisitions, and affiliations—these are terms we hear, read about, and discuss. All organizations, particularly those in healthcare, are experiencing change. In fact, both individual and organizational limits are being tested because of broken systems, inflation, rising pressures on global supply chains, and the resiliency of responding to demands (Colomina, 2022). To continue as leaders in the broken system of healthcare and other environments, nurses must renew their ability to view the broader picture or context; find ways to use resources wisely; adapt to frequent changes or have strong rationales for not implementing recommendations for a change; validate the effects of nursing interventions on patient outcomes; develop strong partnerships; and provide high-quality, safe, and cost-effective care. These goals can be accomplished if nurses focus on health promotion in all types of care settings, encourage multi-disciplinary collaboration, integrate outcome assessment into our daily work as nurses, and embrace a growth mindset so that we can practice autonomously, accountably, and in collaboration with the entire healthcare team. The new leadership science relies on relationships and nurses must lead the healthcare professionals to work synergistically.

To achieve such goals, all registered nurses (RNs) and advanced practice registered nurses (APRNs) must become comfortable with new ways of thinking. Being confident, as well as competent, is consistent with the new view of leadership that will help nurses solidify their roles in the healthcare arena. Indeed, it is time to embrace the problems of organizational change, look at each one of these as a challenging opportunity, and create sustainable solutions. For example, just as technology is facilitating telemedicine and other virtual healthcare delivery methods, so too must nurse leaders gain expertise in leading the interprofessional teams that manage the care of these patients.

> *Do not follow where the path may lead. Go instead where there is no path and leave a trail.* —Anonymous

Consider the following real-life example related to changing our thinking about leadership.

Case Study

Brice experienced working in a pulmonary progressive unit during the COVID-19 pandemic and noticed the breakdown in communication that occurred as a result of visitor restrictions. Nurses in the unit were receiving numerous phone calls each day from concerned family members who wanted status updates. These phone calls were interrupting the nurses during medication rounds and other tasks important to patient care. In addition, if the nurse was busy when the family called, the nurse could not always reach the family member for a return call, and this became a frustrating situation for both the nurse and family member. Nurses tried carrying cell phones, but it was not always possible or safe to answer a call while in another patient's room. Brice and the other nurses in the unit understood that family members wanted to know about the status of their hospitalized relatives, but were also concerned the frequent interruptions would lead to compromised patient care in this busy unit. The nurses' perception of the issue was corroborated by the unit's Hospital Consumer Assessment of Healthcare Providers and Systems (HCAHPS) patient survey scores, which were concerningly low compared with previous scores. After some time, Brice wondered whether thinking about this problem in a new way could lead to a mutually beneficial solution for patients, families, and nurses.

Continued

Case Study—cont'd

REFLECTION QUESTIONS

1. Should Brice be concerned with the low patient satisfaction scores, or is this the administrators' responsibility?
2. What innovative strategies could Brice propose to address the communication challenges arising from visitor restrictions during the COVID-19 pandemic in the pulmonary progressive unit to enhance both family communication and patient care without compromising safety or efficiency?

APPLYING THE NEW LEADERSHIP IN OUR CHAOTIC SYSTEMS

To bring change and new leadership, we must develop new ways of communication and care delivery. Healthcare is currently being transformed by digital technology, and this has expanded nurses' responsibilities in leading the change when compared with their physician counterparts, as nurse leaders are more likely to be responsible for coordinating digital healthcare (Laukka et al., 2022). Advances in information technology (IT) and artificial intelligence (AI) in healthcare require that nurses recognize electronic leadership, or e-leadership as a new way of leading. E-leadership encompasses the ability to influence a team in a digital environment, which often includes virtual teams, advanced technology, and the use of electronic communication tools (Laukka et al., 2022). A few guiding principles of e-leadership that will facilitate more effective virtual team leadership, many of which also apply to face-to-face interactions, include the following:

- Understanding the expectations of followers
- Communicating a clear vision
- Enhancing knowledge of IT
- Being visionary
- Using strategic thinking
- Fully engaging in digital health services to improve implementation (Laukka et al., 2022)

We are certainly in a new age of healthcare. As current nursing research is focused on telehealth and remote patient monitoring, nursing workforce issues, mental health, global health nursing, health disparities, genomics, and technology, healthcare providers, especially nurses, must remain key players in order to improve patient safety and quality care. There are multiple federal and state agencies that provide regulations to promote patient safety, quality care, and access to healthcare, and they have guidelines for nurses to use in order to achieve their goals. The Joint Commission (2023), responsible for accrediting healthcare organizations, has several resources available to healthcare professionals to assist in following the gold standard in delivering safe care.

Currently, many in the United States are focused on culture where fads continuously change and social media often propels these changes. Politics, celebrities, and certain beliefs about wellness, religion, and other significant issues are promoted through social media. Compounding this, much of the information is false and has no authentication source(s). People have little time to think for themselves and have less time to have one-to-one conversations with others. While social media can be an effective method to communicate with individuals, patient groups, and communities, nurses need to be selective with their messages, images, and whom they choose to connect with via Facebook, TikTok, Instagram, LinkedIn, Snapchat, and the like.

PREPARING NURSE LEADERS

Many nurses are not prepared for the role they will need to assume in healthcare settings, and they may become overwhelmed all too quickly. As noted, nurses must rethink the notion of leadership and their roles as leaders so that they can participate more effectively in the new and evolving arena. Leadership skills such as negotiating; collaborating; communicating; networking; mentoring; adaptability; and being passionate, entrepreneurial, honest, credible, accountable, and charismatic need to be taught and will help nurses become successful leaders in the new leadership era.

We are moving from the scientific age, with its emphasis on short- and long-term planning, predicting patient acuity, using formulas to provide staff coverage, and following bureaucratic procedures and policies to get tasks done, to a new science age that stresses empowerment of all, creating while doing, evaluating processes and outcomes, and collaborating as a team. Such change requires us to exercise leadership in an entirely new way.

Covey (2013) described three characteristics a leader must possess for a successful experience in growing and learning: vision, courage, and humility. Having a dream or vision is imperative, but one must also have the courage to continue to define that vision to a group and, at the same time, be humble enough to know when to redefine it to meet the needs of the changing times (both the organization and employees) and prepare for the future. Covey also developed the term *co-missioning*, which suggests that a staff member must have not only a vision or mission but also a way of measuring the outcomes of the vision. This, in turn, will assist in improving the future outcomes. Having the ability to consistently propel a vision in a group or organization takes self-confidence and assertiveness. And, in today's world, being able to facilitate the organization's teams to have a majority of buy-in of the vision will be necessary.

For example, to continue to evolve the nursing task orientation from a task-focused view, which is still present in many healthcare facilities, to a patient-outcome focus, nurses can use leadership skills. If the desired vision was one of nurses working collaboratively with other healthcare members to provide care that best facilitates positive patient outcomes, the monitoring of clients for beneficial or untoward sequelae of nursing, medical, and pharmacological interventions would be done in collaboration with physicians and pharmacists rather than in isolation. Practices that challenge the traditional views of the medical model have to be adopted so that the vision of nursing care takes center stage, and the profession of nursing is recognized as a primary means to achieving positive outcomes.

Nurses need to define what nursing is and wants to be, then work as a unified body to achieve those goals. The current chaotic state of healthcare provides a window of opportunity for the realization of this vision. Nurses need to work to ensure a focus on excellence as well as on cost-effectiveness. Nursing leaders must clearly identify responsibilities of RNs, APRNs, and unlicensed assistive personnel, and they must guide us in creating and strengthening new roles for nurses. With leaders who employ a new way of thinking about leadership, all nurses can be successful in advancing the profession.

CHAOS THEORY

Most nurses acknowledge that the entire healthcare system is in *chaos*, a term meaning to be in a state of confusion and uncertainty. Chaos theory implies the nonlinear randomness of outcomes where cause and effect cannot be predicted due to the complex nature of endless variables; however, certain events can be anticipated (Prestia, 2022). So, if nurses, representing the largest group of professional healthcare workers, can create a culture willing to accept change and use innovative and creative ideas to embrace the unpredictability of outcomes, then nurses can be the leaders in healthcare in these times of uncertainty.

The butterfly effect, an underlying principle of chaos theory, describes the possible chaos a minor, low probability event may induce. The COVID-19 pandemic is a good example of this effect where, much like the flap of a butterfly's wing, a virus outbreak, something that at first appeared inconsequential, created an unpredictable outcome that many leaders were ill equipped to handle (Prestia, 2022). Leaders who relied on linear ways of thinking quickly realized that situations were unique and required creative solutions to adapt to change.

Certainly, each and every nurse has experienced the process of change, either a planned initiative or a spontaneous one in the work setting. What is important for nurses to gain from these change movements is that the innovative and creative thinking that fostered the change must continue to grow and cannot be thought of in an organized, step-by-step linear process. The patterns that emerge during the evaluation process of the change will need to be viewed in the same creative and innovative fashion that triggered the change. By participating in change, allowing time for change to occur, and being aware of the need for more change to evolve, the nurse leaders in the unit or department can create a culture that welcomes continuous change, innovation, and creativity. By creating this culture of uncertainty, the entire staff will bond and work more cohesively. Chaos theory says that nurses must continue to adjust to small fluctuations in a dynamic system (their specific nursing unit), such as with late delivery of medications, limited supplies, and staff shortages. Using chaos theory, nurses can visualize in a creative manner, and perhaps in an autonomous and calm fashion, that the medications will not cause life-threatening problems if they are administered *slightly* later than the prescribed time, that they can creatively use resources to stretch them, and that they can deliver care in a different manner depending on the number of staff and the skill sets available.

Think about the last time you had an emergency patient situation—didn't everyone pitch in? There were no formalities, and if the patient's situation deteriorated, the team probably became more collegial and informal as everyone tried harder. This is easily correlated to what happens in a bureaucratic organization when uncertainty increases. People tend to use more personal and group approaches (Kouzes & Posner, 2017) as they come together for the common good, and this often occurs unconsciously. Leaders can be instrumental at times like this by using the chaos and the changes it ultimately produces as a positive opportunity.

Challenging problems provide people with opportunities for great success. Sweating a bit or being a little anxious about something usually leaves us exhilarated after the problem has been resolved. The healthcare chaos that currently surrounds us is one such problem. This can result in an even stronger role for nurses and the identification of more creative ways to provide high-quality and cost-effective care. An example may help illustrate this point.

Many in nursing bemoan the loss of the 80% professional staff and 20% nonprofessional staff mix we enjoyed in the past and the reality of the current 60% professional staff and 40% nonprofessional staff mix in most hospitals today. It would be contrary to the new science of leadership philosophy, however, to propose a quantitative study measuring cost-effectiveness. Instead, the new science perspective would encourage the emergence of creative leaders who are willing to stray from set formulas and achieve the right mix of staff for their individual units by experimenting until that ideal mix is found. For example, a proposal of gradually decreasing professional staff and increasing unlicensed personnel would be more tolerable than just eliminating RN positions. In addition, having an available RN pool would allow nurses to be called in when the acuteness of the patient's condition justified increased professional care. The previous bureaucratic way of thinking about having a consistent number of staff members for every unit with a certain number of full-time equivalents (FTEs) of professional and nonprofessional staff just does not work in a world characterized by chaos.

The new science philosophy recommends less prediction, prejudgment, and compartmentalization. For example, nurse managers need to try new staffing patterns that acknowledge that a 60% professional and 40% nonprofessional staff mix (or an 80/20, 30/70, or any other mix) is not ideal for every unit but that any number of patterns could work if staff worked with one another in new ways. Also, the idea of using teams of RNs, licensed practical nurses (LPNs), and nurse assistants may need to be reassessed, along with teams of multidisciplinary workers. Leaders need to concentrate first on the people who are working to achieve the goals and establishing positive relationships between and among them. When people have positive working relationships with one another, they are more likely to respect one another and to achieve great things.

Some organizations are calling on nurses to navigate their institutions through this chaotic time, and nursing leaders are using a number of creative strategies to influence change, survive, and even grow. Skills such as creativity, patient-centeredness, coordination, multiple priority management, problem-solving, critical thinking, and system navigation are identified as being necessary for nurses to use throughout their careers. An example of this is using nursing knowledge and machine learning to identify high-need patients, based on chronic illness and social needs, to improve patient outcomes. By avoiding the traditional method of using health utilization costs to classify high-need individuals, nurses can lead the expansion of combining social determinants of health and biopsychosocial features into care models to improve equity in access and patient outcomes (Hewner et al., 2023). Nurse leaders must come to the realization that chaos can be positive and can assist a unit or department to use innovative ideas in leading change.

QUANTUM THEORY

The universe as understood by quantum theory is "a probabilistic, unpredictable, pluralistic, diverse, uncertain and complex universe," compared with traditional views of the universe being uniform and predictable with an absolute perspective (Belgen & Elçi, 2022). The current state of healthcare can certainly be seen as unpredictable, diverse, and complex, which substantiates the need for a new view of leadership. Quantum theory offers a new perspective on leadership, where a leader foresees a constant change in organizations in terms of place, time, and people (Belgen & Elçi, 2022). Focusing on relationships and using a nonlinear approach, in which the real and the potentially real are visualized simultaneously, is a method of thinking that replaces our standard, orderly, task-oriented perspective with a fluid, systems-thinking, goal-oriented approach.

Wheatley (2023) recommends that we approach leadership through the lens provided by the new science and naturally occurring events. For example, after a storm, meteorologists can review storm movements on a computer and visualize a pattern in what initially appeared to be chaos. We can also reflect on the fact that a stream, which initially seems to be little more than a random collection of water, sand, rocks, and silt, actually is not random at all but is a carefully designed system in which all parts work together to allow flexibility and the capacity for change as the natural elements of storms, animals, and humans affect its path.

The new science says that living systems organize themselves by seeking order, but this order is not linear or predictive. Organizations also seek order, but not in a linear, hierarchical way (Wheatley, 2023). Thus, leadership in an organization may best be provided by a social system comprising many leaders, not just one. Those who relate through coercion or with a disregard for others create negative energy, whereas those who are open to others and see others in their fullness create positive energy. Perhaps by focusing on one nonprofessional staff member at a time and allowing a connectedness to occur between that individual and the other staff, a we-versus-they situation can be avoided. If each staff member can be empowered to visualize their own potential as well as that of others, a more positive outlook regarding workload and quality of patient care is likely to prevail.

Quantum theory suggests that an interface among all members of a group is critical. Each person needs to be acknowledged for their talents and potential, and each needs to be helped to grow. Perhaps nurses need to visualize the workforce as germinating seeds in space rather than on earth, where gravity pulls the roots toward it and the stem grows away from gravity. In space, seeds grow every which way because there is no gravity to direct them in only a ground-up direction.

Likewise, people are not fixed entities gravitating toward one spot and able to be predicted by a set of rules and expectations.

People need to be given the opportunity to grow in all kinds of ways—ways that are unknown to anyone until they happen. It is the task of the leader to encourage and facilitate such growth. Perhaps visualizing an organization as composed of figures that stretch and overlap with each other in a three-dimensional, rather than linear, structure would allow for greater diversity and uniqueness and open more avenues for communication and effective outcomes. Work productivity cannot be predicted based on a given number of FTEs, certain types of patient hours, and acuity levels. Such task-oriented thinking is not what patient care is all about. Instead, mindsets need to be more multidimensional and open to new possibilities and things that no one has thought of yet. Leaders are the key to success because they facilitate relationships, encourage growth, enjoy facing uncertainty, and are willing to take risks. Leaders also know how to deal with toxic people or those with whom it is difficult to communicate, develop outstanding leaders, and transform organizations (Albert et al., 2022).

The new way of thinking about leadership in a global and almost limitless fashion, and realizing that each individual has a contribution to make, is necessary if nursing is to succeed in delivering the highest quality care and meet the Institute for Healthcare Improvement (2023) recommendations. Valuing hard work and respecting one another are qualities that need to be revived and that must be pervasive. In other words, the whole culture of the practice settings needs reawakening. A job should be viewed as a piece of an ever-changing plan that affects the overall functioning of the organization. Each person must be respected as crucial to the greater goal. Biases, prejudices, insecurities, and preconceived judgments need to be worked out or left behind. When such an atmosphere exists, communication, mentoring, and collaboration are more likely to occur, and self-empowerment and group empowerment dominate. The change from a task-focused setting to more of a process-focused one allows followers and leaders to propel organizations and the individuals within them forward.

To be effective leaders in constantly changing work environments, nurses must be able to successfully manage and communicate with teams by influencing organizational intelligence, the collective use of all employees' abilities and effective use of information, and creating innovative and safe solutions in response to unpredictable, chaotic environments (Belgen & Elçi, 2022). Another strategy to use in fostering a culture of safety and communication is to apply the Quality and Safety Education for Nurses training (http://qsen.org/) and use root cause analyses with staff to gain additional learning on promoting safety.

The world is moving out of the industrial or Newtonian age in which things were described in a linear way and when we became accustomed to separating every system into parts rather than dealing with the whole. As the world moves toward a greater concern for wholeness, complexity, and interaction, leaders are needed. We must use our imaginations and embrace the idea that there is more to our work than assessing, planning, implementing, and evaluating. Nurses can no longer have tunnel vision and be task oriented. Instead, we need a more in-depth analysis of the data collected before we can decide on what to include in the plan of care, much like the National Council of State Boards of Nurses' (NCSBN) Clinical Judgment Measurement Model (see Chapter 2), in which nurses must first recognize and analyze cues, then prioritize hypotheses and generate solutions before they take action. Our whole philosophy of caring for patients must be broadened, and for most of us, our way of simply moving from one task to another will have to change. Most RNs, average age 52 years (NCSBN, 2021), have worked most of their 20-plus-year career in a very rigid organizational structure, carrying out another profession's orders (e.g., medical doctors, physician assistant, and nurse practitioners). As a result, these nurses will have to reorient themselves to nursing and to leading with a new science of leadership perspective. The quantum mechanics framework of attending to naturally occurring events while also predicting trajectories of potential possibilities appreciates individuals for their knowledge and recognizes that no one person alone can create a sustainable impact in healthcare organizations (Albert et al., 2022).

SUPPORTING PERSPECTIVES AND PERSPECTIVE TRANSFORMATION THEORY

The idea that people and organizations grow and evolve in response to challenges, disequilibrium, and change is not new, nor is it restricted to quantum theory or new science thinking. In fact, it is an idea that has been addressed by psychologists, educators, and nurse theorists. Examples of these follow.

Cognitive Theory

Cognitive and intellectual development occurs through the increasing ability to use complex cognitive skills to analyze issues, manage changing circumstances, integrate multiple points of view, and make sound decisions independently (Perry, 1970). Individuals progress through stages of cognitive development, from seeing knowledge as finite and themselves as absorbers or memorizers of it to viewing knowledge as relative, depending on the situation or circumstance, and themselves as critical thinkers and lifelong learners. Such changes in worldview, similar to any type of growth, occur as a result of disequilibrium. When one's usual way of thinking is found to be lacking, one experiences disequilibrium and is challenged to think in new ways, ask new questions, and develop new strategies. The chaos and disequilibrium with which nurses in practice are challenged, therefore, can be viewed as a stimulus for growth and development. Nurses need to rethink their role in healthcare, the kind of leadership needed in this arena, and their responsibility to provide such leadership.

Developmental Theory

Erik Erikson, a developmental theorist, stated that physical, emotional, and social factors have an effect on an individual's development (Erikson, 1963). He asserted that development is a mixture of maturation (the potential growth a person has inherited) and learning (knowledge to be gained). Most nurses are working in a rigidly structured healthcare system and, without leadership, may not move out of the adolescence or young adulthood stage, when one of the tasks is to master involvement with others. Mastery of these developmental tasks results in intimacy and solidarity, whereas failure results in isolation. Because the new leadership is based on relationships, it is paramount that nurses accomplish the task of young adulthood so that they can be highly effective healthcare team members. The accomplishment of the generativity task (Erikson, 1963) for those more advanced in life leads to productive and creative work. For nurses to experience this generativity, they need to have acquired leadership skills.

Just as our lives can be viewed developmentally, so too can our organizational systems. Only organizational structures that continue to be flexible and adaptable will be able to support the development of people in the organization. Sometimes it is only when a person is pushed, as happens in a chaotic setting or where there is significant conflict with one's peers, that they actually develop and grow. Hence, developmental theory also suggests that disequilibrium is not a negative situation, but rather a positive experience that enhances growth.

Complexity Theory

Complexity theory describes the way life is ordered and emphasizes life is based on the principles of emergence more than it is predetermined by other variables. According to Rusoja et al. (2024), systems are composed of dynamic, often unpredictable interactions, which include continuously changing components that influence our actions, including leading. However, the concepts and principles of complexity theory can be used to improve our continuously evolving healthcare system through transformational leadership, increasing collaboration, and iterative learning (Rusoja et al., 2024). Using complexity science, nurses can note relationships and connections among quantitative and qualitative data. This leads to establishing new patterns of collaboration in contrast to the linear organizational structure in which authority controls the next level and blocks the feedback mechanisms that can lead the organization to grow. The complexity leadership model can help organizations adapt to change and uncertainty and propel the organizations' leaders to succeed. Some examples of this adaptation are discussed in Rusoja et al.'s (2024) article related to the real-world example of the Alameda Health System Vaccine Taskforce in addressing the complex health challenges of COVID-19.

Perspective Transformation Theory

Mezirow's perspective transformation theory postulates people naturally operate from "habitual expectations" known as perspectives, that are developed through the lifelong process of interaction and socialization (Onosu, 2021). Perspectives acquired at an early age, through school, work, or other situations, become the lens through which beliefs, values, and ideas are judged. However, when a disrupting situation is encountered that does not fit into the framework, people must create a new perspective, and then this lens is used to relate self to others and society (Onosu, 2021). A similar process occurs in nursing practice when nurses encounter disrupting situations in healthcare that result in creation of a new lens for judging their ideas, values, and beliefs related to nursing. Fawcett's (1995, pp. 533–534) explanation of perspective transformation depicts how leaders can assist nurses to identify their own ability to lead and hence grow in these chaotic times:

Stage 1: *Stability, which refers to an individual's current cognitive and emotional state,* reflects what many nurses are currently experiencing in their workplaces. Nurses easily maintain the status quo because many were never encouraged to think of themselves as leaders.

Stage 2: *Dissonance* moves one toward the revelation that all nurses can be leaders. It generally means the beginning of a reawakening to one's situation. Nurses experiencing dissonance are aware of the very chaotic times they are in and know they need to start doing something. They may share their feelings with peers and start speaking out when serious staffing problems or unsafe situations occur.

Stage 3: *Confusion* occurs when individuals gain courage from others who validate what they are feeling, speak openly when things are not right in their environment, and decide to strive for excellence rather than accept mediocrity.

Stage 4: In *dealing with uncertainty,* individuals speak out, but they do so sporadically because they may believe that they do not have the ability or strength to change things.

Stage 5: *Saturation* occurs when people feel confident that they have collected the right information and spoken to the right people about a new way of doing things or delivering care.

Stage 6: *Synthesis* heralds the organization of information to formulate a plan to change an unacceptable situation—a plan put into place because individuals care enough to make a change.

Stage 7: *Resolution* indicates that the problems are being solved with the changes that were put into place.

Stage 8: *Reconceptualization* occurs when those who initiated the change continue to work out some of the kinks in the system and empower others to continue to support and pursue new ways of doing things.

Stage 9: *Return to stability* indicates that the change has now become a part of the milieu and is no longer being evaluated and scrutinized extensively.

This framework provides an additional basis supporting why we need to rethink the need for leadership. It depicts a change from nurses practicing in a private way to groups of nurses using a shared model of practice. Perspective transformation is a helpful process to use in assisting nurses to practice more autonomously and could also facilitate nursing receiving a greater portion of the healthcare dollar because it should assist in measuring tangible patient outcomes, which are a direct result of nursing care.

What happened to Brice's dilemma we discussed at the beginning of this chapter? Continue the Case Study to learn how Brice displayed leadership amidst chaos and transformed the unit's perspective.

Case Study, continued

Brice decided this problem required a nonlinear solution. In discussions with unit nurses, Brice uncovered that family concerns for status updates revolved around a few key items and that nurses were usually finished with assessments and medication rounds at certain times during their shifts. After considering the variables, a family update form was created to guide the nurses in the unit in providing standardized daily updates when calling the family member (with patient permission) during scheduled times each shift.

After implementing the form to guide scheduled phone calls, the unit's HCAHPS scores showed a 220% increase in patient perception of staff's consistency in information discussed, which exceeded pre-pandemic scores! Although visitor restrictions in the unit ended after the pandemic, Brice's leadership and new way of thinking helped the unit flourish during chaos.

REFLECTION QUESTIONS

3. How could the outcome have differed if Brice had not been willing to lead change and share the unique viewpoint of knowing both the family and nurse concerns?
4. What aspects of critical thinking and leadership principles contributed to the success of this situation, and how might these principles be applied in other healthcare settings facing similar challenges?

CONCLUSION

We need to change our thinking about what leadership is if we are to survive and thrive in the tumultuous changes in healthcare as well as in the world today. Chaos, quantum, cognitive, developmental, complexity, and perspective transformation theories will assist us in understanding how the disorder and confusion we are feeling in our work settings today are equivalent to what happens in nature. The fact that the natural world we live in can automatically order itself after such turmoil is incredible. We have to realize that adapting the new science of leadership, with its focus on empowering followers and alleviating the bureaucratic organizational structure, will assist us in developing new ideas and new ways of working. Appreciating every individual's capability and contribution instead of seeing them as a mere number on a dashboard will assist us in achieving fearless and brave leadership.

The transformation in healthcare delivery, educational systems, community activism, and a variety of other arenas that nurses are participating in is certainly disorienting and chaotic, but it is necessary to continue to reframe the hierarchical medical model on which the U.S. healthcare system has been based. This major paradigm shift has the potential to improve the quality of healthcare and not merely reduce costs. That will happen, however, only if we have capable nurse leaders willing to take the risks needed to produce such positive outcomes. The theories discussed in this chapter provide evidence that chaos and disequilibrium can be positive instigators for growth and improvement. This new way of thinking about leading will help nurses take a more collaborative and holistic approach to practice and help us achieve our visions for the profession.

CRITICAL THINKING 4-1

1. Explain how the new way of thinking about leadership described in this chapter can affect the way we conceptualize the role of the nurse today. How could you assist others in adapting this perspective? Use some of the resources on Margaret Wheatley's Web site to assist you (https://margaretwheatley.com/).

2. Think about the environment in which you practice. Would you describe it as chaotic? Why or why not? What contributes to the chaos or relative calm? What have been the negative ways that you and others have dealt with chaos in your environment? What positive strategies have been used? What patterns do you see in the midst of all this chaos?

3. Who do you think of as leaders where you practice? What characteristics of the new science of leadership do these people portray? Discuss how appreciating each individual's contribution will assist your organization to be successful.

4. View Sir Ken Robinson's TED talk (2007), *Do Schools Kill Creativity?,* and identify five ways educators could promote individuals' creativity so they can improve their ability to lead in these uncertain and chaotic times. Think about what Robinson says: "Creativity is as important as literacy."

5. Nurses can gain adaptation skills and the ability to be more flexible if they understand the underpinnings of quantum theory. View the YouTube clip *Quantum Mechanics and Chaos* by Daniel Kleppner (2014) and describe how you can be more adaptable and flexible in your work setting and your personal life.

6. Complete the following Garlock & Waters Cognitive Development Related to Complexity Assessment, based on Perry's (1970) theory of cognitive and ethical development, to determine your current development in complex thinking. How did you score? Identify areas for growth in your ability to lead in complex situations, and develop an action plan to advance your cognitive and ethical development to improve your leadership capability.

Directions: Select the answer for each statement you most agree with or that represents your typical thinking. Try not to think about exceptions or special circumstances while answering to get the most accurate results.

1. When it comes to knowing the answer to a problem:

   a. There are right and wrong answers.

   b. There are clearly no right answers.

   c. Some answers are right but it depends on the situation.

   d. Ambiguity and answers both exist.

2. When considering knowledge versus opinion:

   a. The more you know, the smarter you are.

   b. Everyone is entitled to their own opinion.

   c. What is considered true is all relative.

   d. It is important to commit to an opinion.

3. When it comes to truth and viewpoints of truth:

   a. Truth and falsity are easily distinguished by experts.

   b. People who argue their viewpoint of truth are biased.

   c. For each truth, there is an opposite, but equally valid truth.

   d. Commitment to truth is an ongoing, unfolding activity.

4. When considering the value of experts (teachers, physicians, managers, etc.):

   a. The experts should know the right answer to the question.

   b. Experts can research a question to find the right answer.

   c. An expert cannot know everything there is to know.

   d. Knowledge is constructed from expert opinion and my personal experience.

If you answered mostly "a," you are currently an Absolute Thinker:

You consider knowledge and situations in absolute terms, and tend to seek clear-cut answers without questioning or considering alternative perspectives. Characteristics of this stage include rigid thinking, reliance on authority, limited awareness of diverse viewpoints.

If you answered mostly "b," you are currently Exploring Multiplicity:

You are beginning to recognize and appreciate diverse perspectives and interpretations, acknowledging there can be multiple valid viewpoints. Characteristics of this stage include developing openness to ambiguity and recognition of multiple valid viewpoints.

If you answered mostly "c," you are currently a Relativistic Thinker:

You see knowledge as contextual and subjective, and understand that interpretations can vary based on perspective. Characteristics of this stage include embracing the relativity of knowledge and considering different value systems.

If you answered mostly "d," you are currently a Committed Relativist:

You can commit to a viewpoint while acknowledging the relativity of knowledge, to make informed and thoughtful commitments. Characteristics of this stage include balancing commitment with awareness of different perspectives to engage in ethical decision making.

If you answered some of each, you may be in between stages of development. Review the descriptions to see where you feel you currently are.

References

Albert, N. M., Pappas, S. H., Porter-O'Grady, T., & Malloch, K. (2022). *Quantum leadership: Creating sustainable value in health care* (6th ed.). Jones & Bartlett.

Belgen, A., & Elçi, M. (2022). The mediating role of organizational intelligence in the relationship between quantum leadership and innovative behavior. *Frontiers in Psychology, 13.* https://doi.org/10.3389/fpsyg.2022.1051028

Colomina, C. (2022, December). The world in 2023: Ten issues that will shape the international agenda. *CIDOB Notes Internacionals, 283.* https://www.cidob.org/en/publications/publication_series/notes_internacionals/283/the_world_in_2023_ten_issues_that_will_shape_the_international_agenda

Covey, S. (2013). *The seven habits of highly effective people: Powerful lessons in personal change.* Rosetta Books.

Erikson, E. (1963). *Childhood and society* (2nd ed.). W. W. Norton.

Fawcett, J. (1995). *Analysis and evaluation of conceptual models of nursing* (3rd ed.). F. A. Davis.

Hewner, S., Smith, E., & Sullivan, S. S. (2023). Identifying high-need primary care patients using nursing knowledge and machine learning methods. *Applied Clinical Informatics, 14*(3), 408–417. https://doi.org/10.1055/a-2048-7343

Institute for Healthcare Improvement. (2023). *Resources.* https://www.ihi.org/resources/Pages/default.aspx

Kleppner, D. (2014, January 15). *Quantum mechanics and chaos* [Video]. YouTube. https://www.youtube.com/watch?v=BMztKvuI-9w

Kouzes, J., & Posner, B. (2017). *The leadership challenge: How to make extraordinary things happen in organizations* (5th ed.). Jossey-Bass.

Laukka, E., Pölkki, T., & Kanste, O. (2022). Leadership in the context of digital health services: A concept analysis. *Journal of Nursing Management, 30*(7), 2763–2780. https://doi.org/10.1111/jonm.13763

National Council of State Boards of Nursing. (2023). The 2020 national nursing workforce survey. *Journal of Nursing Regulation, 12,* S4–S6. https://www.ncsbn.org/public-files/2020_NNW_Executive_Summary.pdf

Onosu, G. (2021). The impact of cultural immersion experience on identity transformation process. *International Journal of Environmental Research and Public Health, 18*(5), 2680. https://doi.org/10.3390/ijerph18052680

Perry, W. (1970). *Forms of intellectual and ethical development in the college years: A scheme.* Holt, Rinehart & Winston.

Prestia, A. S. (2022). PTSD and the COVID-19 continuum. *Nurse Leader, 20*(2), 197–200. https://doi.org/10.1016/j.mnl.2021.11.001

Robinson, K. (2007, January 7). *Do schools kill creativity?* [Video]. *YouTube.* https://www.youtube.com/watch?v=iG9CE55wbtY

Rusoja, E., Swanson, R. C., & Swift, M. (2024). Using systems thinking and complexity theory to understand and improve emergency medicine: Lessons from COVID-19 in a safety net health system. *Journal of Evaluation in Clinical Practice, 30*(2), 30–336. https://doi.org. /10.1111/jep.13920

The Joint Commission. (2023). *Resources: For nurses.* https://www.jointcommission.org/resources/for-nurses/

Wheatley, M. (2023). *Who do we choose to be? Facing reality, claiming leadership, restoring sanity* (2nd ed.). Berrett-Koehler.

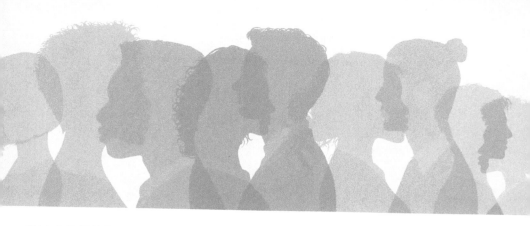

CHAPTER 5

Followership and Empowerment

INTRODUCTION

Due to the complex, chaotic organizational environments previously described, it is clear that leaders need to work collaboratively with followers if any group or organization is to succeed. Indeed, "any organization is a triad consisting of leaders and followers joined in a common purpose. . . . Followers and leaders orbit around the purpose; followers do not orbit around the leader" (Chaleff, 2009, p. 11) (Fig. 5-1). The need for collaboration requires leaders to expand their understanding of followership. The global pandemic in 2020 made it clear that we need to place more emphasis on developing leaders and followers who can lead in complex situations (Uhl-Bien, 2021b).

Despite decades of discussion on followership, a recent literature review revealed the ongoing lack of research on the concept (Honan et al., 2022). These authors explain that "leadership and followership roles are co-constructed, interdependent and synergistic and influence organizational success and patient safety" (p. 69). In fact, without followers there are no leaders (Uhl-Bien, 2021a).

Old Conceptualization of Leader–Follower Interactions

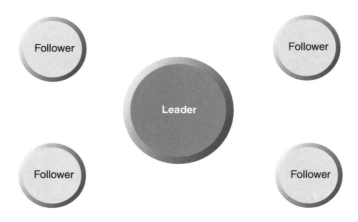

Contemporary Conceptualization of Leader–Follower Interactions

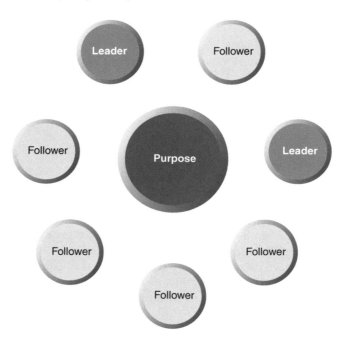

FIGURE 5-1 • Old and contemporary conceptualizations of leader–follower interactions.

The reciprocal nature of leadership and followership was supported through research conducted by Manning and Robertson (2016a, 2016b, 2016c). These researchers developed and tested a three-factor model of followership that illustrates (1) followership and leadership are not fundamentally different, (2) the skills that leaders need in their roles develop out of and build on those needed in follower roles, (3) effective organizations need effective followers as well as effective leaders, and (4) the training of effective followers underpins that of effective leaders.

No one person can know the best strategy, have the clearest vision, or identify the most effective approaches to solve problems. Leadership expert Warren Bennis once noted that the longer he studied effective leaders, the more he was convinced of the underappreciated importance of effective followers. He also claimed that "in our society leadership is too often seen as an inherently individual phenomenon" (Bennis, 2006, p. 130) but acknowledged that "no change can occur without willing and committed followers" (p. 133). Thus, leaders and followers are increasingly important.

As many have noted, *leaders can be leaders only if they have followers.* Indeed, one might say that what defines leaders is that others embrace their vision and want to see it realized. Despite these assertions, however, the concept of followership is rarely addressed to the same extent as the concept of leadership. In an interview at the Wharton Global Forum held in New York City in June 2018, Garrett Reisman, NASA astronaut on a space shuttle Atlantis mission and director of operations at SpaceX, noted that there are many more followers than there are leaders and "having good followers is often much more important than having the one good leader at the top" (Wharton, University of Pennsylvania, 2018). He acknowledged that leadership clearly is important and asserted that followership is something that needs more attention. Why does such a significant role receive so little attention, and why is it not more highly valued? Does our emphasis on leadership "compensate for something in our culture or our organizations that fills us with an exaggerated need to promote leadership and to silence whatever haunts us about the notion of followership?" (Berg, 1998, p. 28).

In her review of her own path to leadership as the president of the American Nurses Association, Dr. Lucille Joel (1999) said she was an "extraordinary follower . . . [who] learned the rules well and followed them exactly . . . [who was] too intimidated to question authority . . . [and who] lacked confidence" (p. 17). Joel concluded that she was, in essence, invisible.

As we will discuss in this chapter the follower role is a powerful one because it is the follower who truly makes the leader–follower relationship work. In fact, "nurses at every level of their career must understand their followership role to contribute to high-functioning teams and proactively add to patient care" (Honan et al., 2022, p. 75).

> *The secret of leadership is . . . the ability to inspire others with faith in their own high potential.* —J. Donald Walters

THE CONCEPT OF FOLLOWERSHIP

Being a "good" follower takes unique talents, just as being a "good" leader does. And "in many ways, great followership is harder than leadership; it has more dangers and fewer rewards" (Bennis, 2008, p. xxvi). Indeed, the qualities of leaders and followers (e.g., being willing to take risks and challenge the status quo, as well as being passionate about a goal) are very similar. Thus, attention must be given to the development of followers, and followership must be cultivated, just as leadership development and the cultivation of leadership are essential. If we fail to remember that followership is voluntary, fail to convey the importance of followership, and fail to cultivate influential followers, leaders will be left without the support needed to realize visions, make changes, and co-create a preferred future. In essence, when the cry goes out to "follow the leader," few will know who to follow or how to follow, and the minimum will be accomplished. Worse yet, teams will not be prepared to identify the leader and may follow the person with the loudest voice or the most charisma.

Followership has been described as the willingness to cooperate in a coordinated way to accomplish shared goals while engaging in collaborative teamwork (Bastardoz & Van Vugt, 2019). Being willing to follow is not about unquestioningly accepting some leader's authority or about abdicating all responsibility for progress, waiting passively for answers to be provided by the leader, or sitting back and hoping to enjoy the ride. Effective followers are much more active and involved than this.

Followership is an art—a skill that can be learned, cultivated, and consciously developed and exercised. Followers need to be "self-directing, actively participating, practicing experts [who work] on behalf of the organization and the mutually agreed upon vision and goals" (Sullivan, 1998, p. 469). They need to trust others and be trustworthy themselves. They need to see themselves as a community, think and act as a team, and invest energy in team building by focusing on the common goal and drawing on the strengths and talents of each team member. Followers need to know their strengths and what their unique contributions to the effort can be. They must complement each other's and the leader's specialties, strengths, and areas of expertise. They need to seek information to have the "bigger picture," which allows them to participate fully and provide significant feedback.

Followers should not invest their energy merely in their or others' agendas. They also should not ally themselves with group members whose goals are out of alignment with those of the rest of the team. They must be counted on to "provide input that focuses on finding solutions, not just on articulating problems" (Sullivan, 1998, p. 478). They are expected to support the leader by asking questions, giving thoughtful feedback, working to achieve group goals, and providing encouragement when the leader takes a risk on behalf of the group. Leaders, in return, are expected to support followers by seeking their input, using their talents entirely, and encouraging them to grow continually.

Followership also involves knowing when and how to assume the role of leader when necessary, a concept illustrated beautifully by geese (Assessment Research and Evaluation—BISD, 2014). Geese fly in a V formation to maximize distance and minimize exertion, and as they do this, the goose at the head of the V will fall back when tired while another goose moves to the front position. In this way, all members of the flock can and are expected to take on the role of leader at some point, and all are expected to be in the follower role at other times. The geese illustration reminds that followership and leadership require interchangeable skills, and team members may move in and out of both roles depending on the context. Similarly, organizations are essentially "communit[ies] of many leaders and many followers, frequently changing places depending on the particular activity that is occurring" (Sullivan, 1998, p. 477).

Honan et al. (2022) explain that effective followers engage in constructive critical thinking, are accountable for their actions, and can step into the leader's role when the situation requires it. The author suggests that ineffective followership can be detrimental to the organization, as demonstrated by low morale, lack of initiative, and lack of trust. Supporting and advocating the ideas and opinions of another demands that the follower think critically about those ideas and opinions, have the skills to advocate for those ideas, and take an active role in providing support to the leader as the ideas are fully developed and advanced.

Consider the following Case Study related to leadership and followership.

Case Study

Helen is a staff registered nurse (RN) in a long-term care facility where the resident population averages 80 years of age. Helen and the nurse manager in the unit have read research showing that increased family involvement in the care of older adults helps decrease their confusion and increase their participation in self-care activities, and they have talked about implementing some strategies in their unit to involve family members more actively. Knowing that many residents could benefit from such interventions, and with the encouragement of the nurse manager, Helen prepares a proposal for the director of nursing about how to increase the involvement of more families in the care of residents at this facility.

REFLECTION QUESTIONS

1. How does Helen demonstrate leadership and followership in preparing and presenting a proposal to the director of nursing for increased family involvement?
2. Consider Helen's role in identifying the need, collaborating with the nurse manager, and formulating an action plan. How might Helen's leadership skills contribute to successfully implementing strategies to enhance family engagement in resident care?

TYPES OF FOLLOWERS

Despite the vital role that followers play in effecting change and realizing visions, negative perceptions of followers and followership still exist. The negative perceptions (passive, dependent, inferior, etc.) of followers and followership suggest that there is only one type of follower. Kelley (1992, 1998, 2008), on the other hand, suggested several types of followers, ranging from those who are vital to the success of the group or organization to those who are passive. Kelley defined the follower types below:

- *Effective or exemplary followers:* These individuals function independently, think critically about ideas that are proposed or directions that are suggested, and are actively involved. They challenge the leader's ideas when necessary, suggest alternative courses of action, and invest time and energy to arrive at the best possible solution for the group.

- *Alienated followers:* These followers think critically about what the leader or other group members suggest, but they remain passive and perhaps even somewhat hostile. They may complain about "the way things are being done," are unhappy, and seem disengaged at times. Alienated followers rarely invest time or energy to suggest alternative solutions or other approaches.
- *"Yes" people:* These are the conformists who are actively involved in the work of the group and enthusiastically support the leader. They are eager to take orders, defer to the leader, yield to the leader's views and opinions, and please the leader. They enjoy a great deal of structure, order, and predictability. "Yes" people are uncomfortable with having to make and live with decisions, and they find freedom almost terrifying. They do not initiate ideas, think for themselves, raise questions, critique the ideas of others, or challenge the group.
- *Sheep:* These are the passive individuals who are dependent and uncritical, going along with whatever the leader tells them to do. They are easily led and manipulated, lack initiative, require constant direction, and never go beyond their given assignment. "Sheep"are not particularly committed to the group's goals and do not invest themselves to any great extent to see that the group continues to move forward.
- *Survivors:* These are passive followers who tend to stay in the background and effectively navigate the organizational politics to maintain their position. They may not actively challenge their leaders or seek to change the status quo.

Types of followers, or followership styles, have also been described by Pittman et al. (1998), who used the dimensions of "performance initiative" and "relationship initiative" to define four followership styles (Fig. 5-2).

Performance initiatives relate to the follower's performance—how an assigned job gets done, how good the person is at what they do, the standards the person sets, how well the person works with others, and how valuable the person is to the organization. *Relationship initiatives* concern the follower's relationship with the leader—how much the person understands the leader's perspective, the person's willingness to give negative feedback or disagree with the leader, and how the person demonstrates reliability and trustworthiness. Each of the four followership styles reflects extensive or limited activity in these dimensions:

- *Partner:* This follower is committed to high performance and building a positive, reciprocal relationship with the leader. The partner may be considered as a "leader-in-waiting" (Pittman et al., 1998, p. 118).
- *Contributor:* This person does the job well, is effective with co-workers, embraces change, and successfully balances work and other aspects of life. The contributor does not, however, try to understand the leader's perspective or promote the leader's vision, nor do they

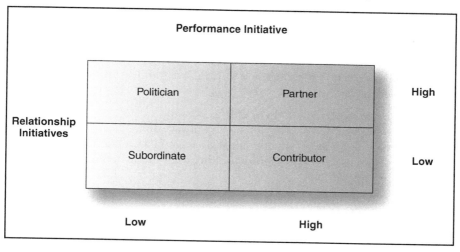

FIGURE 5-2 · Followership styles. (Copyright © 2006 William E. Rosenbach, Robert L. Taylor. Reprinted by permission of Westview Press, a member of the Perseus Books Group.)

negotiate differences maturely, communicate courageously, share expertise and knowledge, or take initiative.

• *Politician:* This individual is empathetic and skilled in interpersonal relationships. The person is willing to give honest feedback and support the leader; however, they may neglect the job and have poor performance.

• *Subordinate:* This type of follower may be competent at assigned tasks and complete work as instructed, but there is no commitment to excellence in performance. In addition, the subordinate is not particularly sensitive to relationships, does not make an effort to support the leader, is disaffected, and is not interested in giving anything extra.

Kellerman (2008) also outlined a typology of followers based solely on one metric: level of engagement. Kellerman outlined a continuum that ranges from "feeling and doing absolutely nothing to being passionately committed and deeply involved" (p. 85). The descriptors used along that continuum are as follows:

• *Isolates:* completely detached, alienated, uninterested, uninformed, and do nothing

• *Bystanders:* aware but deliberately disengaged, choosing to stand by and watch rather than stepping up and participating

• *Participants:* invest some time, energy, or talent to try to have an impact, but do not "go overboard" in doing so

• *Activists:* eager, energetic, and engaged, working hard on behalf of leaders (or to undermine them)

• *Diehards:* deeply devoted to the leader (or ready to remove them) and prepared to do anything for the cause

Finally, Maxwell (2019) offers yet another way to conceptualize the degree of involvement of group members. In the book *Leader SHIFT*, this leadership expert talks about leaders and notes that we all tend to fall into various zones dealing with innovation. These same zones can be applied to followers and leaders, and the situation one faces can be any change, not only innovation. The four zones described by Maxwell are as follows:

- **The Coasting Zone**—to do as little as possible
- **The Comfort Zone**—to do what I have always done
- **The Challenge Zone**—to attempt to do what I haven't done before
- **The Creative Zone**—to attempt to think what I have never thought before (pp. 105–106)

Regardless of the model used to think about types of followers, each type exhibits specific behaviors. Consider the follower's active efforts to do a good job, including actual performance, effectiveness in working with others, serving as a resource for others, and the extent to which change is embraced. One also can examine the follower's working relationship with the leader, including the extent to which one identifies with the leader, active attempts to strengthen the relationship, efforts to build and sustain trust, the ability to negotiate differences, and the willingness to engage in difficult conversations.

Blindly following some leader without question or taking a passive role in one's work setting, community, or professional organization will do little to advance the profession; promote individual growth; or achieve safe, quality patient care. An excellent example of effective followers in healthcare was demonstrated during the global pandemic. Nurses at all levels and healthcare professionals were flexible and adaptable to the everchanging climate, and the effective followers were willing to embrace change and new challenges while contributing to the overall well-being of patients and the community.

The profession of nursing needs followers who have characteristics that are similar to those of leaders: a willingness to serve, assertiveness, determination, a willingness to challenge ideas, courage, an ability to act as a change agent, and an openness to new ideas and perspectives. Indeed, followers and leaders must complement each other (Corona, 1986), as noted in Table 5-1.

An understanding of followership in nursing and its integral relationship with leadership will contribute to a competent and dynamic workforce (Honan et al., 2022). We would do well to accept the similarities, give more credence to the significance of the follower role, and focus *less* on trying to make such distinctions and *more* on developing effective or exemplary followers.

CHARACTERISTICS OF EFFECTIVE OR EXEMPLARY FOLLOWERS

Effective or exemplary followers possess many of the same characteristics as individuals who exercise leadership. Each of us may do well to reflect on the extent to which we are characterized by the following:

- Strength and independence
- Critical thinking

LEADERS	FOLLOWERS
TABLE 5-1 **Traits of Leaders and Followers**	
Study and create new ideas	Test new ideas
Make decisions	Challenge decisions as needed
Assign appropriate responsibilities	Know when to accept responsibility and do so
Create environments of trust, resulting in freedom	Use freedom responsibly
Take risks	Risk following
Are reliable	Are trustworthy and respectful
Are loyal to the followers	Are loyal to the leader
Are self-confident	Know themselves
Assume the leadership position	Follow when appropriate

- Ability and willingness to think for ourselves
- Ability to give honest feedback and constructive criticism, particularly in a timely fashion
- Willingness to be our authentic selves
- Innovation and creativity
- Active engagement in all we do
- Cooperativeness and collaboration
- Being self-motivated
- Exceeding expectations
- Willingness to assume ownership
- Healthy self-esteem
- Attentiveness to others and situations
- Being energized by our work and organizations

Exemplary followers possess their own distinctive voices that leaders typically listen attentively to. They openly express their own ideas, concerns, perspectives, and even conflicting views, and effective leaders pay close attention to these voices. A nurse who proposes to the nurse manager and colleagues how family members can be more involved in planning and, indeed, coordinating or directing the care of patients with serious illnesses—when that is not the norm in the unit—is being bold, not passive, and expressing what may be conflicting views. The colleagues who take this suggestion seriously and consider changing the practice standards in the unit are enriched by this nurse's proposal, and the ultimate goal toward which they are all working—quality care—is more likely to be realized.

A seminal study by Berg (1998) found that an emotional connection exists between leaders and exemplary followers, so that each can reassure the other "during those times when each must show his or her limits and weaknesses to the other" (p. 41). For example, the nurse manager who has been unsuccessful in securing additional staff positions so that nurses can attend valuable professional development training and participate in grand rounds needs to be able to express that frustration. Likewise, staff members need to be able to acknowledge when they do not have the knowledge or skill to care for a particular patient. Showing one's limitations and weaknesses requires mutual trust, emotional intelligence, and a connection between the leader and the followers.

Effective followers stimulate and inspire leaders, challenge their creativity, collaborate with them, complement them, give them feedback, and support them. Leaders may inspire vision, but it is the followers who supply much of the energy to achieve that vision. Followers want *honest* leaders—individuals who are consistent, ethical, and principled. They want *competent* leaders—who know their field of endeavor and know the work that needs to be completed. They want leaders who are *inspiring*—individuals who are enthusiastic, contagious, visionary, and effective in communicating a dream. And they want leaders who are *forward thinking*—oriented toward the "big picture," and able to help followers see their important place in that picture. We might think of these factors in terms of a formula for successful leadership and effective leader–follower relations:

$$\text{Honesty} + \text{Competence} + \text{Inspiration} + \text{Vision} = \text{Credibility}$$

Leaders and followers are interdependent. Theirs is a reciprocal relationship, and they reinforce each other. Indeed, the qualities of leaders and followers are so closely aligned that the same people seen by their peers as effective leaders would also be seen as effective followers. Individuals often move back and forth between leader and follower roles, depending on the situation. They draw on the same skills to be effective in either role. Both have power, but where does it come from, and how do leaders and followers use it to empower themselves and others?

SOURCES OF POWER

The concept of power has both positive and negative connotations and often produces feelings of ambivalence (Albert et al., 2022). Thus, the authors stress the importance of leaders and followers understanding the nature of power and using it effectively.

Often, we think of power negatively, conjuring up images of exploitation and manipulation. Those in authority may abuse the power of their positions when allowing personal feelings for or against a staff member, for example, to influence staffing assignments, performance evaluations, or the awarding of "perks" or benefits (e.g., time off to attend a conference, serving as a preceptor). Power, however, does not derive only from one's position of authority.

In 1960, French and Raven published a seminal work in which they identified five sources of power:

> **Legitimate power** comes from one's title, position, or role in a family or culture.
> **Coercive power** comes from the ability to penalize others.

Reward power comes from the ability to help and get things (e.g., money, praise) for others.

Expert power comes from one's knowledge or competence.

Referent power comes from followers' respect for and desire to be liked and admired by the leader.

Bacon (2011) outlined sources of power that are personal or organizational in nature, as well as arising from one's own will; as can be seen, many of these are comparable to those described by French and Raven (1960), but Bacon explicates the power within to a greater extent. Based on the 11 power sources identified, Bacon developed a 44-item self-assessment tool that provides guidelines on interpreting one's score. The power sources described by Bacon are as follows:

Personal Power Sources
- **Knowledge power:** one's knowledge, skill, and expertise and the extent to which others value it
- **Expressiveness power:** one's ability to speak powerfully, participate actively in discussions, and communicate effectively through various methods
- **History power:** one's ability to develop and sustain close relationships with others, make connections, and be active in groups, committees, and so on
- **Attraction power:** one's appearance and outgoing nature, as well as a way of interacting with others that is not offensive, arrogant, distant, or "pushy"
- **Character power:** one's honesty, integrity, trustworthiness, courage, and follow-through on promises

Organizational Power Sources
- **Role power:** one's formal authority and responsibility in an organization or group
- **Resource power:** the control one has over key resources others need to do their work
- **Information power:** access to information that is not typically available to others
- **Network power:** one's connections inside and outside the group or organization, often including people considered to be important
- **Reputation power:** consistent outstanding performance, being asked for advice or coaching or mentoring, and being held in high regard
- **Willpower:** knowing where one wants to go and being fiercely determined to get there, not easily discouraged, a dreamer, and never wavering

As noted, one gains power by having information that one can control, from the people one knows and can call on, and from a strong sense of self, knowing one's values, being self-confident, being able and willing to take risks, and standing up for that in which one believes. Quy (2019) asserted that people also evaluate their competence and trustworthiness based on their gestures and poses. Although speaking primarily to those who make presentations to groups, the concept of using "power poses" can also apply to leaders and followers. Among the "power poses" discussed, this author includes one's smile (sends message you are genuine, trustworthy, and competent), the use of one's hands (which is viewed as conveying warmth, agreeableness, and energy), and one's posture (which if slumped with the head tucked in is "a low-power pose that does not instill confidence or trust").

To increase one's power base, leaders and influential followers alike would do well to know themselves, develop a strong self-concept, develop and use good communication skills, establish support groups and networks, develop and show their expertise (i.e., market themselves), be willing to take risks, build coalitions, eliminate unnecessary dependence, understand "the system" and how it works, and be politically astute and active. Perhaps completing a tool such as the "Personal Power Profile," developed by Hagberg and Donovan (2007), may help leaders and followers appreciate their sources of power and how effectively they use power.

Liu (2017) asserted that "power is no more inherently good or evil than fire or physics; it just is," and claims that "too many people are profoundly illiterate in power." So that those who *do* understand power and how it operates do not "wield a disproportionate influence and fill the void created by the ignorance of the majority," this author challenges us to change the story and "stir up a new sense of 'us.'" Using the work of Marshall Ganz, a civil rights worker in Mississippi in the 1960s, Liu says we can get power through three nested narratives:

- The story of **self**—how we talk about ourselves, the choices we have made, and the purposes we pursue
- The story of **us**—stepping into the shoes of others to understand their situation and find common interests, which is the most crucial story
- The story of **now**—why the vision we pursue is the "movement moment" when action is needed and possible

A leader in nursing, Rosemarie Rizzo Parse (2008) has proposed another perspective on power, the humanbecoming leading-following model discussed in Chapter 1, which emphasizes that although power may lie in one's position, it is the power that lies within the person that is more effective. The author quotes original work to explain that "power with person is the force emanating from the core of a person who commands the respect of others without the authority or responsibility of a position" (p. 369), thus allowing for both "leaders" and "followers" to have power in various situations.

In a very thoughtful book titled *The Power Tactics of Jesus Christ*, Haley (1989) summarizes what he believes were the strategies Jesus used to realize his vision: Jesus spoke whenever and wherever an audience would listen. He said what was unorthodox. He spoke openly about existing problems or injustices, consistently, publicly, and cleverly. He chose others to join in the "movement." He did not ask more of others than He was willing to give Himself. He articulated long-range plans. He used a flexible strategy, and He put His hope in the young, those who had not yet become entrenched in established ways. Through strategies such as these, Haley claimed, Jesus Christ came to be a powerful force for change.

Nurses, too, can be powerful forces for change in complex healthcare settings. That power comes from their knowledge, the intimate and substantive relationships they develop with patients and families, the holistic perspective they bring to care, and their sheer numbers. Such power is retained by keeping current with best practices, involving the patient and family as part of the healthcare team, serving as an advocate for patients and quality care, not allowing oneself to become too narrowly focused or specialized, and collaborating with nursing and other health-team colleagues to promote excellence in care. Nurses strengthen their power base by speaking up in a knowledgeable, informed manner; calling on networks of colleagues with the expertise that may be needed in a particular situation; and constantly learning.

EMPOWERING SELF AND OTHERS

The idea of empowering an individual, whether self or others, implies that no power or authority existed initially; instead, this power has been granted. Leaders must consider that true empowerment can only occur if both responsibility and authority for the tasks are granted to followers. This distinction is vital because responsibility for a task without true authority related to the outcome of the task is merely delegation of work to followers, not true empowerment. In this situation, followers may resent the leader for "adding work" because no true authority for the task exists. For empowerment to be meaningful, followers must perceive they have the power to positively contribute and have some control over their work (Domínguez-Escrig et al., 2021). Shared leadership and true empowerment create confidence and an innovative mindset in followers, which add value to the team (Cobanoglu, 2021).

Among the tasks of leadership (Gardner, 1989), there are several that, in reality, can be thought of as means to empower oneself and one's followers. By *affirming values*, leaders help followers reflect on and perhaps challenge their values to know clearly what it is they believe and are willing to invest in, thereby instilling a sense of power. By *motivating followers*, leaders unlock or channel motives, promote positive attitudes, and encourage creativity, all of which empower followers to believe in themselves and take action. By striving to *achieve a workable unity*, leaders establish trust, cohesion, and mutual tolerance, circumstances that empower followers to share in leadership and bring innovative ideas. *Explaining* empowers followers through knowledge of the vision, information, and understanding. By *serving as a symbol*, the group's source of unity, collective identity, and source of hope, the leader helps followers seize the power that comes from debate, honest expression of feelings, and sharing in a struggle with others. Finally, through the process of *renewing*, both leaders and followers are empowered to break routines, habits, fixed attitudes, perceptions, assumptions, and unwritten rules, thereby allowing them to grow.

When leaders empower followers—and when followers feel empowered—many benefits emerge. Citing the research of scholars in the field, Yukl (2013) outlines the following potential benefits from empowerment: "(1) stronger task commitment, (2) greater initiative in carrying out role responsibilities, (3) greater persistence in the face of obstacles and temporary setbacks, (4) more innovation and learning, and stronger optimism about the eventual success of the work, (5) higher job satisfaction, (6) stronger organizational commitment, and (7) less turnover" (pp. 122–123). Considering the current challenges in nursing related to burnout and turnover, the effects of empowerment on job satisfaction and turnover alone (Yukl & Gardner, 2020) are enough to justify how critical it is for leaders to share power with followers. However, empowered followers do not materialize simply because a leader has acted to empower them. Followers must accept this power and act on it to transform the organization. Once followers know that change is possible, behaviors and beliefs can become transformed into the spark needed to ignite a revolution of change.

Followers can be helped to believe that change is possible, transform their behavior or beliefs, and start revolutions, if leaders use their power to move the group toward the vision and empower followers. Empowered followers do not materialize simply because a leader has acted to empower them. If the leader can influence a significant majority of the group, then others will follow very quickly (Oliver, 2018). Although it is the ideal that all followers feel empowered, rapid innovation and change are still possible when the leader is committed to fostering an unshakeable belief for a few *exceptional* people.

DEVELOPING EFFECTIVE FOLLOWERSHIP SKILLS

Although there are many opportunities to assume the role of leader, each of us will have countless opportunities to function as a follower. We need to consciously develop followership skills and cultivate and appreciate that role to draw on those skills to assume the mantle of leadership when it becomes necessary. We need to be willing to be the first follower, as pointed out by Sivers (2010); among the points made by Sivers that have relevance for this discussion are the following:

- The first follower is a crucial role, an underestimated form of leadership.
- The follower shows others how to follow.
- New followers emulate the follower, not the leader.
- More followers join in, there is a tipping point, and a movement emerges.
- As more join in, it is less risky to be a follower, and the movement can take off.

These points lead to a "domino effect" and develops leaders and followers within an organization.

Barnum (1987) asserted that "never before has the action of the masses had such potential to influence the direction of our profession" (p. 5), an assertion that is as accurate today as it was decades ago. Nurses practicing at the bedside and nursing administrators collaboratively working as a team, demonstrate quality patient care. The nurse working in the community can influence local legislators with personalized human stories about the pain and suffering associated with polluted environments, lack of food, inadequate shelter, and poor prenatal care, not the statisticians who merely cite numbers and trends without providing a human dimension. The student experiencing the curriculum and the teacher–student relationships can best speak to the quality and effectiveness of the learning environment that exists in a school, not the faculty who designs experiences but do not "live" them. In other words, followers have a significant effect on the future of our profession and the world.

If it is true that the future of our profession and the world will be most significantly affected by the actions of followers, then each of us needs to develop practical followership skills. Nurses who aspire to effective followership and leadership should apprentice themselves as followers by assuming that role, thinking about what it means, reflecting on how they contribute to their organization and the nursing profession by fulfilling that role and *being the best they can be*. In addition, such nurses would do well to study and implement many of the suggested strategies for developing leaders because the roles of leader and follower are so complementary. Among the strategies to help each of us be a more effective or exemplary follower are the following, which have been grouped into two major categories:

Know Yourself and Your Organization and Continue to Grow as a Person and a Professional

- Continue your education, both formal and informal. Knowledge is power and will serve you well as a follower.
- Be committed to something other than your own career development. Find your passion in life and be passionate about what you do.
- Know your organization and organizational politics.
- Know your values and hold on to them.
- Set high standards and expectations.
- Seek mentors or accept an offer of mentoring if it is made.
- Develop your professional networks—within and outside your organization—and use them.
- Remain fully accountable for your actions.
- Share information contagiously.
- Help colleagues grow personally and professionally.
- Be reflective.
- Have a sense of humor and laugh at your own mistakes.
- Develop positive relationships with colleagues, rely on each other, and be responsible to each other.
- Continue to develop a wide array of skills in communication, assertiveness, clinical practice, decision making, and scholarly writing.
- Analyze your performance by asking others for feedback and being honest in your own self-appraisal.
- Give credit where it is due.
- Follow through on your commitments or notify others when unable to follow through. Be credible.

- Be competent, demonstrate your value to the group, and make a difference to the organization.
- Be enthusiastic and spread that enthusiasm to others.
- Be your authentic self.
- Be comfortable with uncertainty and ambiguity.
- Develop self-confidence. Believe in and have faith in yourself.
- Remain calm. Do not be hostile.
- Practice self-care and anxiety reducing techniques often.
- Do not give in to peer pressure.
- Be innovative and creative.

Consider completing the Kelley Followership Questionnaire (KFQ), an assessment tool developed by Kelley (1992) based on an analysis of types of followers and designed to help individuals identify the type of follower they are and whether they need to be more independent and critical in their thinking, as well as more actively engaged. Although this instrument has been used extensively in organizations and research studies, it has not been widely tested and lacks broad empirical support. Ligon et al. (2019) conducted an empirical investigation of the KFQ and concluded that the instrument included a dimension of Attitude and Affect, which appears to be composed of both of Kelley's original dimensions: independent, critical thinking (Attitude) and active engagement (Affect). They suggest that this additional dimension allows for nine types of followers rather than the five proposed by Kelley. They recommend further study of the KFQ and refinement of follower typologies.

Be Involved and Speak Up

- Be involved in your practice setting. Have a sense of ownership and stewardship; do not be merely a spectator.
- Be actively involved in professional organizations.
- Contribute as an equal partner.
- Figure out the steps needed for the group to achieve its goals, then be an integral part of those steps rather than on the periphery of "the action."
- Be cooperative with, rather than adversarial to, the leader.
- Appreciate the needs, goals, and constraints placed on the leader.
- Exercise a "courageous conscience . . . the ability to judge right from wrong and the fortitude to take affirmative steps toward what [you] believe is right" (Kelley, 1992, p. 168).
- Understand the importance of speaking out . . . and be willing to do it!
- Speak up so others can benefit from your views.
- Provide opportunities for the leader to talk about vulnerabilities and concerns, as well as strengths and vision.
- Be open to new ideas and willing to assess and explore them.
- Express skepticism about ideas and proposals in a respectful way.
- Take initiative. Take action without being told to do so.

- Accept a place at the table where decisions are made, or if such a place is not offered, create such a place. For example, agree to serve on a committee when invited or volunteer to revise the admission data form if the one currently being used focuses too much on patient weaknesses and limitations and does not adequately address patient strengths and abilities.
- Be proactive. Advocate and be a catalyst for change.
- Try to solve complex problems and offer solutions.
- Present your position in a forthright manner. Develop excellence in communication by using a variety of channels.
- Provide support for your leader when they are making difficult decisions.

It is obvious that there are many ways in which each of us can be an effective or exemplary follower. It also is evident that it is only with concerted personal effort that we will develop the skills of effective followership. These "keys to effective followership" may be summarized as follows:

- Be a critical thinker, not a "Yes" person.
- Be consistent and dependable.
- Be humble and patient.
- Be able to receive and offer constructive criticism.
- Be a diligent worker.
- Be a disciplined student of study and work (theory and practice).
- Be persistent and consistent at developing leadership (and followership) skills.

Case Study, continued

In preparing this proposal, Helen sought input from several healthcare team members who have worked closely with the residents over time and was pleased that they not only offered perspectives that had not been considered, but they also suggested changes to the ideas Helen had proposed initially. Ideas offered by colleagues in dietary, physical therapy, and social services were included in the proposal. The "menu" of ways in which actual or surrogate family members can participate more actively in the care of all residents in the facility that evolved is now being considered by the nursing director, and Helen is excited about the growing interest in the ideas presented and hopeful many of them will be implemented. Helen realizes that preparing such a proposal was not a job requirement, and that although the nurse manager was supportive of the idea, the nurse manager did not have the time to prepare a proposal. So, Helen is feeling good about following through on the nurse manager's encouragement and support, the positive results of taking the risk to ask for input from others, and the opportunity to participate in leading the family involvement initiative once the nursing director endorses it.

REFLECTION QUESTIONS

3. Discuss specific instances in which Helen exhibited leadership qualities, such as initiative and innovation, and instances where Helen demonstrated effective followership by seeking input from colleagues and incorporating their ideas.
4. How might this balanced approach contribute to a culture of collaboration and improvement within the healthcare team?

CONCLUSION

Followers have more power and more ability to empower others than they may realize. They confer the leadership role, and "the responsibility for making the leader-follower relationship work remains with the 'follower'" (Berg, 1998, p. 33). In fact, Maxwell (2019, pp. 201–202) identifies five levels of leadership that influence why people will follow: because they have to, because they want to, because the leader demonstrates competence, because the leader helps them become competent, and because the leader has a reputation for excellence. Thus, followers can be passive sheep who are not fully engaged in the work of the group, or they can be wholehearted supporters who work to co-create a shared vision.

All of us are both leaders and followers, and most of us are followers more often than we are leaders. That, however, is not anything for which we should apologize or anything about which we should feel regret. "The mark of a great leader is the development and growth of followers. The mark of a great follower is the growth of leaders" (Chaleff, 2009, p. 27). Therefore, when we find ourselves in the follower role, we should rejoice!

CRITICAL THINKING 5-1

1. What makes the follower role attractive? What makes it undesirable?

2. How would you describe yourself in the follower role? How effective have you been in that role?

3. Talk to your peers about followership. What are their views on the concept? Was the concept ever addressed in their educational programs? Do they rate themselves as effective followers? How did they develop the abilities to be effective in that role? With whom do they identify as the most effective followers among their work group? Are these the same individuals they identify as leaders (or potential leaders) among the group?

4. Should we focus more on developing effective and exemplary followers in nursing than on developing leaders all around us?

5. Complete the Followership Style Test that follows. What did you learn about yourself by taking this test? What did you learn about followership and the relationship between followers and leaders?

FOLLOWERSHIP STYLE TEST

This questionnaire includes statements about the type of boss you prefer. Imagine yourself to be in a subordinate position of some kind and use your responses to indicate your preference for the way in which a leader might relate with you.

The format includes a five-point scale: "Strongly Agree" (SA), "Agree" (A), "Mixed Feelings" (MF), "Disagree" (D), and "Strongly Disagree" (SD). Select one point on each scale and mark it as you read the 16 statements relating to followership.

	STATEMENT	SA	A	MF	D	SD
1.	I expect my job to be very explicitly outlined for me.	1	2	3	4	5
2.	When the boss says to do something, I do it. After all, they are the boss.	1	2	3	4	5
3.	Rigid rules and regulations usually cause me to become frustrated and inefficient.	5	4	3	2	1
4.	I am ultimately responsible for and capable of self-discipline based on my contacts with the people around me.	5	4	3	2	1
5.	My job should be made as short in duration as possible so that I can achieve efficiency through repetition.	1	2	3	4	5
6.	Within reasonable limits, I will try to accommodate requests from persons who are not my boss because these requests are typically in the best interests of the company anyway.	5	4	3	2	1
7.	When the boss tells me to do something that is the wrong thing to do, it is their fault, not mine, when I do it.	1	2	3	4	5
8.	It is up to my boss to provide a set of rules by which I can measure my performance.	1	2	3	4	5
9.	The boss is the boss. The fact of the promotion suggests that they have something on the ball.	1	2	3	4	5
10.	I accept orders only from my boss.	1	2	3	4	5
11.	I would prefer my boss to give me general objectives and guidelines then allow me to do the job my way.	5	4	3	2	1
12.	If I do something that is not right, it is my own fault, even if my boss told me to do it.	5	4	3	2	1
13.	I prefer jobs that are not repetitious, the kind of task that is new and different each time.	5	4	3	2	1
14.	My boss is in no way superior to me by virtue of positions. They do a different kind of job, one that includes a lot of managing and coordinating.	5	4	3	2	1
15.	I expect my boss to give me disciplinary guidelines.	1	2	3	4	5
16.	I prefer to tell my boss what I will, or at least should, be doing. I am ultimately responsible for my own work.	5	4	3	2	1

Scoring: Score your followership style by simply averaging the numbers for your answers to the individual items. For example, if you scored item 1 "Strongly Agree," you will find the point value of "1" for that answer. To obtain your overall followership style, add all the numerical values associated with the 16 followership items and divide by 16. The resulting average is your followership style.

SCORE	DESCRIPTION	FOLLOWERSHIP STYLE
Less than 2	Very autocratic	Cannot function well without programs and procedures; needs feedback
2–2.4	Moderately autocratic	Needs solid structure and feedback but can also carry on independently
2.5–3.4	Mixed	Mixture of above and below
3.5–4	Moderately participative	Independent worker; does not need close supervision, just a bit of feedback
More than 4	Very democratic	Self-starter, likes a challenge and likes to try new things by themself

Source: Adapted from Douglas, L. M. (1992). *The effective nurse leader and manager* (4th ed., pp. 25–28). Mosby.

References

Albert, N., Pappas, S., O'Grady, T., & Malloch, K. (2022). *Quantum leadership: Creating sustainable value in healthcare* (6th ed.). Jones & Bartlett Learning.

Assessment Research and Evaluation—BISD. (2014, June 10). *Wisdom of geese motivational* [Video]. YouTube. https://www.youtube.com/watch?v=Vy-QoOTU-Qw

Bacon, T. R. (2011). *The elements of power: Lessons on leadership and influence.* AMACOM/HarperCollins.

Barnum, B. (1987). The need for heros [*sic*] and the need for brave men. *Courier, 54*(5).

Bastardoz, N., & Van Vugt, M. (2019). The nature of followership: Evolutionary analysis and review. *The Leadership Quarterly, 30*(1), 81–95.

Bennis, W. (2006). The end of leadership: Exemplary leadership is impossible without full inclusion, initiatives, and cooperation of followers. In W. E. Rosenbach & R. L. Taylor (Eds.), *Contemporary issues in leadership* (6th ed). Westview Press.

Bennis, W. (2008). Introduction. In R. F. Riggio, I. Chaleff, & J. Lipman-Blumen (Eds.), *The art of followership: How great followers create great leaders and organizations.* Jossey-Bass.

Berg, D. N. (1998). Resurrecting the muse: Followership in organizations. In E. B. Klein, F. Gabelnick, & P. Herr (Eds.), *The psychodynamics of leadership.* Psychosocial Press.

Chaleff, I. (2009). *The courageous follower. Standing up to and for our leaders* (3rd ed.). Berrett-Koehler.

Cobanoglu, N. (2021). The relationship between shared leadership, employee empowerment and innovativeness in primary schools: A structural equation of modelling. *European Journal of Educational Research, 10*(1), 327–339. https://doi.org/10.12973/eu-jer.10.1.327

Corona, D. (1986). Followership: The indispensable corollary to leadership. In E. C. Hein & M. J. Nicholson (Eds.), *Contemporary leadership behavior: Selected readings* (2nd ed). Little, Brown.

Domínguez-Escrig, E., Fermín Mallén Broch, F., Lapiedra Alcamí, R., & Chiva Gómez, R. (2021). Leaders who empower: A gateway to radical innovation. *Journal of Management and Organization, 27*(5), 930–947. https://doi.org/10.1017/jmo.2019.73

Douglas, L. M. (1992). *The effective nurse leader and manager* (4th ed., pp. 25–28). Mosby.

French, J. P., Jr., & Raven, B. (1960). The bases of social power. In D. Cartwright & A. Zander (Eds.), *Group dynamics.* Harper and Row.

Gardner, J. W. (1989). The tasks of leadership. In W. E. Rosenbach & R. L. Taylor (Eds.), *Contemporary issues in leadership* (2nd ed). Westview Press.

Hagberg, J., & Donovan, T. (2007). *Personal power profile.* http://www.janethagberg.com/uploads/3/9/3/4/39346357/personal_power_profile_112710.pdf

Haley, J. (1989). *The power tactics of Jesus Christ.* W. W. Norton.

Honan, D., Lasiuk, G., & Rohatinsky, N. (2022). A scoping review of followership in nursing. *Nursing Research, 35*(1), 69–78.

Joel, L. A. (1999). Life review of an ANA president: The path of leadership. In C. A. Andersen (Ed.), *Nursing student to nursing leader: The critical path to leadership development.* Delmar.

Kellerman, B. (2008). *Followership: How followers are creating change and changing leaders.* Harvard Business Press.

Kelley, R. E. (1992). *The power of followership: How to create leaders people want to follow and followers who lead themselves.* Doubleday Currency.

Kelley, R. E. (1998). In praise of followers. In W. E. Rosenbach & R. L. Taylor (Eds.), *Contemporary issues in leadership* (4th ed). Westview Press.

Kelley, R. E. (2008). Rethinking followership. In R. F. Riggio, I. Chaleff, & J. Lipman-Blumen (Eds.), *The art of followership: How great followers create great leaders and organizations.* Jossey-Bass.

Ligon, K. V., Stoltz, K. B., Rowell, R. K., & Lewis, V. J. (2019). An empirical investigation of the Kelley Followership Questionnaire Revised. *Journal of Leadership Education, 18*(3). 08–112.

Liu, E. (2017, March 28). *To challenge those in power, use stories as a weapon.* Ideas.TED.com. https://ideas.ted.com/how-to-get-power/

Manning, T., & Robertson, B. (2016a). A three factor model of followership: Part 1—Introduction to followership, leadership and the three factor model of leadership. *Industrial and Commercial Training, 48*(6), 277–283.

Manning, T., & Robertson, B. (2016b). A three factor model of followership: Part 2—Research on the three factor model and its application to team roles. *Industrial and Commercial Training, 48*(7), 354–361.

Manning, T., & Robertson, B. (2016c). A three factor model of followership: Part 3—Research on followership, a three factor followership framework and practical implications. *Industrial and Commercial Training, 48*(8), 400–408.

Maxwell, J. C. (2019). *Leader SHIFT: The 11 essential changes every leader must embrace.* HarperCollins.

Oliver, B. (2018, July). 2018's top tech: The year cloud accounting passes the tipping point. *California CPA, 87*(1), 17–18. https://www.proquest.com/trade-journals/2018s-top-tech-year-cloud-accounting-passes/docview/2089814882/se-2

Parse, R. R. (2008). The humanbecoming leading-following model. *Nursing Science Quarterly, 21*(4), 369–375.

Pittman, T. S., Rosenbach, W. E., & Potter, E. H., III. (1998). Followers as partners: Taking the initiative for action. In W. E. Rosenbach & R. L. Taylor (Eds.), *Contemporary issues in leadership* (4th ed). Westview Press.

Quy, L. (2019, March 20). This is how to use power poses to be successful in life. *SmartBrief.* https://www.smartbrief.com/original/2019/03/how-use-power-poses-be-successful-life

Sivers, D. (2010, February). *How to start a movement* [Video]. TED Conferences. http://www.ted.com/talks/derek_sivers_how_to_start_a_movement?utm_source%EF%80%BD%20newsletter_weekly_2010-04-06&utm_campaign%EF%80%BDnewsletter_weekly&utm_medium%EF%80%BDemail

Sullivan, T. J. (1998). *Collaboration: A health care imperative.* McGraw-Hill.

Uhl-Bien, M. (2021a). Complexity and COVID-19: Leadership and followership in a complex world. *Journal of Management Studies, 58*(5), 1400–1405.

Uhl-Bien, M. (2021b). Complexity and leadership and followership: Changed leadership in a changed world. *Journal of Change Management, 21*(2), 144–162.

Wharton, University of Pennsylvania. (2018, May 22). *Wharton to host 52nd annual global forum in New York City, June 13-15* [press release]. https://news.wharton.upenn.edu/press-releases/2018/05/wharton-host-52nd-annual-global-forum-new-york-city-june-13-15/

Yukl, G. (2013). *Leadership in organizations* (8th ed.). Prentice Hall.

Yukl, G., & Gardner, W. (2020). *Leadership in organizations* (9th ed.). Pearson.

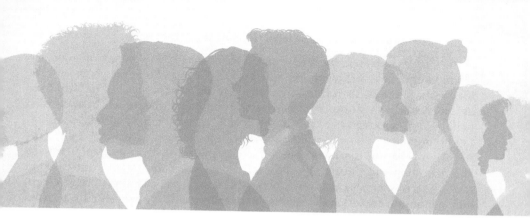

CHAPTER 6

Leadership as an Integral Component of Each Nurse's Professional Role

LEARNING OBJECTIVES
- Identify characteristics of transformational and transactional leaders.
- Compare and contrast the leader–follower relationship in a transformational environment and a transactional environment.
- Explain how transformational and innovative leadership generates growth in individuals, organizations, and groups.
- Discuss how nurse leaders can develop a healthy work environment and empower others.
- Describe how the four components of principle-centered leadership can contribute to an individual's personal and professional growth as a leader.
- Describe how Maslow's hierarchy of needs relates to leadership development.
- Explain how leadership ability is enhanced by emotional intelligence.
- Explain how leadership is an integral component of being a nurse professional.

INTRODUCTION

Professional nurses can no longer think of themselves as "just nurses." Nurses are increasingly expected to provide leadership, whether they hold staff positions or are vice presidents, nurse practitioners, or nurse educators. Nurses must be competent if they are to provide leadership. Grossman (2007) developed a Leadership and Management Competency Checklist to assist critical care nurses in obtaining experiences and gaining competency in leading and managing. Based on Kolb's Experiential

Model (1984), this checklist is recommended for nurses who precept or guide new orientees and nursing students in practicing leadership and management skills. The idea is that individuals learn more if they can integrate what they pick up from an experience with an expert, ideally receive some constructive feedback on their performance, and then have time to process the new learning and reflect on how to improve the next time they are faced with a similar experience. Box 6-1 identifies the major behaviors that nurses need to acquire in order to be competent in leading and managing. Individuals with these strengths will be able to exert leadership in making decisions, collaborating with the healthcare team, adapting to change, providing innovative solutions, facilitating partnerships with other healthcare agencies and healthcare workers, accomplishing goals, and reaching stated visions.

> *All great leaders have had one characteristic in common: it was the willingness to confront unequivocally the major anxiety of their people in their time.* —John Kenneth Galbraith

Consider the following case study about how nurses who use emotional intelligence in leadership can impact their job satisfaction and their patients' care.

COMPETENCE PROPELS NURSES TO LEAD

Nurse leaders know what needs to happen to achieve quality patient care and excellence in nursing education. By following a framework such as the checklist provided in Box 6-1, nurses can assist themselves and other nurses in gaining the knowledge they need to lead their colleagues so that the practice environment will be a positive and exciting place. Individuals will generally feel more collaborative and less competitive if they are empowered with knowledge, are continuously growing, and are feeling competent themselves. This is what Covey (2020) calls

---

BOX 6-1 Components of a Leadership and Management Competency Checklist

Communication: oral and written	**Unit vision and research development:** structure, culture, and quality improvement	**Professional role development and image:** authority, power, and confidence	**Team building and empowerment:** leadership, followership, and group dynamics
Collaboration and networking: interprofessionally and intraprofessionally	**Risk management:** legally and ethically	**Unit management regarding care delivery:** care patterns and patient safety	**Personal and unit specialty skill development:** skills geared to specialty unit
Decision making, problem-solving, and troubleshooting: using nursing models			

Case Study

Cynthia came from one of the urban acute trauma centers to the community hospital to be the nurse manager of the inpatient orthopedic unit and outpatient orthopedic center. She decided to work as a staff nurse 1 day per week in the unit and 1 half-day in the outpatient orthopedic surgery and rehabilitation center. She quickly established rapport with the patients, staff, and physicians in both areas. Her clinical competency with new orthopedic technology and her charismatic manner of leadership were highly respected by the staff. She collaborated with the physicians and members of the units' staff to determine whether the hospital could purchase more equipment in order to expand their services. This was determined to be a definite yes.

However, data showed that most orthopedic patients were waiting up to 3 months for surgery, so some were going to other hospitals far from their homes. The units in both the hospital and outpatient clinics were expanded for surgical procedures, and additional staff were hired to manage the workload. Cynthia felt it would be more cost-effective and satisfying for the nurses and technicians in each area to be able to rotate (similar to the physicians) through the different settings with the new expansion. She set up a committee to explore this option. The committee, under her leadership, found that 90% of the nurses, assistants, and technicians were supportive of the rotations, although 10% were adamant they stay in their current positions and expressed negative emotions about rotating. Cynthia felt upset that not all staff members were willing to try her idea.

REFLECTION QUESTIONS

1. How should Cynthia proceed with her idea considering that 10% of staff do not want to rotate to both areas?
2. What could Cynthia do to support her idea further and obtain staff buy-in?

principle-centered leadership. He suggests that an individual needs to be trustworthy in order to gain trust from others and be able to empower those they lead. In other words, if followers do not perceive the leader as competent or someone in whom they can put their trust, they will not feel empowered or aligned with the goals of the group or organization. Eventually, if principle-centered leadership is embraced at all levels of an organization's structure, the work culture will evolve into a more caring environment where new ideas will be welcomed and used by everyone. It stands to reason that when people are feeling good about their family or personal lives, they can be more effective in their work setting. If the leaders care about their unit and staff, they will push the staff harder to do their best and be motivated to be their best. It is important to create a culture in a practice or unit that not only gives the highest patient care but also allows staff recognition and growth; otherwise, it is probable the unit culture will not be sustainable.

A study of 5,000 employees over 5 years found seven practices that were identified as important to produce a sustainable work environment (Hansen, 2018). The practices included the ability to:

1. Focus specifically on goal attainment
2. Produce highly valued work
3. Support continuous learning
4. Motivate the employees
5. Reinforce peer support
6. Make team members work their very best
7. Collaborate effectively

It is interesting that the first four items are individually focused and the last three are related to fostering team spirit and goal accomplishment (Hansen, 2018). It is important to remember that an individual (in most situations) must be doing their best before they can act as an effective team member. Nurse leaders can gain insight from these findings to propel their unit accomplishments. Additionally, findings from Pink (2018) generate other hints for employees and leaders to understand the scientific secrets of perfect timing for finding one's most productive time of day, when (assessing season, week, month, weekend, or day during the week) a project would be most apt to be successfully started in a unit, and when during one's life is the best time to seek a new job.

A healthy work environment (HWE) is crucial to success with meeting patient outcomes, maintaining staff morale, ensuring patient safety and patient satisfaction, empowering registered nurses (RNs), and implementing monthly interprofessional rounds, and has proved helpful in improving staff communication and collaboration (Mabona et al., 2022). The idea of a healthy quality of work life is another way of viewing an HWE. Improvements in the workplace are needed for nurses to excel in their roles, and nurses must lead the change in creating improvements to positively affect the quality of work life and promote mental health (Maddigan et al., 2023).

Similar to Covey's tenets of principle-centered leadership, Ulrich et al. (2022) describe an HWE as including effective communication, interdisciplinary collaboration, an evidence-based practice environment, the potential for professional advancement, and an atmosphere of empowerment that allows all members to feel confident and competent. Although HWEs for all nurses have declined dramatically since 2018, the American Association of Critical-Care Nurses (AACN) continues to demonstrate evidence of a positive relationship between HWEs, nursing job satisfaction, and nursing retention (Ulrich et al., 2022).

CONFIDENCE, SPEAKING WITH AUTHORITY, AND OTHER QUALITIES OF LEADERSHIP

Nurses who are just beginning their careers can be excellent leaders and make great contributions to the profession. It is important that new nurses become part of the HWE transformation so that they feel comfortable and empowered in their work setting. Nurses, who frequently are working in high-stress situations, could all benefit from "self-leadership," which includes developing feedback mechanisms that enhance well-being, using constructive thought strategies (positive self-talk, visualization, etc.), and employing natural rewards (Mayfield, 2021). Nurses need to know how to best help themselves and feel empowered to succeed in their work and personal life. Kaplan (2019) offers multiple empowerment exercises and ideas to help individuals in spite of themselves. She reiterates that you have to believe a change can happen, that it is never too late nor are you too old, that you should follow your dream and what is important to you, live in the present, get the "bad people" out of your life, and don't forget to manage your financial affairs.

The National Academies of Sciences, Engineering, and Medicine developed recommendations for the nursing profession to improve the health of Americans in the 21st century, with a particular focus on the effects of COVID-19 (National Academies of Sciences, Engineering, and Medicine, 2021). This report, *The Future of Nursing 2020–2030: Charting a Path to Achieve Health Equity*, recommends 10 different role functions for the nurse to assist with, including healthcare access for all, collaborative practices, a diverse workforce, shared decision making, and more nurses working in the community. These recommendations make it apparent that staff nurses must lead. In fact, the National Academies of Sciences, Engineering, and Medicine (2021) emphasizes that leadership is needed at multiple levels in nursing, not only at the top, to address social determinants of health. As nurses increase their skills to achieve these goals, the profession will become stronger and more productive. Now is the time for such action.

When thinking about the leadership that is exercised in a nursing group or organization, it must be realized that every individual, not just the nurse manager, dean, or committee chair, has the potential and the responsibility to assume the role of leader and work with others to fulfill the goals of the group or organization. The individual who happens to be in the appointed, authoritative role (e.g., the nurse manager) may or may not be the person who actually fulfills the role of the leader. As discussed earlier, effective followers have skills comparable to those of leaders, and the effectiveness of the leadership that any individual provides depends largely on the followers. Gardner (1990) said, "Leadership can be distributed among members, and the leader must recognize the needs of the followers, help them see how these needs can be met, and give them confidence that they can accomplish results through their efforts" (p. 149). So, leaders must be able to lead others as well as themselves. If there is a determined and powerful followership, leaders and followers can be successful.

Given the multigenerational diversity in the nursing workforce, all nurse leaders and followers should increase their understanding of each of the generation's beliefs and work ethics. Nurses from different generations can assist one another. For example, Gen Z and Gen Y (millennials) nurses can share their expertise in using technology or with establishing work–life balance with Gen X and baby boomer nurses. The Gen X and baby boomer nurses can mentor others regarding specific nursing techniques, nursing history, and communication methods that have been successful in the past (Tan & Chin, 2023). Leaders can capitalize on the strengths of generational differences in the nursing workforce to create HWEs and improve patient care (Tan & Chin, 2023). Utilizing a One Page Talent Management process can assist the leadership team in choosing new employees according to their skills, education, experience, and talent to achieve a diverse workforce (Effron & Ort, 2018).

Using social media to increase communication with patients, family, and other staff at the hospital or practice can have multiple benefits for both patients and staff because it offers a platform to communicate about health issues and potentially improve health outcomes (Pianese & Belfiore, 2021).

The number of people who engage with social media has tripled in the past decade, and approximately 72% of Americans are social media users (Dean, 2023). Nurses could use social media to advocate for policies at the infrastructure level, engage with patients to provide education to improve patient outcomes, or create a social network of support to overcome burnout and compassion fatigue. Engaging with social media of some type is necessary if nurses want to be active leaders, or successful followers, in healthcare.

It is common, however, for nurses not to be effective followers or leaders. For example, instead of acting as leaders or effective followers, nurses criticize their managers, the institution, the director, the physician, or other people occupying positions of leadership. Instead of suggesting solutions or assuming leadership roles themselves, nurses blame other nurses and fail to collaborate with one another. Nurses fail to challenge physician orders, are often scared to try anything that differs from the "way things have always been," may not wish to become computer savvy, are not interested in using social media, do not have the confidence to capitalize on their extensive knowledge or experience, or claim to be "only a nurse" when talking to a physician or a patient. These examples point to a lack of accountability and willingness to effect change. If nurses are to increase their level of responsibility and if the profession is to survive and thrive, all nurses must exercise their leadership ability. Nursing leadership is a competency that all nurses need to acquire and continue to improve, just as they do with their practice expertise, whether that practice is in clinical, educational, health policy, or other environments. Educators need to integrate this clinical leadership into all of the clinical practice area courses, so nurses are prepared to lead at all levels and in a variety of work environments.

Nurse leaders also need to be authentic leaders—that is, they need to be good communicators and be reflective and have a confident sense of who, what, why, and where they are. In fact, nurses may need to be reminded that the 2022 Gallup Poll (Brenan, 2023) again identified them as the most honest professionals with high ethical standards; such perspectives highlight their authenticity, which serves us well in leadership roles. An authentic leader is someone with self-awareness, transparency in relationships, balanced information processing, and an internalized moral perspective (Duarte et al., 2021). Being able to identify what makes a good leader and to use those skills that demonstrate good leadership would seem to inherently improve oneself. Some lessons about leadership shared by Hennessy (2018) seem helpful and merit review by nurses at every level. He found 10 very attainable qualities that could assist nurses in improving leadership skills: (1) humility, (2) authenticity and trust, (3) leadership of service, (4) empathy, (5) courage, (6) collaboration and teamwork, (7) innovation, (8) intellectual curiosity, (9) storytelling (as described by Stephen Denning [TED, 2011]), and (10) legacy. Perhaps legacy—how you want to be remembered by the practice or hospital you are in now—could be a skill you could begin working on. Do you want the staff and other healthcare professionals and patients to remember you as an organized and caring nurse or advanced practice registered nurse (APRN) who was always empathetic and authentic? Do you want to be thought of as an excellent clinician who really "knew your stuff" and was a great team player? Or maybe you do not care what people will remember about you when you leave this work setting. Your legacy is something you could think about and then decide what is most significant for people to remember about you.

It is important to adopt a main leadership style, but it is difficult to be effective when the challenges and stresses of the environment become overwhelming. In these cases, a different style using other leadership skills might be more beneficial for both the leader and the followers involved. For example, a visionary leadership style may be effective in most situations to advance the team, but an emergency situation with a patient may require a commanding leadership style to keep the team on track, monitor the interventions, and improve patient outcomes. A strategy that may assist leaders to become more effective and to remain true to themselves is to be mindful at work and to pay attention to their well-being and performance. The skill of mindfulness is the ability to be present in the moment, on purpose, and in a nonjudgmental way (Oman, 2023). Nurses who become more mindful should be more reflective and more effective as leaders who can role-model for other health professionals and coach others to obtain a balance between work and personal goals.

Individuals are not born leaders; rather, leaders emerge and continue to evolve as a result of experiences, purposeful self-development, and interactions with a variety of people. Some characteristics that would benefit an individual wanting to increase their leadership ability are discussed by Davis (2010) in his book *The Intangibles of Leadership*. He recommends the following general points:

1. **Wisdom:** View his Wisdom Checklist (pp. 14–15).
2. **Will:** It is possible to motivate others.
3. **Executive maturity:** Do not be defensive and stand back to assess the whole picture frequently.
4. **Honesty:** You must do what you say you do.
5. **Social judgment:** Be open-minded.
6. **Presence:** Garner respect from the group.
7. **Self-insight:** You must be competent and obtain feedback continuously so you remain competent.
8. **Self-efficacy:** Believe in yourself.
9. **Fortitude:** Be courageous.
10. **Fallibility:** You do not have all the correct answers.

All nurses need to practice their leadership and encourage others to get involved, either as effective followers or as leaders. By creating a vision, strategizing how to accomplish the vision, seeking creative ways to implement change, and effectively leading or following in a collaborative manner, nurses exercise the leadership skills that will assist the entire healthcare team in accomplishing its goals, whether they are of quality patient care, are of educational excellence, or are building the science of nursing. In other words, a more positive and passionate outlook must prevail in nurses' work environments.

TYPES OF LEADERSHIP

In a classic work that still has relevance many years later, Burns (1978) described two types of leadership that are used to make change and create new futures: transactional leadership and transformational leadership.

Transactional Leadership

Transactional leadership involves an exchange in which both the leader and the followers get something. The leader gets the job completed or the goal achieved, and the followers get promotions, monetary rewards, or other such benefits. The focus of this type of leadership system is the accomplishment of a task, and it is the type often seen in healthcare organizations. Some even argue that nurses too often focus on tasks and rewards.

Transactional leaders focus on getting the job done and see task completion as the bottom line. Abbas and Ali (2023) describe transactional leaders as more self-concerned, task oriented, and outcome focused. Verbal praise, recognition for employees, and financial incentives are very visible in organizations that consider transactional leadership an important style of leading their employees (Abbas & Ali, 2023). Although there may be some type of connection between these leaders and their followers, this connection often is something other than a common purpose or a shared vision. With such a relationship, both leaders and followers may perceive their work only as a job, and not invest in it as a career.

Transformational Leadership

In contrast, transformational leadership is a process in which "leaders and followers raise one another to higher levels of motivation and morality" (Burns, 1978, p. 20). This motivation energizes people to perform beyond expectations by creating a sense of ownership in reaching the vision. And it is not to say the employees do not have financial incentives and recognition for accomplishments. According to Bass (1985), transformational leadership inspires the team to perform beyond expectations. He cited examples of transformational leadership from a Reserve Officers' Training Corps (ROTC) study, including the following:

- Instilling pride in all
- Building morale through pep talks
- Acting as a positive role model
- Building the confidence of others through personal encouragement
- Complimenting individuals' performances and contributions as a way to instill pride in the group

Bass (1985) characterized transformational leaders as charismatic, able to instill motivation in others, and able to give individualized consideration. Burns (1978) described them as individuals who heighten followers' awareness of what must be done to accomplish the shared goal. Bennis and Nanus (2003) defined transformational leaders as individuals who follow through with getting people to act, assist others to lead, and ultimately facilitate change. Several strategies have been identified (Bennis & Nanus, 2003) to assist leaders to be more transformational: attention through vision, meaning through communication, trust through positioning, and deployment of self through positive self-regard and optimism about a desired outcome. But one merely has to look around and know that although most people can develop into transformational leaders if they choose to, some individuals may be more or less successful. In fact, some research supports a polygenic nature of leadership, meaning genetics may contribute to leadership, and identifies positive genetic correlations between leadership traits and various health indicators (Song et al., 2022). This suggests leadership skills may be inherently more natural for certain individuals. However, nurses must remember that leadership skills are learnable, and maintaining a growth mindset can help improve leadership skills over time.

Transformational leaders emphasize the importance of following a vision and assisting others to participate in making it a reality; they communicate their values and beliefs to others so that they can achieve a common meaning in their work and realize the vision toward which all are striving; they trust others, are honest, and act responsibly; and finally, they use their talents and expertise as a way to express their desire for and commitment to a vision. To realize a vision for a unit, department, or practice, nurses should have an interprofessional collaboration with other healthcare members involved to achieve high-quality, well-coordinated patient care (Sibbald et al., 2021). Nurses can be particularly savvy with interdisciplinary collaboration because they are the professionals who spend the most time with the patient and presumedly would have the opportunity to obtain the most knowledge about the patient. This patient information would be helpful for every member on the patient's professional team. Nurse leaders need to ensure that all interprofessional staff buy into what the nursing staff has chosen for their unit's vision and culture in order to have collaborative, team-based, and exceptional patient care (Sibbald et al., 2021). Stakeholder buy-in, such as from the governing boards, the surrounding community, and regulatory agencies, is also very much a part of achieving a successful vision. If nurses are to be transformational leaders, they must pursue goals, communicate in an articulate manner, be concerned with their own growth and the growth of their followers, establish trusting relationships, and identify their strengths and limitations. They also need to readily accept change and constantly seek new ways of doing things despite the risk (Bass, 1985).

Bass (1985) and Burns (1978) believed that transformational leaders have strong personal value systems and that by sharing these values, they are able to affect and impact followers' beliefs, even without needing to negotiate what's in it for the follower. In essence, transformational leaders have a spirit that creates special leader–follower relationships and promotes individual and group growth. In fact, this spirit, this feeling of mutual involvement, is of greater significance than any isolated task accomplishment. This excitement about a vision or idea that is worthwhile attracts others to follow.

Transformational Leadership and Nursing Practice

Cummings et al. (2021) have suggested that "leadership practices are intricately intertwined with the context in which they occur and do not simply depend on the characteristics of individuals" (p. 10). Nursing leadership benefits significantly from an organizational climate and shared governance structure that encourages nurse empowerment and active participation in decision making (Cummings et al., 2021). By examining nurses' leadership in everyday processes rather than formalized leadership roles (e.g., management positions), it is apparent that nurses' intrinsic motivation to provide quality patient care equips them with the courage to challenge traditions and ideas by proposing new ideas to achieve a desired vision (de Kok et al., 2023). Nurses' intrinsic motivation to do good often outweighs the fear of stepping into a transformational leadership role and rebelling against practices that are no longer effective. However, knowledge, work experience, and patient-driven motivation are necessary for good transformational leadership as an informal leader (de Kok et al., 2023).

Demir and Duygulu (2022) stress the importance of providing transformational leadership development to nurses so that increased safety and quality and improved patient outcomes will occur. Nurses who are transformational leaders set an example, explore innovative approaches for change and development, build relationships founded on trust and cooperation, empower the other nurses, and acknowledge their contributions. These practices of transformational leadership have a positive relationship to nurses' control over practice, and suggest that when nurse managers are transformational, nurses in the unit are able to achieve patient-care goals and provide higher quality care (Demir & Duygulu, 2022). Nurses need to receive leadership development in their academic preparation, continuing education, and on-the-job training so they can be prepared to be transformational leaders. Being able to recognize colleagues' feelings, motivate others, and manage one's own emotions well in relationships serves to foster an environment that facilitates transformational leadership. For example, with the multifaceted problems that healthcare organizations face today, there are numerous crises that demand the entire staff, ranging from the maintenance crew to the chief executive officer, to be able to communicate to the public in a positive and nonthreatening manner. Providing leadership training that encompasses leader-empowering behaviors and formal mentoring is highly correlated with improved leader, staff, and work environment outcomes (Cummings et al., 2021; Richey & Waite, 2019). Some ideas to empower others include the following:

1. Serving the needs of people (employees and patients)
2. Allowing people autonomy in the decision-making process
3. Trusting people with access to needed information
4. Valuing and supporting others' contributions
5. Providing flexibility (Coun et al., 2021)

Creating the vision of a unit, department, or practice and maintaining it are the responsibilities of the whole interprofessional team and are not just the manager's responsibilities. Wang et al. (2022) share some ideas on how empowering leadership stimulates the entire team to work hard on accomplishing its vision, encourages a mindset where individuals are enthusiastic about optimizing success, and fosters behaviors that are geared toward innovation. Additionally, it is key to remember to focus on what one can change on a daily basis. Effron (2018) identifies eight steps to obtaining high performance levels and defines a high-level performer as someone who consistently performs better than 75% of their peers. The eight steps include the following:

1. Develop idealistic goals
2. Control your behavior and actions
3. Attempt to learn all you can
4. Be open and relate to all
5. Maximize your adaptation to the company/unit/practice
6. At particular times fake your feelings and try something new—it might be an improvement
7. Make a firm commitment
8. Try to remain focused (Effron, 2018).

In today's hospitals, clinics, offices, and practice settings, nurses can and should be the high-level performers transforming healthcare delivery to improve patient outcomes, provide cost-effective care, and maximize use of resources.

EMOTIONAL INTELLIGENCE

Goleman (1998) suggested that one of the most important attributes of leaders is emotional intelligence, which is quite different from one's intelligence quotient (IQ). He defined *emotional intelligence* as a group of competencies (self-awareness, self-management, social awareness, and relationship management) that influence the ability to respond to others and manage one's own feelings. Ireland (2022) notes emotions are not just an individual's reactions to something. Rather, it is important to realize that the brain interprets meaning from whatever occurs and then responds. Goleman's research (1998) indicates that emotional intelligence is nearly twice as significant as IQ in becoming a leader. People are born with certain cognitive abilities, or IQ, and that is not likely to change dramatically throughout one's life; emotional intelligence, on the other hand, is something one can acquire and use to improve one's professional behavior. It is essential for nurses to realize the power they have in making positive change in their units, in their agencies, and in the health policy arena. This, coupled with having high emotional intelligence and becoming confident with managing oneself in a highly stressful setting, puts nurses in a position to affect the status quo.

Goleman et al. (2016) recommended that leaders at all levels need the following: self-awareness, self-regulation, motivation, empathy, and social skills. Using these, all leaders can inspire others by effecting change, being creative, articulating visions, helping visions become reality, managing conflict, taking risks, networking, and adapting to new initiatives. Nurse followers and leaders can use their emotional competence to develop an HWE to create a work culture that fosters collaboration. Leaders can maximize their successes as well as facilitate others' achievements by fostering an environment more conducive to using emotional competence, such as by sponsoring staff-recognition days, publishing accomplishments in a unit or agency newsletter, and having peer-evaluated employee-of-the-month designations. Increasing self-awareness, which is an important aspect of emotional intelligence, will most likely help build high self-esteem.

What happened with Cynthia's situation in the Case Study at the beginning of this chapter? Continue the Case Study to learn how Cynthia displayed leadership to promote positive change.

Case Study, continued

Cynthia recognized her emotions and decided she would not allow her feelings and desire to move her idea forward to prevent her from being empathetic toward the 10% of staff who did not want to rotate. Cynthia decided to have a meeting with the units to discuss the findings and use her social skills to explore the staff members' feelings and articulate her vision. After the meeting, Cynthia and her staff unanimously decided that the 10% who did not want to rotate would not have to. The nurses were quite excited about the idea of having a new and expanded scope of practice. Cynthia assisted the committee in setting up in-service training sessions, orientations, and precepting for each individual so that they would be prepared for this rotating unit schedule. Nurses volunteered to present the in-service training sessions and orientations as well as to precept for each other. After the scheduling was set up and piloted, the staff was able to anticipate potential problems and deal with them. Schedules were tweaked, and staff worked in a cohesive way.

One year later, job and patient satisfaction levels were at the highest ever obtained. The average length of stay was the lowest ever measured, and the cost of managing the units was down. Nurses were excited to learn new aspects of orthopedics and were joining the Orthopedic Nursing Society, becoming certified by the American Nursing Credentialing Center, attending conferences and reporting findings back to their unit and colleagues, and conducting two evidence-based practice studies. The nurse manager asked for feedback from her staff every 6 months and found that they were overwhelmingly supportive of her leadership. Using the skills of emotional competence, Cynthia was successful in turning her unit into a cost-generating unit where staff morale and retention increased. In fact, Fosslien and Duffy (2019) found that perhaps emotions do belong in the workplace, because they were found to highly correlate with the ability to work on a team and to be an effective verbal communicator.

REFLECTION QUESTIONS

3. Reflect on Cynthia's leadership in fostering a positive workplace culture and achieving remarkable outcomes in job satisfaction, patient care, and cost management. What specific leadership qualities contributed to the success of the rotating unit schedule?
4. Considering the impact of emotional competence on team dynamics and workplace effectiveness, what are instances in your own experiences where emotions played a significant role in teamwork and communication?
5. How can developing emotional intelligence enhance your ability to work collaboratively with colleagues, and what steps can you take to cultivate these skills in your professional journey?

SELF-ESTEEM AND LEADERSHIP IMAGE

Bennis and Nanus (2003) described transformational leaders as having a good self-esteem. Burns (1978) suggested that Maslow's (1970) concept of self-esteem would be enhanced if it included the concept of positive self-regard. Self-esteem includes the need for achievement, mastery, competence, confidence, independence, and freedom to act. Satisfying one's self-esteem needs tends to result in higher self-confidence and eventually self-actualization (Maslow, 1998). These abilities are congruent with those that define transformational leaders and effective followers, and because individuals who have high self-esteem are able to develop and grow, followers can become leaders. Chapman and White (2019) suggest several tangible ideas to assist in empowering organizations by supporting and appreciating people at the workplace as well as those who are working remotely. Chapman and White (2019) offers advice on specific strategies of appreciation for employees and colleagues, such as giving affirmation (authentic, individualized thanks or praise), sharing time (focused attention and active listening), performing kind acts (helping with small tasks or fielding phone calls), giving gifts (small gifts or food), and physical touch (handshakes, high-fives, etc.). In the current climate of healthcare, where nurses are leaving the profession due to unhealthy work environments and may only get a thank-you gift once a year during National Nurses Week, implementing individualized efforts to show nurses they are truly appreciated can be the first step toward rebuilding a resilient nursing workforce.

Nurses must be self-motivated to change or improve their personal and professional lives. Individuals who are not motivated to change will most likely maintain the status quo and fail to provide leadership to or facilitate others' growth. Therefore, it is important to realize that although transformational leadership tends to increase followers' creativity and ability to be successful, data suggest that a self-regulatory focus shows that followers can increase or decrease their success depending on the situation, both individually and as a team (Van Dijk et al., 2021). Receiving rewards, used in the transactional leadership style, does motivate employees to perform their work. However, it is more and more important for followers to be able to identify their own motivating factors and engage in activities that may also influence their creativity. Nurses, as does anyone, learn what to think from the people they interact with, and are influenced by, so it is important to have strong, positive leaders as role models (Van Dijk et al., 2021). Box 6-2 lists the steps to improve leadership ability.

Many nurses have the attitude that they deserve more simply because they have seniority or have paid their dues. When they do not get more, they perceive themselves to be victims of the system. Circumstances do not change just because people think they deserve special favors (i.e., treatment that ignores system constraints). This idea that experienced nurses have paid their dues only propagates more unhappiness and victimization for the nurses. Kouzes and Posner (2017) note that the unprecedented instability in today's world calls for strong leadership. They recommend that leaders engage in practices to transform followers and help realize visionary goals:

- Model the way.
- Inspire a shared vision.
- Challenge the process.

BOX 6-2 Improving One's Leadership: A Sequence to Follow

- Identify a desire to lead.
- Develop leadership abilities for a specific position.
- Implement new leadership practices.
- Obtain feedback from peers and supervisors.
- Use the feedback and work on improvements.
- Practice new ideas by shadowing a leader role model, especially focusing on new practices.
- Implement the additional new leading behaviors.
- Develop a method of obtaining continuous feedback.

• Enable others to act.
• Encourage the heart.

The first four practices are self-explanatory. The last practice, encourage the heart, highlights the importance of leaders caring deeply about the vision and working hard to accomplish it. It also suggests that people who perform well will be self-satisfied. Kouzes and Posner (2017) strongly recommended that leaders celebrate accomplishments of the people working in the department. Leaders need to feel good about themselves and focus on themselves, but they also need to appreciate their followers' accomplishments. Therefore, it is crucial that leaders enhance their own initiative, self-esteem, assertiveness, and positive self-regard if they are to provide leadership in and advance the nursing profession. Leaders need to have grit (perseverance and passion) but so do followers. Basically, nurses need to have grit to achieve clinical competence and remain in the nursing field successfully (Shin, 2022). Findings suggest that grit boosts clinical competence and has a direct effect on socialization into the nursing profession for newly graduating nurses (Shin, 2022). Nurse leaders should consider programs or strategies to improve not only their own grit but the grit of their followers as well, and nurse education programs should incorporate focus on grit within nursing curricula.

GENDER AND LEADERSHIP

"*Gender* refers to the attitudes, feelings, and behaviors that a given culture associates with a person's biological sex" (American Psychological Association [APA], 2022). Rather than viewing differences between genders as a matter requiring apology or alteration, we should learn to acknowledge and honor these unique qualities. By combining the best of gendered domains of leadership, which includes both the "feminine domain" and "masculine domain," we can create an equilibrium where our visions become lucid and clearly articulated. Leadership attributes that all individuals can strive to demonstrate include being assertive, interpersonal, decisive, and visionary (Boyer et al., 2023). Although there is a good deal of evidence to support clear differences in leadership styles between genders, current research indicates leaders do not adhere to strict gendered roles in their leadership approaches (Boyer et al., 2023). Gender, it would seem, is not a key determinant of actual leadership style but a factor that is likely to influence how the leadership role is implemented. In essence, a shift toward leadership and organizational structures that embrace greater androgyny, integrating the advantages of all genders, may be most effective for the individuals in those groups or organizations, the individuals and communities they serve, and the professions they represent.

WOULD-BE LEADERS BECOME LEADERS

Nurses need to reinvent themselves, much as others have done. Bennis (1993) explains the process of reinventing himself "to avoid accepting roles [which he] was brought up to play" (p. xv). He further describes the significance of being able to invent and reinvent himself so that he would not have to be "content with borrowed postures, secondhand ideas, [or] fitting in instead of standing out" (p. xv).

His warning not to accept stereotypical perceptions offers a lesson for nurses and non-nurses alike: Do not accept stereotypes of nursing. By reinventing themselves, nurses "do not accept the roles we were brought up to play" (Bennis, 1993, p. 2). Nurses are currently facing changes in the healthcare industry, the nursing profession, and opportunities for innovation that did not previously exist prior to COVID-19 (Thepna et al., 2023). These opportunities can be used for nurses to reinvent themselves and focus on larger issues rather than merely day-to-day tasks. If nurses consider entrepreneurial pursuits to improve healthcare, then the issues negatively impacting healthcare could be improved. Nurses who wish to develop their entrepreneurial spirit should surround themselves with people who think differently than they do and who are open to change. To practice entrepreneurialism in nursing, which is a stressful and always-changing profession, nurses need to overcome knowledge gaps related to business, focus on self-efficacy, and leverage existing health systems and policies to initiate change (Thepna et al., 2023). Nurses need to think in innovative ways to best provide nursing care to patients and not wait to be told by other disciplines how to be a nurse. Heyes (2018) and Boyer (2018) remind us that nurses have the knowledge and creativity to develop new and never-before-considered methods of care.

It is imperative to appreciate that nurses complement, but are not subservient to, other healthcare providers, and this perspective develops as one evolves as a nurse. Therefore, nurse educators need to foster leadership in their students, help students integrate leadership as an integral component of their role, and focus as much on the development of leadership skills as on the acquisition of clinical skills. Development of leadership skills must be a part of the student's professional as well as personal journey in life. These skills need to be introduced from birth and reinforced by family, friends, and the community as well as by the individual's school and faculty long before postsecondary education.

LEADERSHIP AS AN INTEGRAL COMPONENT OF EACH NURSE'S ROLE

Nurses are increasingly expected to assume the roles of advocate, teacher, caregiver, disseminator of knowledge, manager, contributor to public health policy development, and leader. Nurses are also expected to be heavily involved in partnering with other nurses and members of other healthcare disciplines to achieve quality patient care. Nurses, therefore, are expected to play a major role in evoking change in healthcare and ensuring their significant role in the restructured care system.

Nurses must acquire principle-centered leadership to be effective in the new healthcare system. Principle-centered leadership involves honoring commitments, cultivating one's own virtues, breaking free from negative habits, being courageous, and having a genuine consideration for others (Covey, 2020). These principles are similar to compasses in that they always point the way and keep us from becoming lost amid conflicting ideas and values. Covey says principles manifest in the form of concepts, standards, values, and teachings that elevate, satisfy, empower, and motivate individuals. Characteristics that exemplify principle-centered leaders include continually learning, having a service orientation, having positive energy, believing in others, leading a balanced life, viewing life as an adventure, being synergistic, and having the ability to self-renew.

Leaders must also possess exceptional communication skills. Nurses, therefore, must be consistent, assertive, and knowledgeable speakers about their role, the state of the healthcare system, and those for whom they care. Likewise, nurses would be more effective leaders if they possessed sophisticated interpersonal relationship skills (e.g., using social media, connecting with staff and managers, and discussing issues in casual situations, such as over coffee) to use with patients, families, communities, other healthcare providers, and the public.

Credibility is another important characteristic that admired leaders possess. Kouzes and Posner (2011) studied people's reasons for respecting, trusting, and being willing to be influenced by others and found the following behaviors as indicative of credibility: supporting, having the courage to do the right thing, challenging, developing and acting as a mentor to others, listening, celebrating good work, following through on commitments, trusting others, empowering others, making time to interact with people, sharing the vision, opening doors, overcoming personal hardships, admitting mistakes, advising others, solving problems creatively, and teaching well. These behaviors reflect the characteristics of a credible, innovative, and transformational leader. The four components that correlated highest with being credible included honesty, competency, inspiration, and being forward looking (Kouzes & Posner, 2011).

Nurses are frequently faced with ethical challenges, and there must be a strong and pervasive culture that supports nurses' ethical decision making. Ethical leaders must actively listen to and invest in their followers to retain exceptionally valuable nurses within the organization. This is critical in the context of the global COVID-19 pandemic, which gave rise to what some economists refer to as "The Great Resignation," during which nurses were leaving healthcare because of unhealthy work environments (Marquardt et al., 2022). Reviewing the American Nurses Association's (2015) *Code of Ethics for Nurses With Interpretive Statements* is a good place to start to understand nurses' ethical code.

Taking a risk to try something new, taking time to dream and imagine how one could make a difference, joining a professional organization and becoming actively involved, and taking courses for personal gain (e.g., public speaking) or to complete a degree or certificate are all activities that nurses should consider as part of their self-renewal. By self-evaluating or using peer evaluation effectively, one can identify strengths and weaknesses, nurture one's strengths, and either work on or work around one's limitations. Nurses also need to become comfortable with trying new things and realizing competency will be achieved. Nurses need to take risks and try something they have never done before if they are interested in a change. For example, just as becoming a per diem employee or cross-trained in another clinical area will expand one's growth, so will taking on a leadership position or participating in a new organizational initiative. Utilizing multiple resources and role models to assist one in developing competency as a leader is critical for transformation of the healthcare system (Brommeyer et al., 2023). As leaders in the healthcare arena today, nurses must embody the qualities discussed in this chapter for nursing services to be accessible to patients, for nurses to be involved in multidisciplinary collaboration, and for nursing care to be identified as the reason for positive and cost-effective patient outcomes. Nurses can and must be leaders.

CONCLUSION

One does not have to be in nursing management to be a true nursing leader; there are unlimited opportunities for nurses to exercise leadership. For many, that may require much self-reflection and reinvention. As Bennis (1993) recommended, "People who cannot reinvent themselves must be content with borrowed postures, second-hand ideas, and fitting-in instead of standing out" (p. 1).

Nurses are increasingly "standing out" and providing leadership as they begin new roles in promoting health in healthcare centers serving people who are experiencing homelessness and in school-based health clinics, and in taking healthcare vans to underserved populations. Nurses are starting satellite outpatient dialysis and chemotherapy centers, cardiac rehabilitation centers, and preoperative learning clinics to assist people in restoring their health. Nurses in acute care areas are developing new nurse-driven protocols; collaborating with other healthcare disciplines in creating critical pathways that focus patient care on meeting outcomes; and participating in teaching stroke awareness, cholesterol lowering, and alternative nonpharmacological programs.

Many nursing leaders are making a difference in patient outcomes and using their leadership to meet their own expectations of self. The profession needs more nurses like this. Some might say that they have true grit, which is the passion and perseverance that help them accomplish their goals (Yeh et al., 2022). Nursing educators must revise curricula to provide students with opportunities to practice leadership as well as clinical roles. Nurse administrators need to create environments that encourage and support open dialogue, peer feedback, innovation, and change. Nurses need to mentor each other and call on the strengths of one another, much like geese who fly in a V formation (Box 6-3). When each nurse sees leadership as an integral component of their professional role, nurses will be able to transform healthcare.

BOX 6-3 Learning Lessons From Geese

Although we may know that geese fly in a V formation, what we may not know is that as each bird flaps its wings, it creates an uplift for the bird following. By flying in formation, the whole flock adds 71% more to the flying range than if each bird flew alone.

A second fact about geese is that when the lead goose gets tired, it moves back into the formation, and another goose flies the point position.

Third, if a goose falls out of the formation, it feels the drag and resistance of trying to fly alone and quickly gets back into formation to take advantage of the power of the bird it follows.

What are the lessons here for leadership? First, leadership must be shared. We all must take our turn doing the work that will help our profession evolve, our organizations grow, and ourselves continue to develop. Second, every member of the group has the potential to "fly the point position" and serve as the leader; we should not limit our expectations of the potential within each of us. Finally, the work we do can stimulate and excite others in our group to also perform better and achieve a level of excellence that was perhaps previously unexpected. There is much we can learn about leaders and leadership from geese. We need only to pay attention and be open to new ideas, perspectives, and possibilities.

CRITICAL THINKING 6-1

1. Describe how you could reinvent yourself, personally and professionally, so as not to merely live the status quo. Using knowledge gained from viewing Edward Tufte's Web site (www.edwardtufte.com/tufte/), design a presentation for your next unit meeting or for a course.

2. How would you describe individuals you think of as leaders? Individuals you do not consider to be leaders? What are some of the differences between these two groups of individuals in terms of courage? Watch Simon Sinek's (2023) video *What Makes a Leader Great?*.

3. How would you describe the image you convey? Look at the way you dress, things you have written, presentations you have made, your participation on committees or in class, and so on. Is this the image you want to convey? If not, what aspects are unsatisfactory to you, and how could you change them? Read *How to Be Successful in Spite of Yourself* by Ann Kaplan (2019). Her book has several exercises on self-empowerment that may be helpful.

4. When you interview for a nursing position, the interviewer may ask you to describe your leadership style. Using the 10 qualities of superior performance (Davis, 2010), describe your leadership or executive practices. (Hint: Do not include democratic, laissez-faire, or any of the traditional leadership styles.) Just expand on how you practice 5 of Davis's 10 qualities of a leader.

5. What can aspiring nurse leaders do to overcome negative stereotypes of nurses and nursing, create a genuinely positive leadership image, and project that image to achieve desired goals? View the TED Talk by Angela Duckworth (2016), *Grit: The Power of Passion and Perseverance,* and practice using some of her strategies.

6. Take some time to reflect on your life—both professionally and personally—and see if you are getting enough time to rest, play, and work. To be the most effective leader who can empower others, it is important for you to have a life of purpose and meaning. Try to align your vision for the future with a happier and healthier you.

References

Abbas, M., & Ali, R. (2023). Transformational versus transactional leadership styles and project success: A meta-analytic review. *European Management Journal, 41*(1), 125–142. https://doi.org/10.1016/j.emj.2021.10.011

American Nurses Association. (2015). *American Nurse Association code of ethics for nurses with interpretive statements.* https://www.nursingworld.org/practice-policy/nursing-excellence/ethics/code-of-ethics-for-nurses/

American Psychological Association. (2022). Gender. *APA Style.* https://apastyle.apa.org/style-grammar-guidelines/bias-free-language/gender

Bass, B. (1985). *Leadership and performance beyond expectations.* Macmillan.

Bennis, W. (1993). *An invented life: Reflections on leadership and change.* Addison-Wesley.

Bennis, W., & Nanus, B. (2003). *Leadership: The strategies for taking charge* (3rd ed.). Harper & Row.

Boyer, P. (2018). *Minds make societies: How cognition explains the world humans create.* Yale University Press.

Boyer, E. J., Reid, R., & Patton, D. (2023). Does gender influence leadership styles? A view from the U.S. nonprofit sector. *Public Organization Review, 23*(4), 1505–1520. https://doi.org/10.1007/s11115-022-00669-y

Brenan, M. (2023). Nurses retain top ethics rating in U.S., but below 2020 high. *Gallup News.* https://news.gallup.com/poll/467804/nurses-retain-top-ethics-rating-below-2020-high.aspx

Brommeyer, M., Whittaker, M., Mackay, M., Ng, F., & Liang, Z. (2023). Building health service management workforce capacity in the era of health informatics and digital health – A scoping review. *International Journal of Medical Informatics, 169,* 104909, https://doi.org/10.1016/j.ijmedinf.2022.104909

Burns, J. (1978). *Leadership.* Harper & Row.

Chapman, G., & White, P. (2019). *The 5 languages of appreciation in the workplace: Empowering organizations by encouraging people.* Northfield.

Coun, M. J. H., Peters, P., Blomme, R. J., & Schaveling, J. (2022) "'To empower or not to empower, that's the question.'" Using an empowerment process approach to explain employees' workplace proactivity. *International Journal of Human Resource Management, 33*(14), 2829–2855. https://doi.org/10.1080/09585192.2021.1879204

Covey, S. (2020). *The 7 habits of highly effective people: 30th anniversary edition.* Simon & Schuster.

Cummings, G. G., Lee, S., Tate, K., Penconek, T., Micaroni, S. P. M., Paananen, T., & Chatterjee, G. E. (2021). The essentials of nursing leadership: A systematic review of factors and educational interventions influencing nursing leadership. *International Journal of Nursing Studies, 115,* 103842, 1–13. https://doi.org/10.1016/J.IJNURSTU.2020.103842

Davis, R. A. (2010). *The intangibles of leadership.* Jossey-Bass.

Dean, B. (2023, November 15). *Social network usage & growth statistics: How many people use social media in 2023?* Backlinko. https://backlinko.com/social-media-users

de Kok, E., Weggelaar, A. M., Reede, C., Schoonhoven, L., & Lalleman, P. (2023). Beyond transformational leadership in nursing: A qualitative study on rebel nurse leadership-as-practice. *Nursing Inquiry, 30*(2), e12525. https://doi.org/10.1111/nin.12525

Demir, O. I., & Duygulu, S. (2022). Relationship between nurses' perception of transformational leadership practices and control over nursing practices. *International Journal of Caring Sciences, 15*(1), 465–475. https://www.internationaljournalofcaringsciences.org/docs/46.pp_456_466-oznur.pdf

Duarte, A. P., Ribeiro, N., Semedo, A. S., & Gomes, D. R. (2021). Authentic leadership and improved individual performance: Affective commitment and individual creativity's sequential mediation. *Frontiers in Psychology, 12.* https://doi.org/10.3389/fpsyg.2021.675749

Duckworth, A. (2013, April). *Grit: The power of passion and perseverance* [Video]. TED Conferences. https://www.ted.com/talks/angela_lee_duckworth_grit_the_power_of_passion_and_perseverance/transcript?language=en

Effron, M. (2018). *8 steps to high performance: Focus on what you can change (ignore the rest).* Harvard Business School Press.

Effron, M., & Ort, M. (2018). *One page talent management.* Harvard Business Review Press.

Fosslien, L., & Duffy, M. W. (2019). *No hard feelings: The secret power of embracing emotions at work.* Portfolio.

Gardner, J. (1990). *On leadership.* Free Press.

Goleman, D. (1998). *Working with emotional intelligence.* Bantam Books.

Goleman, D., Boyatzis, R., & McKee, A. (2016). *Primal leadership: Unleashing the power of emotional intelligence* (10th anniversary ed.). Harvard Business Review Press.

Grossman, S. (2007). Assisting critical care nurses in acquiring leadership skills: Development of a leadership and management competency checklist. *Dimensions of Critical Care Nursing, 26*(2), 57–65.

Hansen, M. (2018). *Great at work: How top performers do less, work better, and achieve more.* Simon & Schuster.

Hennessy, J. (2018). *Leading matters: Lessons from my journey.* Stanford University Press.

Heyes, C. (2018). *Cognitive gadgets: The cultural evolution of thinking.* Harvard University Press.

Ireland, V. A. (2022). Emotional intelligence competencies in the undergraduate nursing curriculum: A descriptive qualitative study. *Nurse Education Today, 119*, 105594. https://doi.org/10.1016/j.nedt.2022.105594

Kaplan, A. (2019). *How to be successful in spite of yourself.* Raincoast Books.

Kolb, D. A. (1984). *Experiential learning: Experiences as the source of learning and development.* Prentice Hall.

Kouzes, J., & Posner, B. (2011). *Credibility: How leaders gain and lose it, why people demand it* (3rd ed.). Jossey-Bass.

Kouzes, J., & Posner, B. (2017). *The leadership challenge: How to keep getting extraordinary things done in organizations* (6th ed.). Jossey-Bass.

Mabona, J. F., van Rooyen, D., & ten Ham-Baloyi, W. (2022). Best practice recommendations for healthy work environments for nurses: An integrative literature review. *Health SA Gesondheid, 27*, 1788. https://doi.org/10.4102/hsag.v27i0.1788

Maddigan, J., Brennan, M., McNaughton, K., White, G., & Snow, N. (2023). The prevalence and predictors of compassion satisfaction, burnout and secondary traumatic stress in registered nurses in an eastern Canadian province: A cross-sectional study. *Canadian Journal of Nursing Research, 55*(4), 425–436. https://doi.org 10.1177/08445621221150297

Marquardt, D. J., Manegold, J., & Brown, L. W. (2022). Integrating relational systems theory with ethical leadership: how ethical leadership relates to employee turnover intentions. *Leadership & Organization Development Journal, 43*(1), 155–179. https://doi.org/10.1108/LODJ-04-2021-0190

Maslow, A. (1970). *Motivation and personality* (2nd ed.). Harper & Row.

Maslow, A. (1998). *Maslow on management.* John Wiley.

Mayfield, M. (2021). Sound and safe: The role of leader motivating language and follower self-leadership in feelings of psychological safety. *Administrative Sciences, 11*(2), 51. https://doi.org/10.3390/admsci11020051

National Academies of Sciences, Engineering, and Medicine. *(2021). The future of nursing 2020–2030: Charting a path to achieve health equity.* The National Academies Press. https://doi.org/10.17226/25982

Oman, D. (2023, March 3). Mindfulness for global public health: Critical analysis and agenda. *Mindfulness.* https://doi.org/10.1007/s12671-023-02089-5

Pianese, T., & Belfiore, P. (2021). Exploring the social networks' use in the healthcare industry: A multi-level analysis. *International Journal of Environmental Research and Public Health, 18*(14), 7295. https://doi.org/10.3390/ijerph18147295

Pink, D. (2018). *When: Scientific secrets of perfect timing.* Penguin Random House.

Richey, K., & Waite, S. (2019). Leadership development for frontline nurse managers promotes innovation and engagement. *Nurse Leader, 17*(1), 37–42.

Shin, E. (2022). An exploratory study on the mediating effect of clinical competence in the relationship between grit and field adaptation in newly graduated nurses. *SAGE Open Nursing, 8*, 23779608221127979. https://doi.org/10.1177/23779608221127979

Sibbald, S. L., Ziegler, B. R., Maskell, R., & Schouten, K. (2021). Implementation of interprofessional team-based care: A cross-case analysis. *Journal of Interprofessional Care, 35*(5), 654–661. https://doi.org/10.1080/13561820.2020.1803228

Sinek, S. (2023, September 14). *What makes a leader great?* [Video]. YouTube. https://youtu.be/NQN4mtTagL0?si=mYmjhTGZ7HjhwTLD

Song, Z., Li, W. D., Jin, X., Ying, J., Zhang, X., Song, Y., Li, H., & Fan, Q. (2022). Genetics, leadership position, and well-being: An investigation with a large-scale GWAS. *Proceedings of the National Academy of Sciences of the United States of America, 119*(12), e2114271119. https://doi.org/10.1073/pnas.2114271119

Tan, S. H. E., & Chin, G. F. (2023). Generational effect on nurses' work values, engagement, and satisfaction in an acute hospital. *BMC Nursing, 22*(1), 88. https://doi.org/10.1186/s12912-023-01256-2

TED. (2011, December 9). *Leadership storytelling | Stephen Denning* [Video]. YouTube. https://www.youtube.com/watch?v=RipHYzhKCuI

Thepna, A., Cochrane, B. B., & Salmon, M. E. (2023). Advancing nursing entrepreneurship in the 21st century. *Journal of Advanced Nursing, 79*(9), 3183–3185. https://doi.org/10.1111/jan.15563

Ulrich, B., Barden, C., Cassidy, L., Varn-Davis, N., & Delgado, S. A. (2022). National nurse work environments—October 2021: A status report. *Critical Care Nurse, 42*(5), 58–70.

Van Dijk, D., Kark, R., Matta, F., & Johnson, R. E. (2021). Collective aspirations: Collective regulatory focus as a mediator between transformational and transactional leadership and team creativity. *Journal of Business and Psychology, 36*(4), 633–658. https://doi.org/10.1007/s10869-020-09692-6

Wang, S., De Pater, I. E., Yi, M., Zhang, Y., & Yang, T.-P. (2022). Empowering leadership: employee-related antecedents and consequences. *Asia Pacific Journal of Management, 39*, 457–481. https://doi.org/10.1007/s10490-020-09734-w

Yeh, Y.-C., Ting, Y.-S., & Chiang, J.-L. (2023). Influences of growth mindset, fixed mindset, grit, and self-determination on self-efficacy in game-based creativity learning. *Journal of Educational Technology & Society, 26*(1), 62–78. https://doi.org/10.30191/ETS.202301_26(1).0005

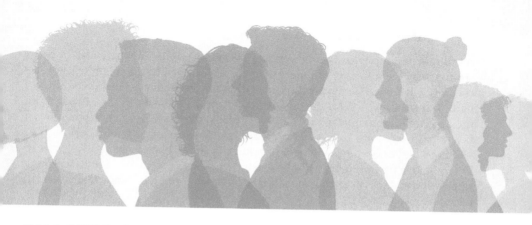

CHAPTER 7

Vision and Creativity

LEARNING OBJECTIVES
- Define the concept of vision as it relates to leadership.
- Describe how a leader or follower can identify, articulate, and communicate a vision.
- Identify strategies that would be effective in making one's personal vision become a reality.
- Formulate a personal vision for the profession or one's particular area of practice.
- Identify characteristics of nursing and non-nursing leaders who are viewed as visionary.
- Describe characteristics of creative persons, processes, and environments.
- Project potential outcomes of using creativity as a nurse leader or follower.
- Examine how incorporating vision and creativity into one's professional role can help vitalize and energize a nurse.

INTRODUCTION

A vital attribute of a leader is possessing a vision for an improved world and thinking on a larger scale, embracing limitless possibilities. Everyday conversations often include terms like *vision, impact, empowerment,* and *facilitation*. It is crucial to go beyond merely saying the words and start taking action to make them integral to everyday practice.

Having a vision and being able to energize followers to join in the effort of making that vision a reality involve credibility, passion, effective communication skills, the ability to maintain momentum, and creativity. Nurses typically are skilled in communication, have high energy levels, and are seen as credible. However, they often do not think of themselves as creative and oftentimes have difficulty sustaining and capitalizing on the momentum of a group. The mere idea of being creative may seem foreign to nurses who are accustomed to following strict protocols for delivering patient care. It is important for the leader to have everyone be a part of creating a vision for the organization (Kouzes & Posner, 2023). In addition, the expectation that nurses have and can articulate a vision also may seem unusual if one has been socialized to expect that only the chief nursing officer (CNO) or vice president or dean has the right or responsibility to have a vision. Being able to incorporate a new philosophy of leadership into one's professional role, accepting responsibility for articulating a vision, and allowing oneself to be creative are all essential.

Leaders do many extraordinary things, but one of their greatest contributions is having a focus or a purpose that emerges from their knowledge and experience, emotional intelligence/competence, and passion. This purpose then guides their actions to engage members of a group to shape a new future. Visionary leadership involves identifying the focus of the organization, department, or group; having a plan that allows the focus to become reality and be sustained; being able to evolve as time goes by; and having an outcome evaluation mechanism that encourages frequent communication among all involved as to whether that focus is to continue or to change.

> *Vision without action is merely a dream. Action without vision passes the time. Vision and action can change the world. —Joel Barker*

Consider the following Case Study about how nurses were able to use their creative abilities and energize themselves and colleagues by following their dream.

Case Study

There was much unhappiness and low morale in the trauma unit where a group of nurses were employed. It was related to strictly enforced role limitations for registered nurses (RNs). Because of the multiple residents rotating through their unit, it was difficult for RNs to gain new skills, communicate with physicians, and collaborate with the intensivists about the challenging cases. The nurse manager was not interested in having an acute care nurse practitioner and constantly blocked any ideas to hire one. The unit was fairly noncollaborative with the physicians. Nurses took orders from the doctors and were not encouraged to discuss their perceptions or share their knowledge about individual patients.

REFLECTION QUESTIONS

1. How is the nurse manager contributing to the low morale, and what specific actions are hindering the unit's growth?
2. What strategies could be employed to overcome resistance and implement positive changes?
3. What potential solutions can be implemented to address the issues of low morale, limited skill development, and lack of collaboration?

THE CONCEPT OF VISION

Leadership is essentially about carrying out a vision and facilitating a group to produce outcomes or deliverables. Of course, the leaders must have meaningful performance, not mediocre performance, and must be successful in promoting staff engagement so that they can continue to propel the staff to follow the organization's vision, or allow for a change in vision, depending on the situation, and accomplish their goals. This type of leadership is needed today in our constantly changing world and is called *authentic leadership*. Giordano-Mulligan and Eckardt (2019) found in their study that authentic leaders are who they are because of their integrity, transparency, and altruism. Additionally, the authors found that these three themes are further characterized by being ethical, self-aware, caring, and able to foster shared decision making, and developing excellent relationships. In some ways, it is being true to their own values that attracts others to work with them and makes them true leaders. Workplace engagement by employees is important in any organization. It facilitates a culture where people strive to follow the vision and further the success of the organization and their own careers. Maylett (2019) studied employee engagement and found that it impacts the bottom line and encourages innovation. Maylett's surveys (n = 32 million) indicate that employee engagement can be learned and measured, referred to as *engagement magic*. Maylett offers the following strategies to accomplish the MAGIC:

M = facilitating **meaning** of the organization's mission and vision
A = **autonomy** in one's position
G = personal and professional **growth**
I = ability to make an **impact**
C = **connecting** with others, including customers and peers

Case studies and examples of how to facilitate the MAGIC and how to attract and retain top-performing employees are discussed in the book *The Employee Experience: How to Attract Talent, Retain Top Performers, and Drive Results* (Maylett & Wride, 2017).

What is vision? A vision is a dream or idea that is "specific enough to provide guidance to people, yet vague enough to encourage initiative and to remain relevant under a variety of conditions" (Kotter, 1990, p. 36). "Based on an understanding of followers' perspectives, leaders need to be able to communicate their own vision to others" (Northouse, 2021, p. 65). A vision for many nurses involves creating a work setting that allows all nurses to develop their leadership potential and collaborate with one another. Creating a culture of innovation in nursing education is a vision for some educators and clinicians; for example, the Ohio State University College of Nursing, Capella University, and the American Nurses Association (ANA) developed a Leadership Institute for Nurses (Ohio State University College of Nursing, 2013) that offers coaching and educational experiences for nurse leaders. Sigma Theta Tau International (2024) has an International Leadership Institute and offers continuing education, self-assessment, mentoring, and a variety of development resources for nurses.

Most educational and clinical leaders realize that the nursing profession needs to have a shared vision for nursing education and practice and to have nurses lead the healthcare team. This echoes the National Academy of Medicine and the Robert Wood Johnson Foundation initiatives on the Future of Nursing (ANA, 2023), which recommend that each nurse, at every level of the profession, be assisted in increasing their ability and skills to do more leading. In 2019, the National Academy of Medicine created a committee to develop recommendations for the nursing profession to improve the health of Americans in the 21st century (https://nam.edu/publications/the-future-of-nursing-2020-2030/). Its report, *The Future of Nursing 2020–2030*, recommends different role functions for the nurse, including serving as change agents and leaders in healthcare.

Indeed, all nurses need more opportunities to practice leadership skills in their educational programs and also during on-the-job training. Nurses can become more involved in health policy changes, formally advocate for their patients' rights, run their professional organizations, initiate change in their unit or department, and mentor colleagues and student nurses. Taking on more responsibilities such as these can assist nurses to become more involved in their organization's mission and to accomplish their own and their agency's vision. It is time for nurses to be more visible in the healthcare delivery system. All nurses must create opportunities instead of waiting for someone else to offer them challenging opportunities.

Kouzes and Posner (2017) report that multiple leaders of large organizations identified vision as a major focus and important for their organization's success. The authors emphasize the importance of creating and maintaining a vision. The authors also ask, If one does not have a vision for the future, why take the lead? A vision overlaps various ideas and values in an organization or group. A vision may begin with an internal orientation and a narrow viewpoint or with an external and broader direction. Either way, it will most likely evolve as more people get involved. For example, developing nurse and unlicensed personnel teams may be a step toward realizing the vision to refocus care to the patient. A nursing unit or clinic may begin by developing or implementing new ways of care delivery by nurses, physicians, and other interdisciplinary staff. As this idea takes hold among all the healthcare providers, word about the positive patient outcomes and cost-effective results of using the new assignment technique spreads to other departments in the organization (e.g., accounting, human resources, staffing). Consumer representatives who had served on the committees to institute the redesign will share the outcomes outside of the hospital, and soon there will be more external community and consumer interest in patient-centered rather than provider-centered care.

DEVELOPING PROFESSIONAL AND PERSONAL VISIONS

One can have both personal and professional visions. Personal vision gives one a purpose in life, and professional vision helps one move work ideas into actions and promote the mission of an organization, group, or profession. Sometimes, it takes a new idea heard from someone else to inspire one to think of "how things could be" before actually investing time to create a personal vision. Too often, one only thinks of career and work life when asked, "What is your vision?"

Developing a Vision

Visions are about hopes, dreams, and aspirations (Kouzes & Posner, 2017). Starting conversations with questions like "What are your professional goals?" or sharing idealistic dreams about work settings can inspire individuals to envision and overcome barriers to realizing their dreams. Reflecting on personal aspirations and recognizing the collaborative potential in projects can lead to innovative ideas that individuals may have yet to consider. Wheatley (2009) supports the use of connector phrases such as the following: "I appreciate how you expressed your goals with illustrations and would enjoy sharing some of my ideas with you" and "Perhaps you could help me illustrate my goals like you did yours" and "My idea about delivery of care seems to be similar to your proposed safety practice regarding patient discharge. Do you think we could combine our ideas and develop a policy for the safety aspect of patient care?" and "I am at a loss for wording to explain my rationale for cost reduction on the IV tubing connectors. Do you think you could assist me in coming up with a procedure so fewer IV tubing connectors would be needed?"

Nurses can improve their practice through reflective techniques, such as reviewing how they managed a particular problem and determining whether they should handle it differently, asking others for feedback on what they perceive would be the best response to a problem and using those ideas, obtaining more information regarding an action they plan to take that will affect other staff and patients, and understanding the importance of taking time to think about ideas and actions in multiple ways.

A vision statement provides a look into the future to create a mental image for others (followers, stakeholders, customers, etc.) of the ideal state the organization desires to achieve. The customer of the product or services being delivered by an organization must be aware of the vision that the agency is following since this vision may be why the customer decides whether to connect with said organization. For example, wouldn't potential patients be more attracted to a healthcare agency that offers the highest quality care with the best access than to one that is open limited days per week and describes their purpose as allowing healthcare students opportunities to gain valuable experience?

Using the Clinical Judgment Measurement Model (National Council of State Boards of Nursing, 2019)—which includes the process of recognizing cues, analyzing cues, prioritizing hypotheses, generating solutions, taking actions, and evaluating outcomes—nurses can learn as much about how to lead just as they can learn about clinical decision making. The Clinical Judgment Measurement Model can be used in developing one's vision in a department, unit, clinic, or professional organization, as well as one's personal vision. During the process of recognizing and analyzing cues, the nurse is continually assessing the situation, gathering data, and identifying patterns of what could be happening or should be happening. By reflecting on their own experiences and observing other effective and noneffective leaders, nurses can compare experiences and know what is occurring. While prioritizing the hypotheses and generating solutions, the leader can prioritize potential issues and what should most likely be included and determine the actual vision.

During the take action step, the nurse can implement the vision, making sure to use effective communication skills and listening to the group's perceptions of what should be included in the vision. Finally, during the evalution of outcomes, the nurse thinks about what went right and what went wrong and makes plans for improving the vision for the future.

The term *co-missioning*, coined by Covey (2004), merges an individual's personal goals and the organization's vision. He describes this process as "the key to unleashing the power of the workforce" (p. 224). Co-missioning is defined as a way of linking mission and vision of a workplace so that there are similarities with the employee's needs. *The 7 Habits of Highly Effective People: 30th Anniversary Edition* (Covey, 2020) emphasizes the importance of taking responsibility for one's life, living with a "carpe diem" mantra, and the need to stop complaining. Covey's (2020) definition of leadership is very clear: Leadership is being able to share others' worth and potential so well that they themselves are inspired.

One must be able to identify opportunities to clarify one's vision and act on incorporating new strategies that will facilitate the implementation of that vision. One also must be cognizant of the potential for barriers that may interfere with the vision becoming a reality. However, in the long run, barriers may assist in mobilizing people to change and accept a new plan or vision. For example, the advanced practice registered nurses (APRNs) at a new nurse-run clinic felt "blocked" by their medical director who insisted that all new prescription orders be cosigned by a physician before the medication could be dispensed. Concurrently, the clinic administrator was negotiating with the director of the adjacent detention center regarding healthcare services needed for inmates. One of the detention center's primary needs was immediate service, including prescriptions for very transient, mobile individuals who might be at the detention center for only 1 to 2 hours per day. A contract with the detention center would generate a large amount of work and a positive community partnership for the clinic; however, this agreement could not be made if the APRNs could not independently dispense medications. The barrier put up by the medical director (e.g., not allowing nurse practitioners to autonomously prescribe new medications) was overturned. The medical director attended a meeting to discuss the role of the APRNs and the state's APRN practice act. This meeting resulted in a better understanding of the APRN role overall and an expanded vision for the nurse practitioner-run clinic, outcomes that never would have been achieved had it not been for facing the barrier regarding autonomous prescription writing.

It is important for each nurse to think positively, speak in possibilities, and not give up. Every nurse must work toward accomplishing an organization's vision and being part of the change initiative in order for a successful outcome to be realized. Evidence suggests that much leadership development of individuals occurs by volunteering to serve on organizational committees, trying a leadership position in one's professional organization, and gradually taking on more responsibility. Additionally, one must be creative when developing a vision because this first vision must be seen as something in process that will evolve into a new vision or expand to include more ideas as time goes by. It seems essential that nurses realize their most promising possibility of accomplishing a vision is to find ways to encourage many people to incorporate some part or parts of this vision into their own trajectory. Individuals want to know that what they are doing can make a profound impact on the lives of their families, friends, colleagues, customers, and communities (Kouzes & Posner, 2017).

Actualizing a Vision

Many leaders have demonstrated the importance of being flexible or being able to accept some unforeseen change in plans to actualize one's vision. Mother Teresa, winner of the Nobel Peace Prize in 1979, founded the Missionaries of Charity in Calcutta, India. She had to make the difficult decision to leave the order of nuns to which she belonged to at the time so she could follow her vision—"helping the poorest of the poor while living among them" (LeJoly, 1983, p. 26). Mother Teresa worked from morning til night, helping the poor and guiding the nuns who joined her to fulfill the vision. She was unsatisfied with her purpose on Earth as a nun in her original order, which felt like the status quo for her, so she took risks, used her creative talent, convinced others, and kept pursuing her dream, even without any funding. Mother Teresa founded a whole new order of sisters, provided exquisite care to the world's poor, and made the world more conscious of the needs of millions of fellow human beings. Such is the power of dreams—of visions.

Kouzes and Posner (2017) describe leaders who can see beyond today's needs and create plans for the future. Nurses can practice consistently with current evidence-based guidelines, and by consistently following guidelines, nurses will be more apt to be prepared for the future. Many (Conger, 1989; Kotter, 2008, 2013) believe that one of a leader's most significant functions is to produce a change that cannot actually be identified as it transpires step by step but is more of a feeling that people grab, attempt to implement, and then share serendipitously! This perspective is most congruent with leadership today, which suggests it would be nonproductive to be too orderly and attempt to implement a vision in a step-by-step fashion because it is unlikely that no change would occur.

Conger (1989) suggested that one positive advantage of having a vision is that it brings people a "sense of contribution to themselves, to an industry or to a society," and "draws workers together as a team" (p. 43). A leader must share and co-create a vision with their followers. A solitary vision not shared by the leader is only daydreaming (Broome & Marshall, 2021). Leaders must recognize followers for their diligent work through an award, public announcement, or financial reimbursement, which may help the followers connect better to the overall vision.

An excellent example of a leader who had a dream, motivated others, and made followers feel as if they owned the dream was Dr. Martin Luther King Jr. His "I Have a Dream" speech, delivered on August 28, 1963, at the Lincoln Memorial in Washington, DC, is a testament to the power of a vision and how it can energize people toward action.

Dr. King's dream was clearly articulated, and the way he conveyed his vision showed his passion and enthusiasm and how they reflected his inner being. Whether a nurse works in administration, education, or a clinical role in schools, homes, hospitals, or clinics—or is a student—there is a reason for choosing a particular area of nursing. That reason may have been to help others, advocate for vulnerable populations, to care for others in need, or develop healthcare programs for all. Perhaps some nurses need to reflect on that original dream and think about how what they are currently doing tends to relate to why they wanted to be a nurse in the first place. It is possible that the motivation to enter nursing is still important and drives the nurse to enjoy their present work, but it also is possible that the nurse is stuck in a "dead end" or a "rut" and feels unfulfilled. For those who get up daily without thinking about why, it may be time for a change; perhaps we need to revitalize ourselves.

By formulating a vision, one can take risks, use creative talents, convince others, and pursue dreams. One can be energized and can make a difference. One may have ideas about how the staffing mix could be more effective, how nurses could better collaborate with healthcare team members, or how technology can be used to better improve patient outcomes. These ideas could be the groundwork for a vision or a dream. Sometimes, an idea that starts out as one person's pet peeve or personal agenda—wireless capabilities in every home or school, helping people with very few resources, or achieving racial equality—can, if communicated effectively, become a group's quest. However one looks at it, one person's dream can empower others to follow or to envision their own separate piece of a larger vision. It seems that people who have dreams want to make a difference and are willing to do whatever it takes to fulfill those dreams. They believe it is better to risk potential chaos or even failure than to accept the status quo. In other words, they are leaders in the fullest sense of the term.

Kouzes and Posner (2017) suggest that potential leaders use the following framework when clarifying a vision (these can apply to your personal or professional visions):

- What needs changing?
- What legacy do you want to leave?
- What is your passion?
- What is the most important part of your life?
- What are your strengths?
- Do you have a role model?
- What is your current vision?
- What are your personal and professional aspirations?
- Do you have a motivating force?
- Do you have one most important part of your work?
- How do people feel about your talents?
- Are you totally focused on any one issue?

For example, a graduate student in nursing decides to apply for a scholarship. The application asks for the usual information about previous work, grade point average, memberships in professional organizations, and so forth. It then requests that applicants share why they should be awarded a scholarship. Using Kouzes and Posner's (2017) framework, this student might focus their application on the following points, emphasizing how obtaining a graduate degree will assist them to grow and make a difference in advocating for healthcare for all. They might describe how their work as a staff nurse led to tangible patient outcomes; note the creative teams of which they were a member or led; describe research with which they assisted and the protocols developed to create improved patient care; articulate clearly their reasons for pursuing the role and for which this particular graduate program will prepare them, specifically relating goals to what they currently do in practice, potential study topics, and what issues in health policy they will be researching that will assist them in accomplishing their goals; and describe how they believe the advanced degree will prepare them to work on their passion, which is health policy. The student then integrates this information into a short vision statement of how this graduate program will prepare them for their ideal job. The student shares insights about the healthcare system and explains how they will make a difference, using examples to maximize viewpoints. The student concludes by writing their goals and expectations upon graduation. Such an application—with a clearly articulated vision—will likely be reviewed positively by the scholarship selection committee as well as serve as a professional guide for this nurse during the graduate program.

WHAT HAPPENS IF THERE IS NO VISION?

When individuals meander without direction in both their professional and personal lives, they often achieve outcomes distinct from those who maintain a clear focus. They may not take advantage of opportunities for professional growth due to a lack of awareness, harbor doubts about their ability to succeed, focus more on short-term goals, or refrain from investing the time and energy needed to succeed.

Manfredi (1995) described what she called the art of legendary leadership by telling a story that depicts what can happen if one does not have a vision: Many years ago, when the long-term mayor of a village passed away, the town elders gathered to select a successor. They asked for volunteers, and after a short time, three candidates were found. There were no job descriptions or selection criteria, so the elders decided to test the candidates' leadership by placing each in charge of the village for 1 month. The most successful candidate would become the mayor. One candidate believed they should keep the village stable and espoused the motto, "No need to grow; support the status quo." The town was so bored, they let this candidate go. The second candidate believed one must create structure to lead effectively, so the candidate developed many rules and regulations to be followed by the people (but not by their leader). Not agreeing with this perspective, the elders had a bonfire and burned all 700 volumes of rules that this candidate had developed. The third candidate believed that leaders know what is best for the people and the villagers cannot be trusted to make decisions or develop ideas, so they made all the decisions and never consulted anyone. After 1 month of such rule, the elders decided this candidate also was not suitable. But what to do? All three candidates were rejected. The elders could not come to an agreement about exactly what the role of a leader should be, so they developed a job description of five functions a leader should be able to do: create visions, climates, conflict, change, and other leaders (p. 62). They finally hired someone who reflected the ideal mayor for their community. Basically, if a person or group does not have a vision, they cannot create a climate for conflict, change, and growth. Without conflict, change, and growth, new leaders will not be able to emerge from the group to inspire further conflict, change, and growth, and the status quo will be perpetuated by the leader who "knows best for the group" and creates many rules and regulations.

Who Should Participate in Vision Development?

Bennis (2009) believed that one can learn how to develop a vision, and Manfredi (1995) made the point that anyone, not just the leader, can initiate an idea that is visionary. In co-creating a vision, everyone needs to integrate their individual goals to create an overall vision for a group or organization. For example, a unit with nurses who are attempting to create more evidence-based protocols, use research-based data, and improve quality of care can form an evidence-based practice committee that meets monthly and an active online communication forum to facilitate participation by all staff in accomplishing the vision of providing evidence-based practice.

Kouzes and Posner (2017) explain that people want to be part of the vision development process and walk alongside their leaders. It is the idea that sparks a vision that is the most significant part of developing a vision, and we all have had creative ideas that have been of great interest to others. Sometimes one individual will express a thought, someone else will add to it, and another person will expand it even further. Soon the entire group is involved in creating the idea. When this happens, change is likely to occur quickly or with minimal barriers. This process can occur when nurses want to develop a new approach to staffing, a philosophy of patient care, or a new nursing-driven protocol. For example, a group of staff nurses is discussing the challenges presented by maintaining the IV lines of patients with hard-to-stick veins. One nurse says how difficult it is to insert a new line every 4 hours, cause discomfort to the patient, and explain to the patient and family repeatedly why a restick is necessary. Another nurse suggests that perhaps nurses should have a voice in determining which patients receive routine IV access and which receive a more invasive line. Someone else then asserts that nurses should insert the peripherally inserted central catheter (PICC) and manage the patients who have these more invasive lines. The entire group then goes on to discuss quality patient care in general. Thus, the idea of providing nurses with more independence regarding IV fluid and medication administration served as the starting point for the even bigger dream of having significantly more nurse-driven protocols so that higher quality, more cost-effective care can be delivered. The nurses who provide direct care are typically most aware of what is best for the patient and what would improve the way care is delivered. Such nurses have ideas, dreams, and visions. Unfortunately, many nurses often feel inadequate to do anything significant about them and wait for administration to solve the problems. A healthier approach is for the leaders in the group to articulate and inspire the vision of a preferred environment and to engage everyone in making that vision a shared reality.

In a classic article on leaders and vision, Zaleznik (1989) suggests two ways to influence people: (1) help them realize that the proposed change will advance their interests and (2) influence them to want to succeed for the group or organization, not just for self-recognition and promotion. Both the leader and the followers, therefore, need to be immersed in the process of formulating the vision and integrating it into the daily work of the group. Throughout this process, the leader needs to be available to followers to help them clarify the vision, see how their efforts contribute to the vision, and be passionate about working toward the vision.

Vision Development Strategies

Positive experiences with trying new innovative ideas, being involved in new opportunities, and being encouraged to take risks will assist with vision development. In 1991, Sarah Weddington, past counsel for *Roe v. Wade*, delivered a keynote address at the National League for Nursing Annual Convention; she shared several ideas on how to gain practice in leading. The major focus of her presentation was that a leader must be passionate about what they do and always strive to accomplish their dream. The dream must be a product of the ideal and what would have the most positive impact on the future (Weddington, 1991). This perspective clarifies that to be effective, a vision must encompass many perspectives and be future oriented. Leaders, therefore, must be proactive and not shy away from challenges or change. Instead, they need to explore different approaches, think in a new way, and have the confidence to encourage others to share the dream.

Cohen (2004) emphasizes the importance of being aware of environmental influences and how it is sometimes necessary to change strategy or components of a plan to fulfill goals. Cohen reminds us that a strategy's success depends on the "judgment and leadership qualities of the individual responsible for the undertaking" (p. vii). He offers 10 essential principles that are helpful when developing and carrying out one's vision:

- Commit fully to a goal: Always invest fully in what you have identified as a goal.
- Seize the initiative and keep it: Grab the opportunity to share your thoughts and maintain the idea's visibility.
- Economize to your resources best: Think twice before spending so you will have enough resources to fill your needs.
- Use strategic positioning: Think carefully about how your new idea or change will affect everyone and how it interacts with every part of the system.
- Do the unexpected: A surprise change (if the change has to occur) is sometimes seen more positively than one that is carefully planned.
- Keep things simple: Following basic policies when introducing a new initiative is always best.
- Prepare multiple, simultaneous alternatives: Allowing participant flexibility will increase buy-in by all.

- Take the indirect route to your objective: Demonstrate how your goal can be accomplished along with several others.
- Practice timing and sequencing: As one says, timing is everything!
- Exploit your success: Be transparent with successful outcomes so that all participants will see the fruits of their efforts.

Cohen's principles provide realistic and relevant steps of strategizing successfully and give ideas on examining one's plan and making changes both midstream and in crises so that a preferred future is the most likely outcome.

One can learn how to communicate a vision in an articulate and persuasive manner. Conger (1989) suggests that the leader use metaphors and analogies to excite others and that the leader stimulate multiple senses (intellect, emotions, values, and imagination) simultaneously. Abraham Lincoln's powerful words in the Gettysburg Address—"government of the people, for the people, and by the people"—had a much greater impact than if he had said, "government of, for, and by the people" (Conger, 1989, p. 169). Franklin Delano Roosevelt tended to use folk imagery to share his ideas with the citizenry, and he used sports analogies in his fireside chats (Conger, 1989, p. 81); both were concepts to which people could easily relate. In a more recent example, the global pop sensation Taylor Swift shares her passion and life experiences through songwriting and music. Her willingness to be vulnerable strikes a chord with her audience and team, making her stand out as an extraordinary leader in a world where many people put on fake personas. In fact, more and more leaders are appreciating the importance of having commitment and passion for work. Robinson (2009) describes reaching one's element or passion in comparison with just reaching the "peak" of one's career or trajectory. Everyone should have their own unique peak, so that over time a bottom-line focus does not take a toll on employees' motivation, loyalty, and performance.

Although some leaders may be inclined to try to convince others with impressive numbers, Conger (1989) suggested brief face-to-face comments as being most substantial in getting people to buy into an idea, pursue a vision, or make a change. Other speech techniques, such as repetition, rhythm, and alliteration, are effective in helping articulate one's vision, as is evident in Dr. Martin Luther King Jr.'s "I Have a Dream" speech. Conger also suggests that one use a loud volume, some body movements, and complete sentences with few pauses between them. It also is helpful to avoid *I think, I guess, please,* and *thank you.* Focusing on the basic message portrays the leader as confident, effective, and someone others would want to follow.

Nurses today are knowledgeable and sophisticated. Therefore, nurse leaders must be able to articulate a clear vision but be open to the team's ideas regarding how the vision can be realized. A framework of skills is needed to be successful and articulate, communicate, and propel a vision. Senge (2006) says that a leader, particularly one in the healthcare arena, must be a systems thinker, have shared visioning, facilitate team learning, and have personal mastery. Champy (1995) agrees with Senge's list of competencies for healthcare leaders and adds the skills of association, collaboration, communication, and mobilizing others, all of which are most important in healthcare. Drucker (1989) reaffirmed these descriptions of a leader when he articulated the skills of envisioning, coaching, knowing technology, and facilitating. All three of these organizational behaviorists agree on the necessity of a leader having and being able to clearly and effectively communicate the dream, the vision.

An analogy serves to summarize these ideas about developing a vision. A sailor returns to port in the middle of a thunderstorm with barely 3 feet of visibility. The best thing the sailor can do is concentrate on the ultimate destination, not on every foot of the sea between the ship and land. This metaphor can describe the journey a group, an organization, or a professional takes to reach a dream. One must constantly look forward, even if it takes a significant amount of time and a great deal of work and energy to get there. To keep on track, the leader must help all team members feel a sense of ownership and be creative throughout the process of moving toward the vision.

CREATIVITY

Nurses must develop foresight and future-thinking leadership skills and advance creative ideas to design innovative 21st-century healthcare systems (Beaudet et al., 2023). Creativity is defined as "the connecting and rearranging of knowledge—in the minds of people who allow themselves to think flexibly—to generate new, often surprising ideas that others judge to be useful" (Plsek, 1997, p. 28). Nurses must reframe how they think about their work so that they are more creative, open to a variety of possibilities, and open to options that might lead to successful outcomes. It is always conceivable that some of our options may not work the way we visualize them, but after observing new methods of providing care and determining they are not feasible, we will discover new options that, with some work and feedback from the team, will be even "better." These new ideas would never have been created if trying different options was not attempted. Creativity "demands intuition, uncertainty, unconventionality, and individual expression" (Conger, 1989, p. 17).

Multiple creativity tests are available online. An example is the Creativity Ability Scale and Activities to Enhance One's Creativity test, developed by Grossman in this text (Fig. 7-1). Most creativity tests include some type of psychometrics on the tool and are free and easily accessible. By taking a creativity screening, one can review what kind of traits are considered creative; perhaps this knowledge will facilitate some individuals to modify their behavior so that they take their time to try to use their creativity and not follow the same routine patterns.

USING CREATIVITY TO MAXIMIZE VISION ACCOMPLISHMENT

Transforming healthcare necessitates nurses to cultivate a forward-thinking approach, harness increased creativity, and broaden innovative perspectives across systems; this is crucial to developing positive changes that advance health (Beaudet et al., 2023). Perhaps nurses need to become more involved in developing outpatient programs, writing grants to obtain funding for healthcare initiatives, creating more flexible staffing schedules based on the unit's and the nurses' needs, developing healthcare policies, serving on political action boards, and any number of other activities that would improve healthcare for people. For nurses to become

CREATIVITY ABILITY SCALE AND ACTIVITIES TO ENHANCE ONE'S CREATIVITY
Part One Pretest Score _____ **Part One Posttest Score** _____
Directions: Take Part One and determine your creativity score using the answer key. This is your Pretest Score. Review Part Two and engage in as many activities as you can over a specific time frame that you have set. If, for example, you set a 1-month time frame, take Part One again after doing the activities in Part Two. This is your Posttest Score. Have you improved your creativity over the last month?

Part One lists statements that are useful in determining a person's perception of their creativity. **Part Two** suggests activities to increase one's creative ability. **Part One:** Answer "SA" to those statements with which you Strongly Agree and "A" to those statements with which you Agree. Answer "D" to those statements with which you Disagree and "SD" to those statements with which you Strongly Disagree. **Part Two:** Put the date you performed an activity.

Part One: Perception of One's Creativity

	STATEMENT	SA	A	D	SD
1	People are born being creative and cannot become creative if they were not born creative.				
2	One can improve one's creative ability by practicing creative activities.				
3	I gain new knowledge about creativity and see potential for increasing my own creativity by interacting with people who think differently from me.				
4	People with a good imagination will be more creative.				
5	Most creative people are artistic and musical and are not good at science and mathematics.				
6	I find that I am very creative and often people mention to me how creative my ideas are.				
7	My presentations are always different and very exciting to audiences.				
8	People who procrastinate and are afraid of failure are most likely not going to be creative.				
9	I feel I am more creative if I am relaxed and in a stress-free environment.				
10	Practicing stress-reducing exercises will relax me and facilitate my creativity.				

Part Two: Activities to Enhance One's Creativity
Dates of Completing Activity _____

	STATEMENT	DATES
1	Becoming more creative is possible, but one should plan to do it over time and in stages. Develop a 1-month plan of how to complete the activities in Part Two.	
2	Practice creative activities.	
3	Interact with diverse people who think differently from me.	
4	Practice using my imagination at work and at home.	
5	Take some classes in something I know little about—this can be anything ranging from painting to astrology.	
6	Set up a 1-hour chat with some friends to analyze how each member of the group will answer a problem. Practice problem-solving and creating solutions to each other's problems.	
7	Ask a few friends to listen to a presentation you are doing at work. Try some new technologies to deliver your presentation. Obtain some critique from your friends on how to be more dynamic and creative with the delivery.	
8	Practice introducing a new and kind of bizarre idea to some coworkers or friends. What is their feedback?	
9	Set up an opportunity to do some out-of-work presentations on topics you are very familiar with so you will not have to do a great amount of preparation for the opportunity.	
10	Take a yoga or meditation class at the gym.	

Continued

FIGURE 7-1 · Creativity Ability Scale and Activities to Enhance One's Creativity test.

Answer Key for Part One
Part One: Perception of One's Creativity

	STATEMENT			
1	People are born being creative and cannot become creative if they were not born creative.			
2	One can improve one's creative ability by practicing creative activities.			
3	I gain new knowledge about creativity and see potential for increasing my own creativity by interacting with people who think differently from me.			
4	People with a good imagination will be more creative.			
5	Most creative people are artistic and musical and are not good at science and mathematics.			
6	I find that I am very creative and often people mention to me how creative my ideas are.			
7	My presentations are always different and very exciting to audiences.			
8	People who procrastinate and are afraid of failure are most likely not going to be creative.			
9	I feel I am more creative if I am relaxed and in a stress-free environment.			
10	Practicing stress-reducing exercises will relax me and facilitate my creativity.			

Very creative = 40
Moderately creative = 20–30
Not very creative = <20

KEEP PRACTICING THE CREATIVITY ACTIVITIES IN PART TWO
AND RETAKE THE CREATIVITY SCALE IN PART ONE LATER.

FIGURE 7-1 · Creativity Ability Scale and Activities to Enhance One's Creativity test.—cont'd

more involved, their leaders will need to inspire creativity and hard work and to challenge the past prologue, recognizing the past is past (Albert et al., 2022).

Reflective practice opens up multidimensional ways of thinking about experiences one has had or will anticipate having. Experts (Bulman & Schutz, 2013; Freshwater et al., 2008) suggest that reflective practice can influence the way one learns and thinks—and perhaps reflective practice can change people's level of creativity and generally improve their leadership ability. By consistently using reflective practice in a consistent fashion, one should be able to use more creative methods of communication and be more successful in making decisions regarding work-related issues, patient care, and even personal ambitions. Schon (1983) found that individuals tend to make decisions based on their experiences more so than on technical rationality. Types of reflective practice have been defined: "reflecting-in-action" means being able to think about what is going on in a situation while in that situation, and "reflecting-on-action" is being able to retrospectively review how one performed in a previous situation. By using reflective practice, individuals can begin to think differently and perhaps in a more creative way. Asking more questions about one's performance, analyzing situations in more depth, applying evidence-based interventions, and conducting more self-evaluation after encounters with colleagues lead to accomplishing the following goals of consistently reflecting on one's practice:

- Focus on increasing one's flexibility and confidence
- Create new ways of delivering health that enhance patient outcomes (Freshwater et al., 2008)

Reflective practice is a result of having more mindful awareness. The underlying neurophysiology behind this process explains that repetitive use of reflective practice techniques will expand emotional circuits in the brain and further develop an individual's prefrontal cortex so one can think in many ways (Siegel, 2007). Those who go on to achieve increased mindfulness will augment their resilience, flexibility, and emotional balance. This will undoubtedly influence their ability to be more creative. The more we can increase our neural circuits with reflective practice, the more neuroplasticity or reorganization of neural pathways occurs (Siegel, 2007). This increased neuroplasticity causes expanded passion and knowledge about our work.

Often, leaders are made, not born, and they accept that the growth process includes making mistakes (Bennis, 2009). This has relevance for the individual nurse who is a leader or an effective follower. It is no longer acceptable for nurses to deal only with the here and now of a specific patient assignment in the clinical setting. Nurse leaders need to partner with the patient and form alliances with family members, friends, community groups, and other healthcare professionals to provide health teaching, promote self-competence for the patient, and gather relevant data to determine whether desired outcomes are being realized. Nurses need to continue changing the belief that what is known is all there is, and how things are done has to be the way things continue to be done. It is important to remember there is no one right answer to most situations. There is no way anyone can plan for all the potential problems that might occur when attempting to institute creative and innovative approaches to reach a vision, and there is no room for an everything-has-to-be-perfect attitude. It makes no sense waiting for everything to be perfect before we act because things will continue to change and some sort of acceptable order will emerge.

As nurses, honing diverse skills is essential for providing comprehensive care and striving to cultivate a balance of analytical and intuitive abilities. This means embracing logical planning and attention to detail while nurturing creativity, intuition, and empathy. Bennis (2009) suggests we become whole-brain thinkers, using both concrete and abstract ideas. For example, the mindmap of creativity (Fig. 7-2) depicts various actions that a creative person uses. Mindmapping is a method of note taking that could be effective in stimulating our creativity, as well as stimulating the flow of ideas. This exercise of illustrating what one reads, sees, or thinks may be helpful in developing the whole brain. For example, a nurse may want to show their colleagues how they can be more creative in care delivery so that they can enjoy an uninterrupted meal during break time. By using Figure 7-2, the nurse can ask each person to write down what they think creative care delivery is. Then, each could describe their ideas to the other team members. This could spark a dynamic discussion, with a creative care delivery model evolving that would be more time efficient.

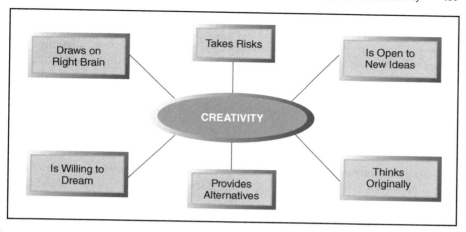

FIGURE 7-2 • Mindmap of creativity.

Nurse educators can assist the profession by designing learning experiences that allow for student creativity and the use of analytical and intuitive abilities. By integrating both sides of our cognitive abilities, we can better adapt to the dynamic challenges of patient care and enhance our effectiveness as healthcare professionals. Also, nurses must focus less energy on and worry less about an unknown future; instead, they should focus more on the opportunities before them today and the possibilities awaiting them tomorrow. Thinking more openly, being more aware of possibilities, and being less structured and more creative will take them a long way.

Case Study, continued

Three nurses in the unit were interested in becoming acute care nurse practitioners so that they could achieve more autonomy in their practice. They were matriculated in the same Doctor of Nursing practice program and were beginning their clinical component. The hospital's policy was that staff should not do their student rotations at their place of employment, if possible, so the students were assigned to the other Level 1 trauma hospital in the city. The three nurse practitioner students observed that the RNs at this other institution had a larger practice scope than the RNs at their original hospital. Because the RNs' role was expanded, their student nurse practitioner role was also expanded and created opportunities for growth that they had never expected. The three students developed and communicated a new vision for their unit with their colleagues, which allowed for an upgrading of the RN role and empowered the RN staff to advocate for changes.

REFLECTION QUESTIONS

4. How might the hospital's policy that discourages staff from doing student rotations at their place of employment influence the professional growth and opportunities for nurses pursuing advanced degrees?
5. How did the three nurse practitioner students develop a new vision for their unit, and what were the key elements of this vision?

In healthcare today, the mergers, affiliations, and partnering are not negatives but rather a natural force—a bringing together of talent, resources, and, one hopes, better patient outcomes. Nurses' ability to be creative and use networking will ultimately allow nurses to thrive. Nurses must foster rethinking, discovery, and curiosity as they support change. This is the new way of thinking about leadership, and nurses must change their way of thinking about their responsibilities. Nurses can support and trust one another and discuss possibilities never thought of before, if they can give up the need to organize every tiny detail, allow themselves to be creative, use their ingenuity, and collaborate with others to maximize creativity.

THE SIGNIFICANCE OF CREATIVITY

Creativity is necessary if nurses are to effectively manage the multitude of changes occurring in healthcare today and that are expected to continue well into the future. *Partnering* continues to be a buzzword that to most nurses means a change in responsibilities or a loss of a job. Perhaps if more nurses thought outside the box, our profession could undergo some serious growth despite the current environment. Being willing to try new things, challenge traditional ways of thinking and behaving, and accept new ways of thinking will broaden our visions. Creativity allows one to accomplish their visions with excitement and enthusiasm. One gets a resurgence of energy when something new and exciting occurs, or when one has an "aha" moment. This energy also comes from change itself, and when that change relates to one's work and what one does, they can experience phenomenal growth. Work, therefore, should not be boring, repetitive, tiring, and frustrating. Instead, it should be and can be energizing, challenging, rewarding, and growth producing.

Nurses have the capacity to use their creative talents to staff units in new ways, research new protocols, administer medications and treatments differently, communicate patient information to other professionals more powerfully, develop materials to market nurses' skills for patients at home, implement support groups for inpatients and outpatients, or build partnerships with clinics or school-based healthcare providers. As new roles emerge and new settings provide opportunities for nurses, there is no need to feel stuck or to be stuck. Nurses are becoming more independent as they practice autonomously and in multiple environments. Today, nurses are vital members of interprofessional teams, willing to do things differently; revising protocols to be more patient oriented; focusing more on measuring patient outcomes; and acting on their concerns about providing quality, cost-effective care. We must be intentional in developing skills to inspire creativity in ourselves and our colleagues. Andiappan and Anih (2022) encourages four team-level interventions (empower employees, adopt a servant leadership model, hire innovators, and schedule a time for innovation) to foster a culture of creativity. These interventions allow the opportunity for individuals and the team to have some autonomy in decision making and the space to offer new innovative ideas. The group culture that develops because of an effective team of nurses working together is a powerful force for success (Coyle, 2018). Nurses need to move away from being reactive and become more proactive and creative both as leaders and problem solvers (Anderson & Adams, 2019).

Zander and Zander (2000) suggest that the way each person sees the world is an indication of whether we see through glasses of scarcity or possibility. If more nurses could use the glass-half-full perspective rather than the glass-half-empty one, they could serve as powerful role models for future nurses. Perhaps nursing courses could build in more shadowing experiences in which students are assigned to work alongside experienced nurses, and these role models could be positive in their thinking, creative in finding new ways to do things, and visionary and goal oriented. All nursing students need more practice leading—it would seem that actually observing an excellent role model would be a most productive growth-producing clinical experience. Additionally, many nurses need to become more independent in their thinking and could benefit from learning how to be more courageous, brave, and daring leaders (Brown, 2018).

McCall (1989) suggests some interesting methods by which leaders can use creative strategies to clarify and achieve their visions. By being "feisty," leaders can deliberately create conflicts to spark new ideas between selected, key people and propel their ideas forward. Creative leaders also are "crafty" in that they are polit-ically astute; know how to increase their power base; and can enlist broad support for creative, different pursuits. If creative leaders are to survive, they must be able to disassociate with failure and associate with success. Being creative puts a leader in a bit of danger because it involves taking risks. Using standards of excellence also characterizes a creative leader because one would have to be very demanding to help everyone involved with the new idea meet the highest, most impeccable standards. McCall (1989) also asserts that a creative leader sometimes must act before thinking, rather than think before acting, and has to be inconsistent so that the leader can keep the system "open" for new ideas and changes.

Finally, creative leaders must use intuition and hunches so that they do not miss a potentially new way to accomplish the vision. Edmondson (2019) offers ideas for providing continuous innovation, effective teaming, and psychological safety in the work setting. He describes strategies for empowering staff, improving engagement, increasing performance, and expanding a creative culture. By using these strategies in any nursing role, it would be difficult to become bored with a job, to burn out, or to feel stuck.

Case Study, continued

The staff, led by the three nurse practitioner students, generated multiple changes and soon had an impact on the culture of the unit to such a degree that the nurse manager transferred to another management position out of the critical care area. One of the students applied and was promoted to the nurse manager position and led the nurses in creating goals, accomplishing them, gaining new skills and responsibilities, creating new acute care nurse practitioner roles, and restruc-turing the unit to become a collaborative practice model. This unit's progress was a result of a team effort, which created a new vision and empowered staff to step up to a new role that eventually involved the entire unit. This is an example of how three nurses' efforts encouraged a whole unit to have ownership in the change process by being energetic, excited, and enthusiastic. They also used what Quibell et al. (2019) described as deep creativity to spark creative spirit and, con-sequently, morale. Components of this model of increasing one's ability to think and act creatively include the following ideas: love, nature, the muse, suffering, practice, the sacred, and art. As the nurses prevailed in leading the unit to a more dynamic and creative culture, the nurses and physicians began to collaborate more, and patient outcomes improved.

Continued

Case Study—cont'd

REFLECTION QUESTIONS

6. How can the positive cultural changes within the unit be sustained over the long term?
7. What lessons can be drawn from this case study for other healthcare units looking to initiate positive cultural changes?

CONCLUSION

There is no doubt that leaders must be passionate about their visions, their dreams of making a significant difference, or bettering the world. It is also crucial that leaders be able to persuade and influence followers to share the vision and become involved in creating change. As Zaleznik (1989) noted, "One cannot be successful without using one's imagination and without being more comfortable with disorder and chaos. In other words, nurses need to avoid the 'If it ain't broke, don't fix it' way of thinking" (p. 62). Change will occur no matter what we do to try to maintain the existing order. If nurses have articulated worthy visions, become comfortable with the notion of creativity, and use creative strategies to achieve their vision, they will thrive from this change, grow personally, and be effective leaders who shape a better world.

CRITICAL THINKING 7-1

1. What is your vision for nursing in general? What is your vision for yourself in your current or future practice setting? What goals do you have for your own growth as a nurse and for the nursing profession? Which of these goals can be achieved by nurses themselves, and which need external support or action? How can you use Wheatley's (2009) conversation starters to assist you in connecting with others to help you accomplish your vision?

2. Think about your current leadership abilities. Read *Better Decisions. Better Thinking. Better Outcomes: How to Go From Mind Full to Mindful Leadership* by Steven Howard (2018). This book will give you advice on how to manage stress and protect your brain.

3. How can you maximize your leadership skills so that you will be able to accomplish your professional goals and increase your impact on the healthcare system? Using reflective practice, describe an example of when you recently succeeded in making a measurable difference in your unit or in the organization.

   - Explain your plan, using at least three objectives, to promote and implement your professional vision.
   - Validate your growth over the past 6 months regarding your leadership skills. Are you where you want to be? How can you facilitate more growth in promoting your vision?
   - Describe your evaluation outcomes for use in determining whether your vision is successful.

   To assist you with this exercise, view Simon Sinek's TED Talk (2009), *How Great Leaders Inspire Action*.

4. Take the Creativity Ability Scale Part One pretest and determine your creativity level (see Fig. 7-1). Practice improving your creativity with activities from Part Two of the scale for about a month and then take the Part One posttest. Has your creativity level improved? If not, consider additional creativity-enriching activities (e.g., attend a nursing conference on creativity).

References

Albert, N., Pappas, S., O'Grady, T., & Malloch, K. (2022). *Quantum leadership: Creating sustainable value in healthcare* (6th ed.). Jones & Bartlett Learning.

American Nurses Association. (2023). *Future of nursing reports: The future of nursing 2020–2030.* https://www.nursingworld.org/practice-policy/iom-future-of-nursing-report/

Anderson, R., & Adams, W. (2019). *Scaling leadership: Building organizational capability and capacity to create outcomes that matter most.* John Wiley & Sons.

Andiappan, M., & Anih, J. (2022). Seven ways to inspire innovation in the health technology industry. *Biomedical Instrumentation & Techology, 56*(1), 1–7.

Beaudet, O., Pesut, D., & Lemberger, O. (2023). The ANA innovation engine: Activating innovation through education and communities of practice. *Online Journal of Issues in Nursing, 28*(2).

Bennis, W. (2009). *On becoming a leader: Leadership classic—Updated and expanded* (4th ed.). Perseus Books.

Broome, M., & Marshall, E. (2021). *Transformational leadership in nursing: From expert clinician to influential leader.* Springer.

Brown, B. (2018). *Dare to lead: Brave world. Tough conversation. Whole hearts.* Random House.

Bulman, C., & Schutz, S. (Eds.). (2013). *Reflective practice in nursing* (5th ed.). John Wiley & Sons.

Champy, J. (1995). *Reengineering management.* Harper Business.

Cohen, W. (2004). *The art of the strategists: 10 essential principles for leading your company to victory.* American Management Associates.

Conger, J. (1989). *The charismatic leader: Behind the mystique of exceptional leadership.* Jossey-Bass.

Covey, S. (2004). *The 8th habit: From effectiveness to greatness.* Free Press.

Covey, S. (2020). *The 7 habits of highly effective people: 30th anniversary edition.* Simon & Schuster.

Coyle, D. (2018). *The cultural code: The secrets of highly successful groups.* Penguin Random House.

Drucker, P. (1989). *The new realities: In government and politics/in economics and business/in society and world view.* HarperCollins.

Edmondson, A. (2019). *The fearless organization: Creating psychological safety in the workplace for learning, innovation, and growth.* John Wiley & Sons.

Freshwater, D., Taylor, B., & Sherwood, G. (2008). *International textbook of reflective practice in nursing.* John Wiley & Sons.

Giordano-Mulligan, M., & Eckhardt, S. (2019). Authentic nurse leadership conceptual framework: Nurses' perception of authentic nurse leader attributes. *Nursing Administrative Quarterly, 43*(2), 164–174.

Howard, S. (2018). *Better decision. Better thinking. Better outcomes: How to go from mind full to mindful leadership.* Caliento Press.

King, M. L., Jr. (1963, August 28). *I have a dream.* American Rhetoric. http://www.americanrhetoric.com/speeches/mlkihaveadream.htm

Kotter, J. (1990). *A force for change.* Free Press.

Kotter, J. (2008). *A sense of urgency.* Harvard Business Press.

Kotter, J. (2013). *Management is still not leadership.* Harvard Business Press.

Kouzes, J., & Posner, B. (2023). *The leadership challenge: How to make extraordinary things happen in organizations.* Jossey-Bass.

LeJoly, E. (1983). *Mother Teresa of Calcutta.* Harper & Row.

Manfredi, C. (1995). The art of legendary leadership: Lessons for new and aspiring leaders. *Nursing Leadership Forum, 1*(2), 62–64.

Maylett, T. (2019). *Engagement magic—5 keys for engaging people, leaders and organizations* (2nd ed.). Greenleaf Book Group Press.

Maylett, T., & Wride, M. (2017). *The employee experience: How to attract talent, retain top performers, and drive results.* John Wiley & Sons.

McCall, M. (1989). Conjecturing about creative leaders. In W. E. Rosenbach & R. L. Taylor (Eds.), *Contemporary issues in leadership* (2nd ed., pp. 111–120). Westview Press.

National Council of State Boards of Nursing. (2019, Spring). Clinical judgment measurement model and action mode. *Next Generation NCLEX News.* https://www.ncsbn.org/public-files/NGN_Spring19_ENG_29Aug2019.pdf

Northouse, P. (2021). *Leadership: Theory & practice* (9th ed.). SAGE.

Ohio State University College of Nursing. (2013, June 27). *ANA, Ohio State launch leadership institute.* https://nursing.osu.edu/news/2019/12/10/ana-ohio-state-launch-leadership-institute

Plsek, P. (1997). *Creativity, innovation, and quality.* American Society for Quality Press.

Quibell, D., Selig, J., & Slattery, D. (2019). *Deep creativity: Seven ways to spark up creative spirit.* Shambhala.

Robinson, K. (2009). *The element: How finding your passion changes everything.* Penguin Group.

Schon, D. (1983). *The reflective practitioner: How practitioners think in action.* Basic Books.

Senge, P. (2006). *The fifth discipline: The art and practice of the learning organization* (2nd ed.). Doubleday Currency.

Siegel, D. (2007). *The mindful brain.* W. W. Norton.

Sigma Theta Tau International. (2024). *Sigma Academies.* https://www.sigmanursing.org/learn-grow/sigma-academies

Sinek, S. (2009, September). *How great leaders inspire action* [Video]. TED Conferences. https://www.ted.com/talks/simon_sinek_how_great_leaders_inspire_action/discussion

Weddington, S. (1991, June). *Leaders are made not born* [Novello Lecture]. Presented at the National League for Nursing Convention. Nashville, TN, United States.

Wheatley, M. (2009). *Turning to one another: Simple conversations to restore hope to the future* (2nd ed.). Berrett-Koehler.

Zaleznik, A. (1989). Why managers lack vision. *Business Month, 8,* 59–64.

Zander, R., & Zander, B. (2000). *The art of possibility.* Harvard Business School Press.

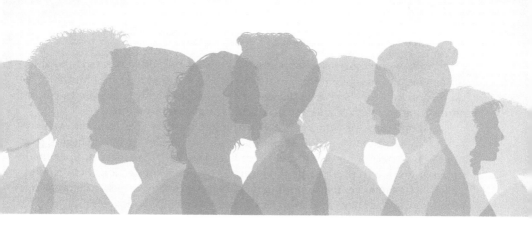

CHAPTER 8

Shaping the Desired Future for Nursing

INTRODUCTION

Nurses continue to be the largest healthcare workforce, with 5.2 million registered nurses (RNs) and 89% employed in the United States (American Association of Colleges of Nursing [AACN], 2024). With these numbers, nurses have the potential to be a powerful force in envisioning and shaping a preferred future. In fact, the government predicts that more than 203,000 new RN positions will be created each year from 2021 to 2031 (AACN, 2024). Leaders in nursing have the responsibility to prepare today for tomorrow's challenges. Although nurses must be fully aware of the past so that they can learn from it and be fully aware of their present so that they can thrive in it, it is perhaps most critical that they have some sense of the future so they can plan and shape it to their desired future. Leaders are responsible—through their vision, creativity, ability to facilitate change, and ability to manage and navigate uncertain times—for articulating a desired future for the profession and for those who engage in its practice, whether they are in clinical, administrative, educational, research, health policy, or other roles.

Contemplating the future is not something to postpone. As John Maxwell says, as leaders, we need to see more than others, and we need to see before others; planning is predetermining tomorrow's results today (2019). Leaders in the nursing profession can effectively shape the future by fostering connections between individuals who empower them, shifting their focus from routine tasks to embracing a broader purpose. They can do this by taking on several different roles:

- **Leaders as integrators:** Leaders must see beyond the differences of various groups or team members and seek synergy to use divergent talents and perspectives to benefit the group.
- **Leaders as diplomats:** Leaders must help people overcome their conflicts and facilitate their collaboration.
- **Leaders as motivators:** Leaders must bring out the best in each group or individual and allow those attributes to be shared with the entire team.
- **Leaders as emotionally intelligent thinkers:** Leaders must be creative and open to new possibilities that have not been previously conceptualized.

In essence, leaders foster collaboration among individuals, develop far-reaching networks among multiple interprofessional groups, and keep lines of communication open among all group members to best secure goals with the available resources. There is a continued need to improve interprofessional collaboration in healthcare to maximize patient outcomes and also to increase the providers' morale. The bundling of treatments for specific diseases and patient-care problems is already decreasing healthcare delivery costs and improving care. Continuous improvement of pathways for a variety of frequently occurring problems is being implemented to prevent negative patient outcomes. For example, at one hospital, nurse practitioners started a mandatory post-hospitalization clinic visit for all hospitalized heart failure patients. They found that if the patients made a clinic visit within 7 to 14 days post-discharge (setting up an appointment prior to discharge), patients followed the discharge orders (e.g., medication compliance, adherence to diet, modified exercise). They had better outcomes (e.g., fewer rehospitalizations, no additional weight gain, less shortness of breath, less fatigue) than if they did not have a clinic visit within 7 to 14 days (Waters & Giblin, 2019). Nurse leaders may find a post-discharge clinic visit would benefit many patients.

Rosen et al. (2019) explain that the coordination and delivery of safe, high-quality care demands reliable teamwork and collaboration within and across organizational, disciplinary, technical, and cultural boundaries (p. 433). Recognizing the importance of organizational adaptability, it is crucial to be more dynamic and allow for flexibility between various care environments rather than solely focusing on the individual employees. Multiple similarities in the care environments would benefit collaboration; employees can be cross trained to work in various care environments.

An orientation toward the future involves having an idea of societal trends and awareness of the social, political, economic, technological, and organizational forces that create, influence, or are influenced by those trends. Certainly, anyone would agree that it is very difficult to predict how these forces will transpire. With the continuing upheaval of governments in many countries in the world, the ever-changing nature of healthcare in the United States and globally, and the volatile international economic markets, it seems that much of the future is difficult to imagine, let alone attempt to predict. It is, however, imperative that the nursing profession be included in the group charged with making predictions and decisions about healthcare and policy.

The nursing profession needs to be a leader in providing ideas and creative solutions so that healthcare reform will evolve successfully. Leaders, however, cannot shape the future alone; they must engage others to achieve this goal. In Miami, Florida, at Nicklaus Children's Hospital, nurses are working with the hospital healthcare system's venture capital group to identify innovative solutions for everyday clinical problems. The nurses are closely involved in this arm of the healthcare system since they identify the problem, offer solutions, test the solutions, and evaluate the solutions in their "living laboratory"—the hospital (Lopez et al., 2019). More nurses can get involved in this type of business or start their own entrepreneurial business because they are spending extensive amounts of time with the patients (at the bedside in the hospital, in the home, long-term care facility, etc.) and are most knowledgeable of patient needs. Nurses could obtain financial backing and advice from a financial consultant. They can sell their product/process to other healthcare systems and disseminate their ideas to a wider audience. Nursing leaders and followers must analyze scientific, technological, and healthcare trends and identify innovative strategies to maximize the nurse's role in leading change in healthcare delivery.

It is time for each nurse to get involved and make a difference in their practice area and in the profession as a whole, engaging in more reflective practice, which will (hopefully) improve morale and increase quality of care, as well as increase measurements such as patient satisfaction scores to reflect positively on nurses. This, in turn, will assist nurses to have the confidence and voice necessary to lead change initiatives in healthcare reform. For example, the patient satisfaction survey assessment scores are a meaningful benchmark for institutions to use to market their successes. These outcome measurements are also significant for a successful Magnet application, which recognizes nursing's contributions and provides a reason for senior leadership to assess how nursing contributes to the overall reputation of the healthcare system. Nurses must use their emotional competence, critical thinking, negotiating skills, and vision to co-create a desired future. One study measured the unit nursing leader's characteristics, the work environment, and their relationship to the frequency of patients' adverse events. Researchers used the Leadership Influence over Professional Practice Environments Scale and the Hospital Consumer Assessment of Healthcare Providers and Systems to collect data. Results showed fewer adverse events with a strong leader and work culture than with a leader who had fewer leadership characteristics (Adams et al., 2018).

An example of leading excellence with evidence-based research in healthcare is the Magnet Model—Creating a Magnet Culture. developed by the American Nurses Credentialing Center (American Nurses Credentialing Center, 2023), which includes five model components:

1. **Transformational leadership:** Leaders must reshape their organization's core values, beliefs, and behaviors. While guiding individuals toward desired destinations may be straightforward, a transformational leader must steer them toward where they must be to address tomorrow's challenges.
2. **Structural empowerment:** Strong professional practice flourishes where the mission, vision, and values come to life to achieve the outcomes believed to be important to the organization.
3. **Exemplary professional practice:** This involves a thorough grasp of nursing's role; its implementation with patients, families, communities, and the interprofessional team; and the integration of evidence-based knowledge.
4. **New knowledge, innovations, and improvements:** This is the redesigning and redefining of current systems and practices to be successful in the future.
5. **Empirical quality results:** These are the results and outcomes to be obtained once the initial four components are established.

> *There is only one direction for a leader: FORWARD.* —Advertisement

Consider the following Case Study that illustrates how nurse practitioners made significant differences in their practice setting.

Case Study

At a student health clinic, nurses are continuously improving their practice by implementing new initiatives. The clinic provides primary healthcare services, counseling, and wellness education. Recently, the clinic has encountered a significant increase in the number of students seeking medical assistance, leading to longer wait times and difficulty triaging concerns effectively. Upon discussion, they are considering implementing a chatbot system to assist with initial call triage and provide basic health information to students.

REFLECTION QUESTIONS

1. How can the clinic ensure that the chatbot addresses the most common health concerns of the student population?
2. What potential challenges might arise during the integration of the chatbot with the existing health information system?
3. What strategies can be implemented to encourage students to use the chatbot rather than calling the clinic directly?

ANTICIPATING, PREPARING FOR, AND SHAPING THE FUTURE

When listening to someone talk about things they expect to see in the future, it is often difficult not to chuckle and dismiss the ideas. Ideas that sounded like science fiction years ago—mobile apps for anything, ambient furniture, interplanetary Internet, neurotechnology, human brain emulations, virtual animals with digital minds, geoengineering techniques to reverse carbon emissions, anti-aging rejuvenation therapies, laboratory-grown organs to transplant into humans, three-dimensional (3D) mapping capabilities, exponential technologies, artificial intelligence (AI), and intelligence augmentation procedures are very real in today's world. Mike Walsh (2019) explains that we must reinvent ourselves and stay ahead of technology. He offered guiding points to help us with our transformation for the future, and the principles correlate well in guiding nurses in any situation. Walsh calls them his 10 principles to try to achieve success in an algorithmic world:

1. Imagine the future and work backward, not forward, toward the future.
2. Maximize growth in every sector continuously.
3. Strategize like a computer.
4. Try to be less wrong but do not strive to be always right,
5. Be human.
6. Engage all and insist on their input for decisions.
7. Foster reinvention of everyone—you cannot always get the best results.
8. Always look beyond the answer and think about what else it could be.
9. Obtain fresh ideas and opinions.
10. Attempt to accomplish the purpose with profit as a lower priority.

Nurses are constantly creating solutions to everyday problems, and these nurse-identified solutions are, in fact, part of the future. Nurses can do trendspotting or forecasting while caring for patients, such as identifying the most effective method for teaching patients how to test their blood sugar, do a specific exercise, self-administer a subcutaneous medication, or operate an IV pump. Just by analyzing how the various patients perform these tasks, the nurse can develop an easy-to-use protocol for any of these interventions that will work to save time, increase patient compliance, and be more effective than just letting patients muddle through coping with their health interventions. These findings can be published and disseminated to assist other healthcare professionals with their clinical patient teaching and thus help nurses and patients both now and in the future.

In healthcare, multiple trends are shaping a new future: virtual healthcare assistants, 3D printing for organs, insurance or healthcare payment reform related to patient indicators, convergence of mental and physical healthcare delivery, improved team handoff communication, and lower healthcare costs. Nursing leaders need to be aware of these trends so that the profession will be influenced positively and be a leading force in creating the future of healthcare, not merely reacting and adapting to those changes. Nurses need to seek and develop new leadership skills that include identifying workplace issues, educating teams to collaborate and respect others, and creating continuous evidence-based practice initiatives. The aims of such efforts are as follows:

- Execute the innovative unit, staff, department, and patient initiatives.
- Increase the use of social media networks to connect with patients, families, the community, new staff, and the entire healthcare team.
- Improve the work environment, decrease workplace violence, and decrease the potential for patient safety threats.
- Embrace technology and create work projects utilizing AI.
- Set the highest possible expectations and vision for the unit, department, or practice.

Kouzes and Posner (2023) recommend that nurses think of the future as a time for great possibilities and that, in most instances, things will improve. These authors found that terms such as *foresight, focus, forecasts, future scenarios, perspectives*, and *points of view* are common in discussions of visions of the future among leaders. It is important, however, that leaders and some followers be able to translate these terms into detailed descriptors as much as possible when sharing the vision so that the team can better understand what the vision represents and more fully participate in making it a reality.

There are methods that futurists use to try to determine future happenings. Leaders must know a particular area well and continue to study it, understand how certain occurrences in this area developed and evolved, and be knowledgeable about how patterns of related happenings might affect the area currently and in the future. This kind of information will assist the leader in knowing how and where to notice trends and determine whether they are indicators of future patterns. What does this mean for nurses? Certainly, the profession is moving forward in leaps and bounds, as evidenced by a significant patient impact made by nurses in all areas of practice, and this trend seems to be growing. Additionally, the National Institute for Nursing Research (NINR) reports that nursing science continues to make significant contributions to patient care and will continue to address health equity, social determinants of health, population and community health, prevention and health promotion, and systems and models of care (2024).

Futurists recommend that leaders read what is new and predicted for the future, review the histories of significant developments, maintain a global perspective on new issues and economic growth, and review information from sources like the U.S. Census Bureau and U.S. Bureau of Labor Statistics. Every individual and every profession or group needs some context within which successful plans for the future can be made, and resources such as these help a leader create that context. Small groups of nurses can create various scenarios to increase their ability to visualize future possibilities and strategize how they can create the future they desire for nursing. This might occur in a retreat setting where nurses engage in strategic vision planning, or it can begin at staff meetings or during intentional discussions over coffee.

By analyzing changes in societal values, public policies, and individual behaviors that are significant to the future of health, rather than dwelling merely on medical breakthroughs, nurses can significantly influence the general welfare of humanity. For example, if society does not improve social determinants of health, which are related to illness, for all people, more people will use hospital emergency departments for their basic health needs, thereby increasing costs; less emphasis will be placed on health promotion and disease prevention; and the populations with the least resources will be likely to have more illness complications. If nurses become involved in developing health policy that mandates health promotion for people who are uninsured, whose incomes are below the federal poverty threshold, or who have gaps in health literacy, the long-term health of such populations will likely improve dramatically.

Nurses can make strong contributions to improving healthcare in multiple areas and can significantly change the quality of life for many, as well as enhance cost savings. The following strategies can be effective in meeting such goals:

- Informing and educating the public
- Advocating for adjustments in healthcare policies
- Offering wellness and holistic care to everyone, especially those in need
- Establishing nurse-led programs and initiatives to enhance quality outcomes and foster patient-centered healthcare

Most nurses would probably agree that the preferred future depicts a healthier, more educated population. Health promotion will reign, and wellness-focused health centers will populate the country and outnumber disease-management clinics. Nurses, as leaders of health, must propel their visions forward and begin thinking in a future-forward frame of mind so that they can have more input into how the future will transpire. Nurses in every aspect of care have the power, for example, to spearhead a massive campaign by educating all people and empowering them to make healthy choices. Who better than nurses to teach the population how to manage health, prevent illness, reduce complications of illness, and choose health resources?

In addition to nurses understanding how health promotion and education impact the future, they must also acknowledge the unknown. The science of leadership makes us more open to the unknown becoming a reality and to accepting that the future holds endless possibilities for us. Despite this unpredictability, however, the nursing profession must attempt to shape the future by creating a workforce that is agile, diverse, sustainable, talented, and able to collaborate with other healthcare professionals and succeed (Canton, 2019). Canton recommends that organizations change their organizational culture and vision to align more with new talent, new ideas, or both and not do the opposite of having employees totally adapt the company's vision and culture. Most importantly, the vision and culture should be dynamic and able to change or, at least be modified, as time evolves.

A desired future does not just happen. We dream about it and shape it to some extent every day. Whenever a change is proposed, no matter how small, it influences the future and can contribute to the growth of the organization or profession. Change of any type ultimately will have ramifications for any number of people.

An example from clinical practice may help illustrate this notion of interdependence and how a change can have a ripple effect. A nurse practitioner in the primary care clinic recommended to the medical director after seeing so much noncompliance from patients not having their blood work done before their appointments that they should change to having a hemoglobin A1C (HbA1C) along with fingerstick glucose obtained a few minutes before the patient's visit with the primary care provider. The medical director had the advanced practice registered nurse (APRN) provide a rationale for the proposed change at the next clinic monthly meeting for all staff. Everyone agreed it was worth piloting this new process because it would improve how the providers could manage the care of patients with diabetes. Outcome evaluation 6 months later proved that the new process was assisting providers in being able to care for their patients with diabetes, and the patients stated that they understood what the HbA1C and fingerstick results indicated now that they had the immediate results and an estimate from the past 3 months. The new blood draw process was instituted throughout the clinics, and findings were published in a diabetic management journal. This is an example of how one idea, tested by one nurse practitioner, then acted on and followed through by other providers, can generate a significant difference for patients and have a positive impact on both patient outcomes and costs.

Nurses are currently in an opportune position, and each nurse needs to propel themself further so that the profession will be a strong contributor to the healthcare system. Additionally, making local, regional, national, and international partnerships between universities and healthcare institutions is essential, and must be established as a priority during resource allocation. The nursing profession needs to network with nurses and healthcare workers globally. Withers et al. (2019) offer advice on how globalization is changing higher education in their seminal report, "Establishing Competencies for a Global Health Workforce: Recommendations From the Association of Pacific Rim Universities." The report covers competencies (e.g., knowledge of issues, cultural awareness, identification of global diseases, international governance structures, diplomacy, leadership, ethics, human rights, and project management) for the majority of healthcare professionals. Not only can the profession gain an exponential number of ideas for improving nursing/healthcare provider education, but it can also garner innovative ways to reshape the world by using culture- and country-specific healthcare delivery with the opportunity to connect electronically for global access to patients.

GENERAL PREDICTIONS

It is difficult not to be slightly pessimistic when considering some of the current issues and predictions about the future: climate change and ecological deterioration, nuclear and biological warfare, terrorism, cybersecurity attacks, AI, increased violence, economic demise, and infectious diseases that are resistant to antibiotic therapy. Such challenges and predictions, however, also can serve to challenge us to plan proactively to minimize these possibilities and their negative effects. Challenges can promote enthusiasm for countering negative trends, for example, by developing super-antibiotics and gene therapies, connecting to space exploration, increasing the quality of life and life span, benefiting from the ability to map all the genes in human DNA, strengthening the total world infrastructure, and using solar power and other renewable energy sources.

Continued advancements in consumer electronics will facilitate greater communication, easier access to services, remote jobs, less traveling time, global travel, space travel, increased leisure time, and new education avenues. These changes will impact global communication, influence how people interact with one another and spend their time, and possibly assist people in living a more productive life.

In addition to infrastructure changes, dramatic changes in family structures and population demographics will continue to occur. The family unit is undergoing great change. There are more single-parent families, grandparent families, and blended families than ever before. The total U.S. population stands at approximately 339,665,118. About 18.15% are younger than 14 years, 63.72% are between the ages of 15 and 64 years. and 18.12% are older than 65 years. Currently, the median age in the United States is 38.5 years, and the life expectancy is 78.5 years for men and 82.9 years for women. It is accurate to say a large portion of the healthcare business is and will continue to be caring for older adults (Central Intelligence Agency [CIA], 2023). The United States is not growing in population the way many other countries are growing. There will be fewer young people, and the United States will have less of a voice regarding global issues.

With more older adults and a lower percentage of young people, the United States may focus more on issues affecting seniors over those impacting the young. If this shift happens, nurses could contribute to it in the following ways:

- Spearheading programs to support older adults in living independently.
- Advocating for insurance coverage for self-care and encouraging seniors to take charge of their health.
- Organizing volunteer opportunities, mentorship programs, and part-time jobs for seniors to stay active in their communities.
- Creating healthcare policies tailored to safeguard the rights of older adults when it comes to their health.

Although general predictions are made and prepared for, one can never fully prepare for the future. This requires the leader to be proactive in leading and co-creating a shared vision for the future, knowing changes will be made along the way.

Case Study, continued

The student health clinic implemented the chatbot system. The pilot of the chatbot system initially presented challenges regarding the technology's use in relaying messages and streamlining student concerns. The nurses promptly contacted the vendor and inquired about additional training to ensure proper use of the technology.

REFLECTION QUESTIONS

4. What training will the nursing staff need to effectively use the chatbot and integrate it into their workflow?
5. How could the clinic support nursing staff during the transition period and during the challenges related to the implementation?

PREDICTIONS ABOUT THE FUTURE OF HEALTHCARE

Between 2018 and 2027, national healthcare spending is predicted to increase at a rate of 5.5% per year, reaching $6 trillion (Centers for Medicare & Medicaid Services [CMS], 2024). Healthcare costs in the United States are predicted to consume about 19.4% of the gross domestic product (GDP) in 2027, which will be a 0.8% faster growth than the GDP (CMS, 2024).

In 2010, the Affordable Care Act (ACA) was passed, which allowed 32 million Americans to obtain health insurance who had previously never been able to afford it. The purposes of the ACA were to increase patient access to healthcare, increase quality of care, and decrease the expense of healthcare. While this healthcare reform provided some improvements in access to care, the debate about how to reform the healthcare system effectively is ongoing. Options range from national health insurance for all to continued revisions of Medicare and Medicaid for the future. Nurses need to lead with health policy changes that transform how healthcare is delivered and how it could be improved in their communities.

Many governmental and corporate organizations are importing their members' drug prescriptions and imaging interpretations from other countries to attempt to decrease costs. Some individuals even have surgeries outside the United States to save costs. Outsourcing to cheaper healthcare resources will be expanding, as will workforce-centered care that offers employer-based on-site healthcare, which may decrease or eliminate the role of third-party insurance markets.

Value-based healthcare is a framework for identifying the goal of value for patients; healthcare organizations are focusing their attention and resources on measuring and marketing their patient outcomes and costs, which equals value-based care. The American Nurses Association (ANA) offers various resources—such as the toolkit *Guidelines to Prevent Catheter-Associated Urinary Tract Infections*—on their Web site (2024). The ANA Web site provides multiple quality guidelines to assist nurses and evidence-based data to support the guidelines. Monitoring nursing-sensitive quality indicators in acute care settings and home care has been a long-standing practice, contributing significantly to nursing's leadership role in healthcare. The focus on delivering high-quality services at reasonable costs yields the following advantages in today's landscape:

- Enhanced consumer awareness and education
- Accreditation and certification of healthcare professionals
- Expanded options of healthcare providers (e.g., nurse practitioner, nurse anesthetist, nurse midwife, physician assistant, and physician)
- Facilitated interprofessional collaboration through advanced technology
- Strengthened healthcare partnerships
- Increased autonomy for nurses and other nonphysician providers
- Expansion of telehealth and telemedicine
- Establishment of outcome-driven, cost-effective healthcare systems
- Enhanced care outcomes for patients, families, and communities

The emphasis on quality, cost, and the measurement of outcomes requires that all healthcare professionals be accountable and responsible for providing competent interventions that generate positive patient and population-based outcomes. The Hospital Value-Based Purchasing Program (VBP) under Section 1886 (o) of the Social Security Act measures several indicators that are used to evaluate quality healthcare, such as clinical care efficiency, safety, costs, and patient experience (CMS, 2024). Nurse leaders can use the annually collected data along with other quality indicators to identify problems/challenges and create new solutions to prevent recurrence.

Currently, and as we move further into the future, healthcare will focus increasingly on the prevention of illness and the promotion of health. More care will be provided in short-stay units, urgent-care centers, subacute facilities, work sites, schools, and homes. Healthcare has moved from independent, freestanding agencies to integrated networks that focus not only on primary or tertiary care but also on the entire continuum of healthcare delivery. It is expected that all healthcare agencies will continue to develop affiliations with other hospitals, home-care agencies, rehabilitation centers, detoxification clinics, subacute care facilities, community centers, long-term care facilities, retail store clinics, workplace clinics, schools, and laboratories, as well as satellite centers in the community, to provide primary and secondary care.

Advances in mobile medical devices and diagnostics development are becoming increasingly available, and results are readily accessible for patients and healthcare providers. Medications such as anti-aging antidotes, ribonucleic acid–based therapy, prediabetes medications, vaccines, anti-obesity remedies, and gene therapy are being developed and continuously improved. These advancements are important, and nurses must be involved in advancing healthcare and how it directly impacts patient care. AI will continue to impact the world with big data analytics, robotics, and different teaching/learning deliveries (Sahota & Ashley, 2019). Robotic surgery and telemedicine will continue to become a more frequently used invasive technique in most diagnostics, interventions, and surgeries.

PREDICTIONS ABOUT THE FUTURE OF NURSING

The expanding role of the RN and the APRN, value-based care, and post-COVID-19 implications are the most significant issues facing nursing now and in the future. Employment of RNs and APRNs is expected to grow as the older, baby boomer RNs continue to retire and more healthcare is administered by nurses. Additionally, with a shortage of 124,000 primary care and specialty physicians predicted for 2034, APRNs will have to become more autonomous in states where they do not have full practice privileges (Association of American Medical Colleges, 2021). Employment for RNs is expected to grow by 6% from 2022 to 2032 (U.S. Bureau of Labor Statistics, 2024). In 2022, 59% of nurses were employed in hospitals, 18% were employed in ambulatory care services, 6% worked in long-term care facilities, 5% worked in government, and 3% worked in educational services (U.S. Bureau of Labor Statistics, 2024). In March 2022, the American Nurses Foundation and the ANA released the results of its COVID-19 Impact Assessment Survey, which found that 52% of nurses were considering leaving their current position due primarily to insufficient staffing, work negatively affecting health and well-being, and inability to deliver quality care. In addition, 60% of acute care nurses reported feeling burnt out, and 75% reported feeling stressed, frustrated, and exhausted (American Association of Colleges of Nursing, 2024).

Many elements of the chaos in healthcare, such as the provider shortage, consolidating healthcare institutions and agencies, the value-based care paradigm, and the global pandemic all have had an impact on nursing. In addition, many demographic changes, such as the increasing population of older adults, single-parent families, people who experience homelessness, immigrants, refugees, and people with few resources needing healthcare in their communities, provide increased opportunities for delivering care outside the hospital. To meet the ongoing challenges posed by the pandemic and shifting patient demographics, the healthcare system will require additional nurses in fields like telehealth, home healthcare, long-term care, rehabilitation, and outpatient care centers (ANA, 2024).

The nursing workforce needs more nurses who practice autonomously, use evidence-based nursing interventions that generate positive patient outcomes, implement quality improvement initiatives, provide input on the development of health policy, and participate fully in interprofessional healthcare teams. To create a desired future for nurses, they must be responsible for identifying problems, implementing solutions, and seeing them through to a positive patient outcome. The future of the profession depends on nurses following through, taking responsibility, being accountable, and documenting the outcomes of their research-based interventions. Only then will nurses truly be able to negotiate with colleagues from other healthcare disciplines and be involved not only in predicting the future but also in creating the future they desire.

In *The Future of Nursing 2020–2030: Charting a Path to Achieve Health Equity*, the National Academy of Medicine and the Robert Wood Johnson Foundation (2021) collaborated toward promoting a culture of health for all by strengthening nursing capacity and expertise. The report is available online and provides recommendations to achieve health equity through nursing and the desired outcomes (National Academies of Sciences, Engineering, and Medicine, 2024). The following list contains common themes shared within the report and recommendations:

1. Create a shared agenda to focus efforts of all nurses to address the social determinants of health and eliminate barriers.
2. Support nurses with robust education, resources, and autonomy.
3. Promote the health and well-being of all nurses.
4. Capitalize on nurses' potential to help people live their healthiest lives.
5. Pay for nursing care.
6. Use technology to integrate data on social determinants of health into nursing practice.
7. Strengthen nursing education and prepare nurses to respond to disasters and public health emergencies.
8. Build the evidence base.

Nurse leaders are essential to changing healthcare, and this perspective helps explain why nurses need to start leading as soon as they graduate and develop their leadership skills as they grow and evolve throughout their professional careers. Additionally, nurses should be recognized for their vast contributions and be well positioned to lead and make more positive changes in healthcare.

The use of AI—including patient-monitoring systems, conversational interfaces, computerized medication administration, telehealth, interactive computer communication, data analytics, and computerized patient data storage—is a good example of how nursing can benefit from change. Technological advances such as those just mentioned maximize the potential for nurses to spend more time with patients, allow more independent clinical judgments, provide immediate communication with other members of the healthcare team, and help nurses manage patient data for quick retrieval when they analyze patient outcomes.

To shape a desired future for nursing, all nurses should be involved with developing health policy, networking with legislators and political groups, and spearheading changes in the delivery of healthcare to consumers by participating on boards and taking on leadership positions in policymaking organizations. To accomplish these actions, however, nurses need to understand how to advocate for a change in health policy and how to initiate a new health policy. They also need to learn the politics of healthcare and the value of being a member of their state nurses' association. Gaining some experience during undergraduate and graduate nursing programs in observing and participating on a board, developing health policy, stepping up to the leadership position on a taskforce or committee in their work setting, or volunteering in a community health project by writing a grant for funding of an aspect of the project would assist nurses in shaping a preferred future for nursing. Such actions will enable nurses to influence necessary changes in healthcare that will improve the profession's image as a competent and powerful contributor to the health of all people.

No longer can nurses focus solely on their particular unit or specialty area, because nurses need to be versatile to work in multiple units. Many nurses who work in acute care institutions will need to be educated to work in outpatient delivery units. Nurses will need to constantly engage in learning new techniques and methods to communicate and document. They must be aware of the larger arena of healthcare, continue their education, and remain flexible. Nurses also will do well to focus on measuring nursing care outcomes, being attuned to cost-effectiveness, ensuring high-quality nursing interventions, participating in ethical debates, providing access to healthcare for all, working collaboratively with one another and with other healthcare professionals, increasing educational preparation standards, and being a vital voice in healthcare policymaking.

Furthermore, all nurses need to be knowledgeable about multiple views of issues facing healthcare, nursing education, and the nursing profession, and they must be flexible and capable of making decisions and executing decisions when the need arises. For example, a staff nurse directs the care of patients and reviews, and in many instances, determines or coordinates what transpires between the healthcare team and each patient. In addition, the nurse plays a negotiator role regarding what the patient should receive, what type of services, and when. The nurse also oversees ancillary workers, builds consensus to successfully implement patients' plans of care, ensures patient safety and high-quality care are given, and empowers patients and other staff to advocate and be counted among those who will make a difference. Nurses need to be knowledgeable about the healthcare delivery system in which they work, as well as about the newest knowledge on which their practice is based to perform these tasks.

It is important to realize that no single individual can determine what the future will be, but nurses can shape their own future by being cognizant of multiple possibilities and being open to trying new and innovative changes. Nurses cannot be passive and accept everything the future hands them; instead, they must create a desired future for nursing. The following discussion is intended to help nurses become more effective in increasing their ability to shape the future for the profession and for healthcare.

Approaches to Shaping a Desired Future and Perception of Nursing

Nursing education must prepare graduates who are able to participate as full partners in healthcare delivery and shape health policy. Nursing curricula should emphasize patient safety, value, and population-based care; patient education; use of interprofessional teams; health promotion; rehabilitation; self-care; alternative methods of healing; informatics; and palliative care while maintaining the concern for acute and tertiary care. Nursing education accreditation bodies recommend that nursing educators, along with nurse executives and clinicians in practice settings, shape practice. All curricula should include, at appropriate levels, case management; healthcare policy; research; quality indicators; outcome measures; value-based care; financial management; legislative advocacy; diversity, equity and inclusion; and data management. The notion of lifelong learning for all nurses to maintain competency must also be continually addressed, perhaps through mandatory continuing education or certification.

Improving the perception of nursing for the future involves enhancing public understanding. Nurses must clearly define what they do and communicate it to the public with education and awareness campaigns, media representation, community engagement, and professional development opportunities so that consumers will be able to understand the role of the RN and APRN.

Influencing and Co-creating Change

To influence and co-create change, nurse leaders need to promote and educate others regarding alternative practice models (e.g., community health centers and mobile units to provide comprehensive primary care to underserved populations, telehealth to provide healthcare remotely by technology, and nurse-managed health clinics) in order to maximize resources and conserve costs. These changes in care delivery are already happening and aim to improve access, efficiency, and patient outcomes while adapting to changing healthcare needs and preferences. In addition, nurses can influence one another to visualize that many nursing activities could become a part of the patient's own care process. For example, nurses could have monthly group meetings to check blood pressure, weight, and blood work and offer a 15-minute interaction time between patients with similar problems regarding their best hints for managing their health problem. The uncertainty that exists at present regarding the future provides nurses with an opportunity to create and pilot new care models that increase the accountability of patients and families for their own health. At the same time, nurse leaders must be sure nurses and other interprofessional healthcare staff are involved in hospital initiatives. Small advances lead to big advances.

Nurses also need to receive ongoing education regarding knowledge and technical expertise to help prepare them to care for their patients. A concern regarding time devoted to professional development is having enough nurses available full-time to teach other nurses. One would think there will continue to be a need for centralized staff development; however, there is a trend for more of the nursing support functions, such as orientation, training nurses on new equipment, and annual competency-based learning evaluation, to be conducted by unit-specific staff or online. This continues to be a controversial issue, and although some acute care institutions do maintain a small, centralized staff of nurse educators, other institutions feel that all nurses should be practicing direct patient care in order to maintain competency.

It would be excellent for the profession of nursing if each nurse were also involved in a nursing organization that was actively working to create an optimal future for the profession. Sigma Theta Tau International and other organizations (e.g., American Association of Critical-Care Nurses, ANA, and National League for Nursing) are committed to creating a positive future by offering leadership institutes, helping members to expand their networks, and offering recognition through awards and citations as a way to motivate nurses to work at their highest level. Whether working at the local or chapter level as a committee member or officer, serving on a board of directors, working on an international committee, or reviewing manuscripts for an organization's journal, nurses are working to advance the future of nursing and are shaping that future by leading health policy change, volunteering in the community to provide pro bono healthcare or knowledge, and keeping the image of nursing visible to the public.

Nursing Research

Research must be conducted to determine the extent to which evidence-based research is implemented and if cost-effective patient outcomes are generated. Nursing science must continue to be developed, so that nurses can provide care that will increase positive healthcare outcomes (Melnyk & Fineout-Overholt, 2023). Nurses and interprofessional staff conducted a national 20-month, collaborative study where they implemented the **A**ssess pain, **B**oth awakening and breathing trials, **C**hoice of medications, **D**elirium, **E**arly mobility, and **F**amily (ABCDEF) bundle for caring for critically ill ventilated patients who were being weaned off support. They were most interested in ensuring pain, agitation, and delirium assessments were made and the outcomes managed effectively. Their findings supported use of the entire ABCDEF bundle to improve patient outcomes (Balas et al., 2019). More units can follow their lead and adapt using the bundle to provide best practices to this patient group. A group of pediatric nurses and medical residents developed a laboratory specimen checklist and used it at daily interprofessional rounds to ensure discussion on what laboratory values were needed and not needed. They found a significant decrease in blood draws post-checklist implementation that generated better patient outcomes, nurse satisfaction, and cost-effectiveness (Geaman et al., 2019). Nurses are making great strides in using evidence-based practice and quality improvement initiatives and will continue if nurse leaders model this behavior and empower others to participate.

Hesselbein and Goldsmith (2009) share multiple examples of how organizations that provide work environments that foster commitment and pride can be pivotal in creating long-lasting and positive organizational change for the future. Their book gives suggestions on what they believe are imperative steps for organizations to follow to secure a desired future:

1. **Strategy and vision:** One must be able to identify and follow a vision that is not stagnant but continuously evolving and relates to positive patient outcomes.
2. **Organizational culture, values, emotions, hope, ethics, spirit, and behavior:** Each organization needs to incorporate its values, emotions, hopes, spirit, and behavior and ethically create an organizational culture that transforms its employees and collaborative communities.
3. **Designing the organization of the future:** A group of leaders must be able to identify and plan for new socioeconomic shifts so their organizations will survive the impact of these changes.
4. **Working together:** To have successful organizations, it is paramount that there is a team spirit, and that leaders and followers are working together.
5. **Leaders:** Leaders of the future will need to share how they plan to execute their new actions and share suggestions for what leadership styles work best.

Nurses must study the effectiveness of what they do and provide leadership, perhaps using Hesselbein and Goldsmith's (2009) suggestions regarding the nursing aspect of interprofessional research. They must continue to study the healthcare practices of various groups, as well as patient responses to specific interventions. Such patient responses might include pain management and understanding of one's health status, stress level, and ability to perform self-care to maintain or enhance function. In other words, nurses must measure the specific effect of nursing care and not merely describe problems that exist in healthcare or nurses' perceptions of what the problems may be.

Some potential future research topics for nursing include telehealth and remote monitoring, nursing workforce and well-being, integrative and complementary therapies, technology in nursing education, and environmental health and nursing. Results should be disseminated in publications and presentations, including those that are multidisciplinary in nature and those accessed by the public. There must be a commitment to using research results as a basis for practice, and being involved in the conduct of research must be integral to every nurse's ongoing practice.

Nursing Teams

The uncertainty and challenges of the world require high-performing teams to work together to solve problems and seek numerous solution options. Leadership is not a position but a process and a role that everyone can and must assume at some point. Consider the light switch, which turns a light on or off, and a dimmer switch, which allows a light to vary in degrees of brightness. The light switch has two options, but the dimmer has many. Leaders must remember to look at the range of options and beyond the simple binary.

In essence, everyone has something to offer; there is a place on the team where each person can make important contributions. Perhaps if the strengths of all individuals were appreciated and they were empowered, members of a team would develop the self-confidence to do their very best and make significant contributions to shaping a desired future. This attitude of people working hard, feeling good about themselves, and having their contributions acknowledged can significantly affect the accomplishment of a once seemingly distant vision.

The U.S. Department of Health and Human Services' Agency for Healthcare Research and Quality funded the TeamSTEPPS training program for healthcare professionals (Agency for Healthcare Research and Quality, 2023), which assists all healthcare staff in gaining increased knowledge and experience working as a team. This team model fosters point of care and decision making at the bedside, horizontal organizational structure, shared governance, and leadership. Using principles of teamwork such as equity, accountability, and ownership, each member contributes a unique set of talents to achieve the common goal (e.g., quality patient care); each partner is patient centered, and no one tells the other partner what to do or when to do it. The paradigm supports collaboration, dialogue, patient participation, freedom of expression, and empowerment, all of which are crucial to success. Nurses must take pride in the responsibility that they have to monitor patients and provide health surveillance in all healthcare settings. Nurses must take pride in the leadership they provide as case coordinators and the role they play in holding the system together. This is what nurses do, and it is their unique contribution to healthcare.

CHARACTERISTICS OF NURSE LEADERS NEEDED TO CREATE A DESIRED FUTURE FOR NURSING

Leaders of tomorrow must be transformational with the ability to use various skills given the challenges they face. We cannot think of change as a one-time occurrence; rather, it will be continuous. Arussy (2019) reinforces the idea that "change is no longer the exception, it's the rule" (p. 2) and advises people to develop "change resilience" not "change resistance" by following these steps:

1. Identify the facts.
2. Review and make sense of the informative facts.
3. Reinvent the information to work for you.
4. Learn the new facts and adapt it to you/yours.
5. Take it and run with it.

Transformational leaders are those who can propel a vision, recruit the new generation of nurses, empower followers to work enthusiastically to realize a vision, meet change head-on and grow from it, harness conflict to ensure people are thinking in different ways, and keep harmful stress at a minimum for themselves and the organization. They must be designers, teachers, and stewards (Senge, 2006). Senge defines *designers* as those who assist in developing the vision; *teachers* as those who help followers develop the skills and gain the knowledge to work toward making the vision a reality; and *stewards* as those who act as spokespersons for the group, keep the group focused on the vision, and facilitate the long-term growth of all followers. Using these role descriptions facilitates teaching leadership skills and coaching nurses to design, teach, and successfully steward.

Leaders have ideas about what the future can bring and what it could be like, but they do not just sit around and wait for things to happen. In fact, Bennis (2007), who has interviewed multiple leaders and identified common talents they possess, concludes that exemplary leaders have six skill competencies that define them as leaders:

1. Create a sense of mission.
2. Motivate followers to work with them on the mission.
3. Develop a social ambience for their followers.
4. Create trust and optimism.
5. Develop others to lead.
6. Obtain results.

Being able to envision the future and create a sense of vision separates leaders from others. To accept the challenge of leading is a decision each of us must make. When nurses accept that challenge, they also accept responsibility for shaping a preferred future for nursing. Nurses may be more successful in shaping a preferred future if they incorporate the following guidelines (Kouzes & Posner, 2023):

- Be ready to embark on the vision.
- Maintain your credibility, integrity, and competence and think of the future.
- Stay grounded but think *big*—try something new but be realistic!
- Be aware you cannot do it by yourself—you need a team.
- Every individual needs to use their leadership abilities.

As long as a person has a vision, articulates it clearly, enlists others to help make it a reality, is aware of factors that influence it, and is able to keep the vision on course, that individual really is a leader and is shaping the future. Johansen (2012) suggests the following characteristics, still discussed and used today, for leaders to acquire to be well-prepared to lead in the future:

- **Maker instinct:** Try to create your own vision (using as many ideas from the organization as possible) and connect with everyone you can.
- **Clarity:** Think logically and present a plan to manage the complications and hard times that may present—remain motivated and on track.

- **Dilemma flipping:** Turn dilemmas, which are problems that cannot be solved and just have to be accepted, into challenges and opportunities.
- **Immersive learning ability:** Immerse yourself in the digital environment and gain new skills.
- **Bio-empathy:** If you try to see issues and problems through nature's patterns, you will gain new and successful solutions.
- **Constructive depolarizing:** Assist all from diverse backgrounds to connect with one another.
- **Quiet transparency:** Be open and authentic with everyone and be humble.
- **Rapid prototyping:** Try out your new ideas spontaneously and see if any catch on—if not, try another one.
- **Smart mob organizing:** Always network, even when you think there is no use.
- **Commons creating:** Be sure to have a common asset that is respected and generates competition between the group members to work a little harder.

It is much more exciting to help determine what the future will be than to merely react to it as it happens around us. So, it is imperative that all nurses acquire more leadership skills and learn to be dynamic with their communications. True wisdom and true leadership typically come from learning from the past, developing new ideas, enjoying and growing in the present, preparing for the future, and creating the future. Johansen believes "our past shapes our future" but that "there are opportunities to break out of your old patterns" (2012, p. 210), so one can have a more positive, volatile, uncertain, complex, and ambiguous future world. This point of not always thinking our past shapes our future is extremely important—we absolutely cannot rely totally on the past to shape our future.

Case Study, continued

Inspired by overcoming the challenges of the implementation and learning new technology from this experience, the nurses decided to permanently implement the chatbot system and features for the student population. This initiative serves to decrease the volume of calls handled directly by nurses, ensure that urgent cases are prioritized, and provide students with accurate and timely health information. By being willing to explore and implement new technology, the nurses provide better care to the student population.

REFLECTION QUESTION

6. What long-term impacts might the implementation of a chatbot have on the clinic's operations and student health outcomes?

This Case Study of a common situation illustrates how nurses in any practice setting can choose to exercise their leadership. Recognizing an issue, detecting patterns, and finding alternative methods to resolve it helped these nurses make a difference in the care they provided. These nurses were empowered to take the time and make a difference because they cared enough to discuss their intuitive thoughts. Nurses have much to share and can lead others in providing improved care to patients if they use their leadership competencies. Some nurses would greatly benefit by expanding their knowledge base and using new leadership skills to assist them in changing the way they practice.

CONCLUSION

The world around us is changing dramatically, and the role of the nurse will continue to expand and evolve. Considering this, nurses must decide how they want the role to develop and then act to make that happen. Nurses will need to become more visible and disseminate how the profession impacts the health of the nation in such an exceptional way; AI networks will facilitate this development. All nurses can embrace the vision of providing quality healthcare to anyone in need, but they will have to be prepared so they can adapt readily to new information. What they need to do now is work collaboratively to make this vision a reality. They must think critically, not on a linear trajectory but with a multidimensional perspective. They will need to communicate effectively with their interprofessional partners on the healthcare team to determine and implement the evidence-based interventions that will result in the highest value-based care. Nurses will need to determine what nursing tasks can be performed by digital technology and what new avenues the profession can create.

Leadership must be everybody's business. That means each nurse must believe that every nurse has the power to make a difference in maximizing the health outcomes of patients. Just like nurses work with experienced nurses to gain clinical expertise, nurses need to shadow expert leaders and be mentored by someone who can help an individual nurse grow. Every nurse must stand up for a cause, bridge a gap, network with others, and do what needs to be done to move the profession forward toward *the future they desire*.

 CRITICAL THINKING 8-1

1. Imagine that it is the year 2035 and you will be interviewed about the significant difference you have made and will make to the nursing profession. What will you talk about? What significant differences have you made? How will you respond when the interviewer asks what you plan to do this year and in the next 5 years to continue to make a difference?

2. Describe how you, a nurse leader, would motivate and inspire your healthcare team (composed of all members of the healthcare disciplines) that is assigned to manage the healthcare of 100 people in 2035. These patients were exposed to an unknown infectious agent, requiring them to be quarantined for 30 days. Your governing organization has equipped you with a state-of-the-art "Disaster Healthcare Module" to use for managing the situation, and you can ask for resources for any potential emergencies.

3. Given the predictions about the future in general, the future of healthcare, and the future of nursing, what kinds of nurse leaders will the profession need to shape a desired future? Are these same qualities needed today? Why or why not? How is globalization affecting these predictions?

4. Informally interview a variety of people (e.g., child, older adult, healthcare provider, nurse colleagues, new college graduate) about the future of the healthcare system. Ask them what they think things will be like in the year 2035 and beyond. Also, ask them what they think we need to do now to achieve the positive things they envision and avoid the negative things they think could happen. Are the views of nurses different from those of other groups? Are there differences in the views of nurses from different cultures?

5. List the top five opportunities you wish to be challenged with as a nurse leader so you can develop your leadership capacity to prepare yourself for a successful career. Analyze how you will be able to obtain these experiences in the next 5 years.

6. Often people ask nurses to explain healthcare issues. To best be prepared for these situations, choose two healthcare issues about which you are most interested in gaining more knowledge. Use factcheck.org, an excellent nonpartisan Web site that will provide the facts—not the site's opinions—about multiple issues so that you can be well prepared for current, past, and future discussions. Plan to spend at least 30 minutes a week reviewing this site for information sources about the healthcare issues most important to you.

7. With the multiple issues impacting public health in the United States and globally today and in the future (e.g., opioid crisis, climate change, increasing older population, immigration, refugees, violence, infections with little known interventions, and pandemics), nurses need to have strong communication, technology, and leadership skills, as well as clinical acumen, in order to promote health. Imagine additional issues we are not totally aware of yet and try to identify what will be expected of the nursing profession. What are some new experiences nursing educators need to teach students? How should working nurses prepare for the future?

References

Adams, J., Djukic, M., Gregas, M., & Fryer, A. (2018). Influence of nurse leader practice characteristics on patient outcomes: Results from a multistate study. *Nursing Economic$*, *36*(6), 259–267.

Agency for Healthcare Research and Quality. (2023). *TeamSTEPPS: National implementation.* http://teamstepps.ahrq.gov

American Association of Colleges of Nursing. (2024). *Nursing fact sheet.* https://www.aacnnursing.org/News-Information/Fact-Sheets/Nursing-Fact-Sheet

American Nurses Association. (2024). *ANA CAUTI prevention tool.* https://www.nursingworld.org/practice-policy/work-environment/health-safety/infection-prevention/ana-cauti-prevention-tool/

American Nurses Credentialing Center. (2023). *Magnet Model—Creating a Magnet culture.* https://www.nursingworld.org/organizational-programs/magnet/magnet-model/

Arussy, L. (2019). *Next is now: 5 steps for embracing change—building a business that thrives into the future.* Simon & Schuster.

Association of American Medical Colleges. (2021). *New research shows increasing physician shortages in both primary and specialty care* [Press release]. https://news.aamc.org/press-releases/article/workforce_report_shortage_04112018/

Balas, M., Pun, B., Pasero, C., Engel, H., Perme, C., Esbrook, C. L., Kelly, T., Hargett, K. D., Posa, P. J., Barr, J., Devlin, J. W., Morse, A., Barnes-Daly, M. A., Puntillo, K. A., Aldrich, J. M., Schweickert, W. D., Harmon, L. Byrum, D. G., Carson, S. S., . . . Stollings, J. L. (2019). Common challenges to effective ABCDEF bundle implementation: The ICU liberation campaign experience. *Critical Care Nurse*, *39*(1), 46–60.

Bennis, W. (2007). The challenges of leadership in the modern world. *American Psychologist, 62*(1), 2–5.

Canton, J. (2019). Are you future-ready? *Institute for Global Futures.* https://www.globalfuturist.com/

Centers for Medicare & Medicaid Services. (2024). *Hospital value based purchasing program.* https://qualitynet.cms.gov/inpatient/hvbp

Central Intelligence Agency. (2023). *CIA world factbook.* https://www.cia.gov/the-world-factbook/countries/united-states/#people-and-society

Geaman, M., Brennan, K., & Vanderway, J. (2019). Quality initiative to decrease laboratory draws for hospitalized pediatric patients. *Pediatric Nursing, 45*(3), 115–121, 141.

Hesselbein, F., & Goldsmith, M. (Eds.). (2009). *The organization of the future: Visions, strategies, and insights on managing in a new era.* Jossey-Bass.

Johansen, B. (2012). *Leaders make the future: Ten new leadership skills for an uncertain world* (2nd ed.). Berrett-Koehler.

Kouzes, J., & Posner, B. (2023). *The leadership challenge: How to make extraordinary things happen in organizations.* Jossey-Bass.

Lopez, E., Gonzalez, J. L., Cordo, J. A., Janvier-Anglade, M., & Fitzpatrick, T. A. (2019). EntrepreNurses: Nursing's evolving role in innovation strategy. *Nursing Economic$, 37*(3), 159–163.

Maxwell, J. (2019). *Leadershift: 11 essential changes every leader must embrace.* HarperCollins.

Melnyk, B., & Fineout-Overholt, E. (2023). *Evidence-based practice in nursing and healthcare.* Wolters Kluwer.

National Academies of Science, Engineering & Medicine. (2024). *The future of nursing 2020–2030: Charting a path to achieve health equity.* The National Academies Press.

National Institute of Nursing Research. (2024). *The National Institute of Nursing Research 2022–2026 strategic plan.* https://www.ninr.nih.gov/aboutninr/ninr-mission-and-strategic-plan/research-framework

Rosen, M., DiazGranados, D., Dietz, A., Benishek, L., Thompson, D., Pronovost, P., & Weaver, S. (2019). Teamwork in healthcare: Key discoveries enabling safer, high-quality care. *American Psychologist, 73*(4), 433–450.

Sahota, N., & Ashley, M. (2019). *Own the artificial intelligence revolution: Unlock your artificial intelligence strategies to disrupt your competition.* McGraw-Hill.

Senge, P. (2006). *The fifth discipline: The art and practice of the learning organization* (2nd ed.). Doubleday Currency.

U.S. Bureau of Labor Statistics. (2024). *Occupational outlook handbook.* https://www.bls.gov/ooh/healthcare/registered-nurses.htm#tab-3

Walsh, M. (2019). *The algorithmic leader: How to be smart when machines are smarter than you.* You Two Publishers.

Waters, S., & Giblin, E. (2019). Acute heart failure: Pearls for the first posthospitalization clinic visit. *Journal for Nurse Practitioners, 15*(1), 80–86.

Withers, M., Lin, H. -H., Schmidt, T., delos Trinos, J. P. C. R., & Kumar, S. (2019). Establishing competencies for a global health workforce: Recommendations from the Association of Pacific Rim Universities. *Annals of Global Health, 85*(1), 47.

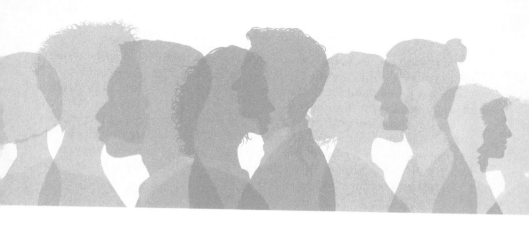

CHAPTER 9

Developing as a Leader Throughout One's Career

LEARNING OBJECTIVES
- Describe ways in which individuals can develop as leaders.
- Describe characteristics of environments that facilitate the development of leadership skills in oneself and others.
- Relate the concept of empowerment to the development of leaders.
- Analyze the process of mentoring as it relates to the development of leaders.
- Propose a personal plan for leadership development that attends to empowerment, mentoring, role-modeling, networking, self-assessment, and continued renewal.

INTRODUCTION

One of the early leadership theories, the Great Man Theory, espoused that leaders were individuals who had been born into the "right" family at the "right" time. As noted earlier, this theory has been challenged over the years as being far from useful in understanding the multifaceted nature of leadership, and there is now widespread agreement that leaders are made, not born. The question remains as to how an individual can be "made" into a leader.

Individuals who are acknowledged as leaders do not simply declare that they will be leaders and expect that others will accept such a declaration. In addition, being successful in one role (e.g., student) does not guarantee success in a leadership role (e.g., project director) because different skills may be required (Ruben et al., 2023). Instead, as demonstrated in our own profession (Houser & Player, 2004, 2007), individuals who are acknowledged as leaders often are nurtured and guided by others, seek and function in environments that encourage leadership behavior, test the role, and study others who have been leaders. In addition, leadership is a practice and series of actions (Raza et al., 2024) that can be developed throughout one's nursing career.

Thus, the development of oneself as a leader is a purposeful process that is enhanced by guidance and support from others. But what are the ways in which one can develop leadership skills? This chapter explores numerous approaches to leadership development, and several of the strategies that have particular relevance for nurses are examined in depth.

> *Knowing is not enough; we must apply. Willing is not enough; we must do.* —Goethe

Consider the following Case Study about how nurses can develop as leaders throughout their careers and can use mentors to further future career possibilities to leave a lasting legacy.

Case Study

Marty and Josh were classmates during their nursing program, and immediately after graduation, both went to work at the local medical center. Although they both enjoyed successful careers in nursing, each evolved to a very different place in terms of leadership and the extent of influence in the field.

Both Marty and Josh identified Dr. Richards as one of the best professors they had in nursing courses. She was knowledgeable in the subject she taught but admitted to not knowing things and thought through those situations out loud so that students could benefit from her thinking processes. She used innovative strategies to facilitate learning and actively engaged students in designing their own learning experiences. Dr. Richards published extensively in her area of expertise, completed research that influenced patient care, was inducted into the American Academy of Nursing, received numerous awards for her work, consulted with schools of nursing across the country, was invited to speak at national and international conferences, was actively involved in her specialty organization, and most recently was inducted into the National League for Nursing's Academy of Nursing Education. Although she did not brag about these accomplishments, Dr. Richards kept her students informed about her activities and the directions in which her career took her.

Neither Marty nor Josh thought they would pursue an academic position, but they were impressed with Dr. Richards's accomplishments and contributions, and they often talked about their desire to have a career as exciting and productive as hers. Marty took steps to make that happen. Josh did not.

REFLECTION QUESTIONS

1. Do you have a teacher or professor you consider to be the best and if so, what attributes does this individual exhibit to make you think they are the best?
2. What are some reasons that Josh may not have taken steps to pursue his desire and do you see any of these barriers in your own life?

GENERAL APPROACHES TO LEADERSHIP DEVELOPMENT

Emergence as a leader is a developmental learning process in which capacities, insights, and skills gained through one experience or at one level serve as the basis for further growth; thus, leaders go through stages in their development. It also is generally acknowledged that one learns to be a leader by serving as a leader. Merely talking about being a leader or observing others in that role does not make one a leader. Someone is a leader when they act and exercise leadership.

Based on past performance or promise of future performance, one often is expected to provide leadership to a group. As a person has success in that role, increasing leadership is expected of that individual; thus, one may continually be promoted to higher levels of leadership responsibility.

Finally, leadership development is a lifelong process. As nurses progress throughout their careers, they will face new challenges. The need for change will always exist, and groups will need leaders to help them weather the forces of change. Conflict also will always exist, particularly as resources become more scarce and new healthcare workers challenge traditional roles; groups will need leaders to help them manage those conflicts. New visions will continually need to be articulated as previous visions are realized or changing societal expectations demand new directions; groups will need leaders to help them see and realize those new visions. Thus, as the circumstances of our lives are constantly altered, our leadership skills also need to be refined, renewed, and further developed.

Lecture and Discussion: Formal Coursework

Perhaps one of the most common and easiest ways to develop leadership skills is through participation in lectures, discussions, or formal course work on leadership. Such experiences provide information about the phenomenon, facilitate a formal examination of individuals who have demonstrated leadership in the past or in contemporary society, and stimulate thinking about the nature of leadership and followership. Participation in an effective discussion group also provides experience in working with others to reach decisions and helps one develop an awareness of the need for more than single, simple answers to complex problems.

Nursing curricula often include courses related to leadership and management, though they often focus more on the latter concept than on the former. However, the success of nursing as a profession has been affected by the COVID-19 pandemic and now requires nurses to demonstrate greater leadership capabilities (Vuorivirta-Vuoti et al., 2023). This necessitates a shift in nursing education to enhance clinical judgment through integrating leadership concepts throughout curricula, in addition to teaching this as a separate course.

In response to requests from employers, expectations issued by the Institute of Medicine (2021), and *The Essentials* from the American Association of Colleges of Nursing (AACN, 2021), many nursing education programs have incorporated leadership courses and threaded leadership competencies throughout the curriculum. Nursing educators must continue to develop curricular approaches to address the complex challenges that health systems currently face and develop transformational practices to equip the next generation of nursing leaders (Bernhardt et al., 2023).

In response to such calls and challenges, purposeful efforts are under way to help learners develop as leaders. Faculty are designing learning experiences to help students achieve such goals, and many are even using creative strategies, including games, case studies, simulation, and role-playing games (RPGs) to help leadership concepts come alive for students (Egan, 2024; Lasley, 2024; Leal et al., 2022). Lasley (2024) asserted that educators must incorporate play and creativity into education for leadership development to be conceptualized within a social context. Involving students in a co-creative educational process equips students to confront adaptive challenges and creates social justice. Although Lasley (2024) is not speaking specifically to nursing educators, the insights and recommendations offered for improving education in leadership are equally applicable to nursing programs. In order to fully develop students as leaders, learning experiences need to encompass conflict management, teamwork, advocacy, and self-efficacy in progressing complexity throughout the curriculum (AACN, 2021). There is no question that faculty in many schools of nursing have taken to heart recommendations to integrate leadership concepts throughout a program and not merely include a leadership and management course at the end of a program.

Individuals who want to learn more about the complex concept of leadership and the effective exercise of leadership, particularly in nursing and healthcare, may benefit from enrolling in additional courses or programs, including continuing education courses, such as those offered through the Center for Creative Leadership (www.ccl.org/open-enrollment-programs/) and other groups or organizations that focus on the topic. However, it would be wise to study the course description carefully before enrolling to be certain that it does, indeed, focus on leadership rather than on management.

Role-Playing, Simulation Exercises, and Games

Although it may be uncomfortable, participation in role-playing, simulation exercises, or games is an excellent way to develop leadership skills. By being expected to play the role of leader, one must be articulate, forward-thinking, and creative; one also must be able to manage conflict and resolve differences among group members, acknowledge and build on the strengths of followers, and help the group move forward. Role-playing also can serve as a diagnostic technique, through which one's strengths and areas needing improvement become apparent. For example, it will be evident if the individual playing the role of leader cannot articulate a vision clearly; the individual will then know that this is a particular skill needing more development.

Role-playing or simulation also can serve as a way to test various solutions to problems before actually being in those problem situations. For example, a group might construct a scenario in which one of its members plays the passive "sheep" follower role (Kelley, 1992), and the leader must figure out ways to help that follower become more effective. Knowing that reality often presents leaders with many sheep followers, being able to address this situation through role-playing gives leaders an opportunity to generate a number of approaches to dealing with such a situation before finding themselves actually faced with it. In addition, this kind of experience provides other participants with an opportunity for vicarious learning in which they have observed which strategies were successful and which were not.

Students have been helped to develop their leadership skills through the use of simulation (Dopelt et al., 2023), which offers yet another way of learning to be a leader. The study conducted by these researchers showed that healthcare students who participated in simulated situations learned more about functioning in a leader role compared with traditional lectures. Simulation had a positive influence on the learning process and addressed unpredictable situations to improve management and leadership abilities. Students progressed in leadership knowledge and skill acquisition through simulations and they thought their own teaching–learning needs were better met through simulation, in part because simulation resulted in deep personal reflection on individual leadership and management skills (Dopelt et al., 2023). Thus, simulation, which appears to be an effective strategy to develop leadership skills as well as an effective learning experience, is another way one might develop skills as a leader.

Zhao et al. (2023) discuss how virtual reality (VR) and augmented reality (AR) are viable venues for education and can bring information to life by enabling learners to experience leadership encounters that would not be feasible in a traditional setting. Learners are also able to react to the virtual or augmented reality, instead of simply discussing a scenario. Although VR/AR leadership scenarios are more immersive learning experiences, they should be utilized concomitantly with discussion groups or one-to-one instruction because learning is inherently a social experience (Zhao et al., 2023).

One other opportunity to reflect on one's leadership abilities is to participate in a game using the "Be a Leader Thumball" (www.trainerswarehouse.com/be-a-leader-thumball.html). In this activity, a group of individuals tosses around a ball that contains 32 thoughts or questions, such as the following: "I'd be a better leader if I spent more time on . . ." or "Am I a good follower? Why?" or "I am least effective when . . ." When individuals catch the ball, they are expected to share their reaction or response to whatever prompt lies under their thumb, and this leads to a discussion of what leadership and followership are all about, as well as the individual's strengths, areas needing improvement, and ideas for how to develop in those weaker areas. Such an exercise combines movement, fun, and learning and can be quite effective in helping individuals develop as leaders.

Thus, it can be seen that in-person or virtual games, role-playing exercises, and simulations all can be used to help individuals think about and develop their leadership abilities. It is important to keep in mind, however, that such exercises must be carefully designed, implemented with precision, and followed by effective debriefing sessions during which participants are helped to reflect on what has been learned and what personal insights have been attained.

Sensitivity Training

Sensitivity training sessions led by expert facilitators provide participants with an opportunity to focus on openness, how hostilities and defensiveness may be exhibited within a group, and one's personal feelings, perceptions, and biases. Participation also increases one's sensitivity to others' needs and helps one appreciate the significance of shared decision making. Finally, such sessions also assist group members to reflect on the inner workings or processes of the group itself: who assumed what kinds of roles, who emerged as the leader, who was most effective in moving the group forward and why, and so on. Such insights are invaluable for those who will provide leadership in their work settings, professional associations, or communities.

Role-Modeling

Effective leadership skills can be developed by carefully observing individuals who are successful as leaders. By studying what such people do, how they communicate, how they motivate followers to join in the cause, their level of energy and personal investment, their ability to keep the group focused on the vision despite conflicts and challenges along the way, and how their careers have evolved can be extremely helpful to the novice leader.

Role-modeling occurs whether or not it is planned or purposeful. In other words, many individuals pattern themselves after others even though they may not be aware of such unconscious "decisions" and may find that they have adapted the negative or unhelpful behaviors exhibited by others, as well as the positive or helpful ones. Therefore, role-modeling is much more effective when it is done consciously and with deliberation.

Conscious or formal role-modeling may be enhanced by attending professional conferences and conventions where one observes how participants conduct themselves, deal with "hot" issues that are open to debate, express opinions, and connect with members of the audience. It also can be achieved by being more observant during meetings. Who is typically able to convince the group that their point is the one that should be supported, and what does that person do that makes them so convincing? Conscious role-modeling occurs when one reads articles or editorials written by nurse leaders and reflects on their communication style, their willingness to address controversial topics publicly, and the fact that they use media to convey a strongly held viewpoint or to articulate a vision.

Leadership can be facilitated by reading biographies about leaders in nursing, such as the 23 leaders presented by Houser and Player (2004, 2007). Listening to the journeys of the 13 nursing leaders spotlighted in the Betty Irene Moore Leadership speaker series on YouTube (https://www.youtube.com/playlist?list=PLop RJPO6GaifsYPGP_jcWXZzU10H3AaX7) also can help you reflect on your leadership qualities. In fact, Saeed et al. (2024) use a sense-making process that involves organizing data until the environment is understood well enough to enable reasonable decisions. This helps individuals tap into the knowledge and wisdom of past and current leaders as a way to help them reflect on what effective leadership is and why it is so critical in today's complex and ever-changing environment. Finally, learning more about contemporary or historical individuals outside nursing and studying what they did and how they did it can also be quite informative to those who aspire to leadership (Box 9-1).

Institutes and Fellowships

Other, more formalized approaches to leadership development occur through participation in institutes and fellowships. Such opportunities are announced in professional publications and are open to a wide variety of individuals, although some are limited to members of a particular organization.

BOX 9-1 **Studying Our Leaders**

The analysis of individuals who have been effective leaders can be a valuable way to help individuals think about leadership and their own skills. Often the subject of the case is someone who has come to be quite well known (e.g., Florence Nightingale or Joan of Arc), but by stepping back into that person's history to appreciate factors that influenced them to emerge as a leader or to better understand what ignited their passion and vision, one can learn about how individuals develop as leaders.

Of course, more contemporary figures—including those in one's own field or organization—also can be used for a case study. Although it may be difficult to identify influencing factors without knowing the outcome of the person's leadership or without the benefit of hindsight, exploring specifics of those providing leadership in the culture and context that are more relevant to a current situation can enhance individuals' understanding of how they might need to develop.

In 1992, the National Student Nurses' Association (NSNA) developed an independent study module that was intended to serve as a model for schools to involve students as active participants in learning about leadership, developing leadership skills, and enhancing professional socialization. Through individualized learning contracts with faculty members, students used their local, state, or national NSNA experiences to learn more about leadership, study their own leadership style, gain confidence when leading groups, appreciate the many facets of group decision making, and understand the legislative process. This has now evolved into the NSNA Leadership University (https://www.nsna.org/leadership-university.html), a cooperative initiative between the NSNA and individual schools of nursing that are constituents of that organization.

The American Nurses Association (ANA) offers a collection of online, self-paced modules and books designed to help nurses develop as leaders. Under the Leadership and Excellence section, this collection of resources is available to nurses who desire to become effective nurse leaders (https://www.nursingworld.org/continuing-education/ce-subcategories/leadership/).

Sigma Theta Tau International Honor Society of Nursing (STTI), which has as one of its major goals the development of leadership among its members, also offers many programs and opportunities to help members develop their leadership abilities and bring about transforming change (www.sigmanursing.org/learn-grow/sigma-academies). Acknowledging that nurses function at different leader levels (i.e., emerging, experienced, expert, and legacy) and have diverse scopes of influence (i.e., local, regional, national, and global), STTI now offers four distinct programs for individuals in practice and educational settings: Nurse Leadership Academy for Practice, Nurse Educator Development Academy, New Academic Leadership Academy, and Experienced Academic Leadership Academy.

Similarly, the National League for Nursing offers several leadership development opportunities through its Leadership Institute (https://www.nln.org/education/education/leadership-institute). The LEAD program is designed for nurses in education and practice who have recently been challenged with rapid transition into leadership positions, those in leadership positions who desire a formal leadership program, and those emerging and aspiring to lead. The Leadership Development for Simulation Educators program is designed for the experienced simulation nurse educator who wishes to assume a leadership role in simulation and advance simulation initiatives in nursing education and practice.

The American Organization for Nursing Leadership, formerly the American Organization of Nurse Executives, offers several leadership development programs, particularly for those who are in or aspire to management positions. The Emerging Nurse Leader Institute (www.aonl.org/education/enli) prepares staff nurses with leadership responsibilities, assistant managers, or nurses who aspire to be leaders of tomorrow. Additionally, several programs and fellowships (www.aonl.org/education/nursing-fellowships) are available for those who hold nurse executive positions and wish to strengthen their leadership skills.

The Wharton School at the University of Pennsylvania is the business school division that offers a number of intensives related to the development of leaders, including one designed specifically for nurses, particularly those in executive positions in hospital settings. Designed to help participants be more effective nurse leaders by providing tools to better manage resources, be more responsive to stakeholders, and optimize performance of the institution's nursing staff, the Wharton Nursing Leaders Program (https://executiveeducation.wharton.upenn.edu/for-individuals/all-programs/wharton-nursing-leaders-program/) is a week-long experience.

The University of Maryland School of Nursing sponsors a Leadership Institute that offers a year-long Leadership Development Program to prepare nurses to assume leadership positions and participate as full partners in developing healthcare delivery models that improve health outcomes for Maryland residents. Information about this program can be found at www.nursing.umaryland.edu/academics/pe/nli/.

Finally, several prestigious leadership programs are sponsored by nonprofit foundations, including (1) the Kellogg Leadership for Community Change program, which evolved into the national Community Learning Exchange, where communities share learning and support one another in the development of local collective leadership and community change, and is now offered through their Center for Ethical Leadership (http://www.ethicalleadership.org/community-learning-exchange.html); and (2) particularly for nurses who practice in the community, the Institute for Sustainable Communities Leadership Academy (https://sustain.org/program/sustainable-communities-leadership-academy-scla/), which offers a series of intensive, peer-learning and training workshops that advance, accelerate, and scale up urban climate and sustainability solutions. In addition, the Center for Creative Leadership (North Carolina) is a well-established program that offers research-based workshops, books, and other resources to positively transform the way leaders, their organizations, and their societies confront the most difficult challenges of the 21st century (www.ccl.org/), and the Center for Courage & Renewal (www.couragerenewal.org) helps participants reflect on "reconnecting who you are with what you do" through programs and retreats that focus on, among other topics, the courage to lead.

All these and many more programs are designed to enhance leadership development. When combined with on-the-job training and extensive reflection and self-assessment efforts, individuals can be most effective in developing as leaders in their organizations, communities, and professions.

On-the-Job Training

One very effective way to develop as a successful leader is to use such skills on the job so that one can learn from experience. On-the-job training may include temporary job rotations to positions that require the use of new skills, assignment as an assistant or apprentice to someone in a leadership role, serving as the chair-elect of a committee, or participation in some leadership internship, such as those described previously or those offered through one's employing agency. On-the-job training also may occur through a mentor relationship, a concept discussed in more depth later in this chapter.

Reflection and Self-Assessment

Reflection is generally viewed as having two dimensions: reflection-on-action and reflection-in-action. Reflective practice is an important approach in which an individual persistently and actively reflects on their actions, and also systematically and thoughtfully reflects in their actions through consistent self-inquiry (Rozimela et al., 2024). Reflective practice involves learning from everyday experiences and gaining insights about oneself and one's actions. By thinking deeply and honestly about your vision; your character; your passion; your ability and willingness to share power; the way you communicate; your persistence; the extent to which you embrace and celebrate differences; and other qualities of effective, transformational leaders, you can identify the strengths you wish to enhance and the limitations you wish to improve as a leader.

Such insights also occur through serious and thoughtful completion of self-assessment tools (some of which are listed here) and careful reflection on what they reveal about you:

- The Leadership Framework Self-Assessment tool (www.leadership academy.nhs.uk/wp-content/uploads/2012/11/NHSLeadership -Framework-LeadershipFrameworkSelfAssessmentTool.pdf) challenges individuals to reflect on their strengths in five core leadership domains: demonstrating personal qualities, working with others, managing services, improving services, and setting direction. It also challenges individual leaders to reflect on their contributions to creating the vision and delivering the strategy. This tool has been designed particularly for individuals involved in health and care services and may be of particular interest to nurses or nursing students.
- The How Good Are Your Leadership Skills? tool (www.mindtools .com/pages/article/newLDR_50.htm) helps individuals analyze their performance in specific areas of leadership, identifying where they

already lead effectively and exploring where their skills need further development. The analysis of individuals' responses is then used to direct them to the resources that can help them be exceptional leaders.

- The Leadership Self-Assessment Tool (www.zerotothree.org/resources/413-leadership-self-assessment-tool) focuses on components of reflective leadership, which is characterized by self-awareness; careful and continuous observation; and respectful, flexible responses that result in reflective and relationship-based programs. It includes a series of statements and reflective questions that offer insight into one's leadership style to help the individual identify their strengths and opportunities for growth.

- The Leadership Competency Inventory (Yoon et al., 2010) has two parallel forms, one that is completed by followers and one that is completed by the leader. Among other factors, this valid and reliable tool asks respondents to comment on the leader's teamwork and cooperation, flexibility and resilience, coaching, conflict management, vision, creative thinking, interpersonal competence, and external awareness, all of which are elements of effective leadership as discussed throughout this book.

- Another helpful self-assessment tool is the CliftonStrengths assessment, formerly known as StrengthsFinder (Rath, 2009). The extensive research conducted by the author with 20,000 leaders and 10,000 followers led to three key findings about the most effective leaders (pp. 2–3): (1) they are always investing in strengths, (2) they surround themselves with the right people and then maximize their team, and (3) they understand their followers' needs. The author concluded that "the path to great leadership starts with a deep understanding of the strengths you bring to the table" (p. 3). They developed this self-assessment tool to reflect four domains of leadership strength: *executing* (the ability to "catch" an idea and make it a reality); *influencing* (the ability to speak up, take charge, and make things happen); *relationship building* (the ability to serve as the glue that holds a team together); and *strategic thinking* (the ability to keep the group focused on what could be and continually stretch thinking for the future). More information about the tool, which has been used by more than 21 million people, can be found at https://www.gallup.com/cliftonstrengths/en/254033/strengthsfinder.aspx.

- The Situational Leadership Self-Assessment tool is based on Hersey's (1985) situational leadership model and helps users consider their ability to make sense of information and identify problems; communicate information and ideas; take action, make decisions, and follow through; take risks and be innovative; and manage conflict. It is available at www.scribd.com/doc/299936677/Situational-Leadership-Self-Assessment.

- One other popular self-assessment method is based on Keirsey's personality theory of four temperaments (https://keirsey.com/temperament-overview/): artisan, guardian, rational, and idealist. This test helps users appreciate if they are more of a teacher or promoter, inventor or performer, inspector or mastermind. It can help individuals understand if they are expressive, probing, tough-minded, or introspective, so they can better understand who they are and how they relate to others, both of which are critical for effective leaders.

Thus, reflection and self-assessment are important strategies for leadership development and should be integral to the ongoing development of any leader. In fact, one could argue that this is an essential practice for nurses because approximately 50% do not view themselves as leaders (Booher et al., 2021; Frilund et al., 2023). Seeking feedback from peers and potential followers also is useful in assessing your leadership qualities. Self-reflection and input from others can help you assess your qualities as a follower, which is important because followers act either as a resource "contributor" or a "predator" for the leader, where the contributor followers engage mutually with the leaders, and predator followers consume the leader's energy and resources on unproductive interactions (Zheng et al., 2024). Do you embrace the role? Do you have a servant mentality? Do you make the leader look good? Do you actively support the leader's vision (which is essential if you want to be an effective leader)? Self-reflection and input from others also can help you determine whether you are "contributor" or a "predator."

Continue the Case Study to learn how Marty pursued activities and self-reflection to foster resilience, lifelong learning, the acquisition of nursing expertise, and assertion of leadership.

Case Study, continued

While still a student, Marty took advantage of the opportunity to talk with Dr. Richards and other faculty about their careers, how they balanced professional development activities with work responsibilities, and how they got where they are. He asked for advice about jobs, how to get involved in professional organizations, who the movers and shakers were in his area of interest (rehabilitation), how to get the most out of conferences one attends, and whether Dr. Richards would mentor him, particularly at the outset of his career. He wrote goals for where he would like to be at 5 and 10 years after graduation and began to outline steps to achieve those goals. As a registered nurse (RN), Marty volunteered to serve on several committees at the rehabilitation center where he worked, proposed innovations in patient care that evolved from research reports he read, submitted abstracts for presentation of those patient care innovations at the national convention of the nursing rehabilitation organization, sought feedback from peers and supervisors about his practice, challenged ideas presented by others and offered alternative solutions, and worked with his mentors to advance professionally. Ten years after graduation, Marty was well known in the field of rehabilitation nursing, was collaborating with experts in that field to design and implement research projects, and was reporting the findings from their research in journal articles and at conferences. Rehabilitation nurses across the country knew of Marty's work and used his research findings and ideas about innovative practices as the basis for their own practice. Without question, Marty was a leader in the field, and his work influenced the work of others and helped shape a preferred future for rehabilitation nursing practice.

Continued

Case Study—cont'd

Josh, on the other hand, never sought out his teachers while he was a student or afterward. He was dedicated to providing excellent care to people experiencing homelessness, but he made no effort to actively shape that practice or advocate for the population he served daily. When asked to attend a meeting about care of people experiencing homelessness, Josh accepted, listened attentively, and prepared a comprehensive report of what took place during that meeting; however, he made no special effort before the meeting to be best prepared for it, did not contribute to the discussion, did not take risks to offer different perspectives (even though he disagreed with some of what was being proposed), did not influence the thinking of those at the table, and did not bring back to his own practice environment what he had learned in order to improve care and nursing practice. Although he knew of several organizations that worked diligently on behalf of people experiencing homelessness, Josh did not join or actively participate in any events sponsored by those organizations. He also did not attend professional conferences on the topic, attempt to incorporate research findings into his practice, challenge his colleagues to continually strive for excellence, seek out a mentor, or expand his professional networks. The care he provided to individuals was exceptional, but his sphere of influence was extremely limited, and his plan to advance as a leader was essentially nonexistent.

REFLECTION QUESTIONS

3. Compare the impact of Marty's and Josh's different approaches on their respective spheres of influence within the nursing profession. How did Marty's proactive engagement with mentors, participation in professional organizations, and dedication to research contribute to his recognition as a leader? Contrast this with Josh's limited involvement and lack of proactive steps to advance professionally.
4. Reflect on the importance of active engagement, networking, and continuous learning in shaping one's career and influence within the nursing profession. What are three ways you can apply what you have learned to your own education and future career path?

Summary

In essence, nurses who are seeking to develop or enhance their leadership skills and abilities would benefit from attending thoughtfully to those in their work and professional environments (e.g., as potential role models) and considering becoming involved in some type of formal leadership training program. In selecting such a program, one should look for opportunities to examine the complex phenomenon of leadership in depth, be certain one chooses carefully between leadership development and management training programs, and choose a program that provides opportunities to actually experience the role of leader; receive thoughtful, critical feedback on one's performance in that role; and receive guidance in building on areas of strength and developing areas of weakness. Potential and effective nurse leaders also would be best served by practicing in an environment that facilitates their development as leaders. The Case Study illustrates how one can purposefully pursue development as a leader, as well as how lack of planning can result in missed opportunities and delayed or limited development in the role.

ENVIRONMENTS THAT FACILITATE LEADERSHIP DEVELOPMENT

Aspiring leaders may not be in a position to create an environment that facilitates leadership development. However, they may be in a position to choose to practice and participate in such environments. What do such environments look like? What should nurses look for in such environments?

Much like those that promote creativity (see Chapter 7) and human develop-ment in general, environments that promote the development and enhancement of leadership skills and abilities are open, trusting, and dynamic. In such environ-ments, individuals feel free to raise questions about what is being done, how it is being done, why it is being done in a particular way, and why it is being done at all. Not only is a questioning attitude accepted, but it is also encouraged and expected.

Environments that promote the development of leadership do not maintain the status quo and do not put individuals into boxes, but they do encourage each person to reach their maximal potential. A spirit of competitiveness that constantly pushes members to achieve excellence may characterize the environment, but group members are not in competition with one another. Indeed, environments that facilitate the development of leadership recognize the strengths and talents of each member of the group; find ways to build on those strengths; and expect group members to guide, encourage, and support one another as they continue to grow. They are, in essence, environments in which leaders are allowed to emerge and followers are seen as valuable, contributing members of the team.

Individual members of the group are encouraged and expected to take risks and try new roles, even though they may fail. For example, a relatively new nurse may be asked to head up an ad hoc committee that is charged to look at how the work-ing relationships between licensed and unlicensed personnel can be enhanced. With the guidance and support of the nurse manager or more seasoned nurses in the unit, this new nurse would be expected to take the lead in working with group members to formulate the goals for this group, suggesting ways the group could go about achieving those goals; maintaining open communications with other nurses not directly involved in the project about the progress of the committee; and keep-ing the group focused on preparing a timely report that includes realistic, feasible recommendations for how working relationships can be enhanced. Along the way, this nurse may make some mistakes, but they have been provided with an oppor-tunity to develop leadership skills and to become a leader.

An environment that facilitates leadership development does not "recycle" the same people over and again, giving only a limited number of individuals an opportunity to grow. Although reusing previous leaders does allow organizations to make the best use of people who have proved themselves to be effective and ben-efit from the experience and history of these individuals, repeated recycling with limited opportunities for involvement of inexperienced nurses does not serve the profession well in the long run because it does little to contribute to the ongoing development of leaders.

Finally, a leadership development environment is characterized by good chan-nels of communication and a sense that all members are free to suggest ideas (e.g., they do not merely wait for the person in charge to generate ideas). Such an envi-ronment forces members to address issues of significance to them and the profes-sion, and it encourages the sharing of information, rather than the hoarding of it. The Leadership Environment Assessment Survey (Box 9-2) can be used to help analyze the extent to which one's work settings or professional organizations can facilitate the development of leadership.

BOX 9-2 Leadership Environment Assessment Survey

Think about your place of employment or a professional organization in which you are involved (e.g., your state nurses' association, your clinical specialty group, your local honor society). With that organization in mind, consider each of the following questions about the nature of the general environment or culture. YES responses to most questions suggest that the organization supports, encourages, and expects leadership among its members. NO responses to most questions may suggest that the organization's priorities do not include leadership development.

QUESTION	YES	NO
Is this organization open to new ideas and new ways of doing things?		
Do members of the organization feel free to raise questions about what is being done? How things are being done? Why things are being done at all? Why things are done in a particular way?		
Is a questioning attitude accepted, encouraged, and expected in the organization?		
Does the organization prevent putting individuals into "boxes"?		
Does the organization push members to strive for excellence?		
Is competition among group members healthy and productive?		
Are the strengths and talents of individual members recognized?		
Are the strengths and talents of individual members built upon?		
Are group members expected to guide, encourage, and support each other as they continue to grow?		
Are leaders allowed to emerge in the organization?		
Are followers seen as valuable, contributing members of the group?		
Are individual group members encouraged to take risks and try new things?		
Are mistakes accepted as part of the learning process for group members?		
Are different group members given opportunities to develop as leaders?		
Are channels of communication clear and open?		
Are group members allowed and encouraged to address issues that are of significance to them and the profession?		
Is information shared?		
Are accomplishments of group members acknowledged and rewarded?		

EMPOWERMENT

An environment that encourages, supports, and expects leadership development can be thought of as an empowering environment. Empowerment is a process through which individuals feel strengthened, in control, and in possession of some degree of power. It often is "given" by someone in a position of power or authority (e.g., a nurse manager, the home health agency supervisor), but it also can be "taken" by an individual.

Instead of using power over people, servant leaders inspire team efficacy by empowering and supporting followers (Zheng et al., 2024). Empowerment occurs when leaders encourage followers to take charge and be proactive instead of being fearful that such proactivity will result in the leader losing power. In fact, empowering followers to take charge and be proactive thinkers improves team dynamics and results in decreased workload and mental exhaustion of the leader (Zheng et al., 2024).

When someone in a position of power empowers others, it is through the sharing of that power. People are empowered by others when they are invited to participate in making decisions that will affect their lives, their work, and their futures. Rather than having "the boss" make all the decisions because "they know best," the people who will have to live with the consequences of decisions are involved in making them. It is clear that this model has relevance for the administrator–staff nurse relationship, but it also has relevance for the nurse–patient relationship, the teacher–student relationship, the parent–child relationship, and any other relationship in which one person typically has more power than others.

Nurses are empowered in their organizations when they are held accountable. Rather than being in a position in which blame can be placed on someone else or "the system" for less-than-ideal outcomes, empowered nurses know that the quality of care they deliver is their responsibility and that they are accountable for their actions and inactions. By being held accountable, nurses actually have more power in the practice arena.

Nurses are empowered when a shared governance or "shared leadership" (Broome & Marshall, 2021) model is in place. In this environment, nurses set their own schedules, formulate goals for their unit or agency, set standards of excellence, participate actively in peer review, and support one another. The structure is more open and interactive than limiting and hierarchical, and the success or failure of the group is the responsibility of all members, not only the nurse manager or supervisor. Such a model requires that nurses are adequately prepared to assume such responsibility and that there is a mix of skills and experiences in the group to implement the model most effectively.

Although we tend to think of empowerment as something someone in power does for those who have less power, that is far from the only means to empowerment. Nurses who find themselves in work or professional environments that are not designed to be empowering can still feel strengthened and in control by their own actions.

Empowerment or strength comes from a number of sources. Among the most significant of those sources is knowledge! Nurses empower themselves when they are knowledgeable and expert in their area of practice; when they know the structure, dynamics, and culture of the organizations in which they work; and when they know how to use resources effectively. They also empower themselves when they know themselves: their strengths and limitations, their values and biases, and what motivates them.

Empowerment also comes from having a sense of control over one's life. This may take the form of choosing where one will work; the level of excellence toward which one will strive, regardless, perhaps, of the standards held by others in the setting; and the degree to which one will accept being spoken down to, taken advantage of, bullied, or criticized unjustly. To some extent, it is related to self-esteem, self-worth, personal pride, and one's sense of identity.

Participating actively in one's work setting, professional association, or community also gives one a sense of having control over one's life and is empowering. By serving on committees, for example, nurses are in a better position to influence decisions that are made, and they are able to ensure that nursing's voice is heard; this is empowering. Holding office in a professional association or engaging actively in the debate of issues presented at a convention of that association is empowering because it gives nurses an opportunity to shape the future of the organization and, perhaps, the profession. Meeting with local legislators and community leaders about ways to enhance the resources available to children and the elderly in one's community is empowering because it reinforces one's ability to advocate for and help improve the lives of those who cannot speak for themselves.

Thus, empowerment need not occur only when someone in a position of power or authority decides to give some of that power away. Each nurse can take some power by their own actions. Perhaps one needs to return to school for an advanced degree, attend a workshop on assertiveness, volunteer to serve on a committee, run for political office, or review and reaffirm their values related to excellence and quality patient care. Perhaps one also can feel more empowered by entering into a relationship with a mentor.

MENTORING

Mentor was a figure in Greek mythology who served as the wise and faithful guardian and tutor of Telemachus during the 10-year absence of his father, Odysseus, who fought in and struggled to return home from the Trojan War. The words *mentor* and *mentoring*, therefore, typically refer to an experienced individual who befriends and guides a less-experienced individual.

Although the word *mentor* is often overused today—with anyone who shows the slightest interest in a person or offers the slightest amount of assistance being referred to as a "mentor"—a true mentor invests a great deal of time and effort in the advancement and growth of a protégé. Such a relationship is conscious, is purposefully designed, and typically extends over a number of years.

What Is a Mentor?

Mentors are close, trusted, experienced counselors or guides. They are accomplished and more experienced individuals, usually, but not always, in the same profession of the neophyte, and they offer neophytes advice, teach them, sponsor them, and guide them through significant points in their careers. As such, they help protégés establish themselves in the profession.

By serving as a mixture of good parent and good friend, mentors provide counsel during times of stress, encouragement during risk-taking endeavors, intellectual challenges, and assistance in the development and enhancement of professional skills. They encourage, cajole, test, teach by example, advise, model, act as a partner, sponsor, and give honest feedback, both positive and negative.

Mentors see some potential in a neophyte, which the neophyte often does not see in themselves, and then they do something about that potential. The "something" mentors do is commit themselves to the neophytes, often for a number of years: helping them develop a clearer professional identity, fostering their growth in personal and professional power, supporting and facilitating the realization of their dreams, and acting as an energizer and a sounding board.

Mentors also inspire neophytes and challenge them to achieve a level of professionalism they may not have known otherwise. By representing a point of development to which neophytes aspire, mentors invite their protégés into a new world, as peers and colleagues, and open doors for them. They help their protégés learn the ropes within a broadened community of colleagues so that they can sense the political climate, spot the behind-the-scenes actions, gain insights into the profession, expand their networks, and eventually spread their wings and fly.

Myths About Mentors and Mentoring

Mentoring often is thought of as a panacea for solving the problems of nurses in the healthcare arena or executives from underrepresented groups aspiring to climb the corporate ladder. Nurses, however, would be wise to be alert to a number of myths surrounding mentors and mentoring (Cantalupo, 2023):

- *Myth:* Being a mentor takes too much time. *Reality:* Mentoring is not as demanding as people assume it is, and one way to ensure time is well spent is to set expectations for the relationship and determine goals.
- *Myth:* Mentoring is a one-to-one relationship. *Reality:* Although one-to-one mentoring is certainly an option, other mentor relationships could be one-to-many (group) mentoring, mentoring circles, or reverse mentoring. A mentoring circle is a form of group mentoring that enables participants from various areas and experience levels to connect collaboratively and receive guidance from others in the group. Reverse mentoring involves the person with less experience mentoring the person with more experience and can facilitate connections across generations; promote diversity, equity, and inclusion; identify promising talent; and foster a culture of learning.
- *Myth:* Mentors have to be older and more experienced than the mentee. *Reality:* It is quite possible that the more experienced, accomplished individual in the relationship is younger chronologically. Mentorship is a symbiotic relationship in which a less experienced person may have insights or a creative perspective for the topic that can benefit a more seasoned individual. Mentorships should not reinforce power dynamics, but instead should foster growth and positive relationships.

- *Myth:* Only mentees benefit from the mentoring relationship.
  Reality: Many people wrongly assume that mentoring is a one-way benefit. However, the true benefit of mentoring is its potential to create collaborative relationships, enhance critical thinking, and develop mutually beneficial growth for both the mentor and the mentee.
- *Myth:* Mentoring is a feel-good thing, but it is not measurable.
  Reality: People may recollect how a mentor positively influenced them, but lack data to prove the benefit of the mentor relationship. However, it is possible to measure both qualitative and quantitative benefits of mentoring, including improved engagement, development, and retention.

Additionally, mentors and mentees should work to overcome myths surrounding "model behavior" and be culturally sensitive to racial and ethnic backgrounds (Vierra et al., 2024). The evolving leader would do well to be aware of these myths about mentoring, challenge them as needed, and not allow oneself to stop pursuit of such a relationship.

What Mentors Look for in Protégés/Mentees

Mentors and leaders look for novices who have the potential to move the profession ahead. They then invest the time, energy, and caring to create what they believe will be a future leader in the field. With this kind of investment expected of mentors, it is no wonder the mentor will choose a novice who shows they are worth investing in and are likely to show some measure of reward for the investment made.

Specifically, mentors often seek protégés who possess certain qualities. Box 9-3 presents characteristics that may serve as a guide to determine whether you are the kind of individual in whom a mentor might invest. In essence, mentors look for protégés who are beginning leaders or who have the potential to be leaders. They then work to help those individuals develop the knowledge, skills, and savvy needed to be effective leaders.

Mentors also look for protégés who, they believe, will "weather the storms" of the various stages of the relationship. Such stages have been named and described in various ways, but Clutterbuck's model (National Institute for Health and Care Research, 2022) provides a comprehensive understanding of five predictable phases:

Rapport-building: deciding whether there is a common group and desire to work together and negotiating expectations of the relationship
Directions-setting: achieving clarity about the goals of the mentorship and milestones for the mentee to achieve
Progress-making: working to achieve the goals through meetings, discussions, and suggestions—this is where most of the work of mentoring is done

---

BOX 9-3 What Mentors Look for in Protégés

Mentors often seek protégés who possess certain qualities. The following characteristics may serve as a guide to determine whether you are the kind of individual in whom a mentor might invest:

- Intelligence
- A self-starter: someone who is internally motivated
- Someone who is looking for new challenges
- Good interpersonal and communication skills: someone who is articulate
- A risk-taker
- A hard worker
- Someone who has and understands ideas and is always open to new perspectives and possibilities
- Integrity
- Someone who presents themselves professionally: in appearance, through the written word, and so on
- A sense of humor
- Someone who is willing to invest in themselves
- A curious mind: someone who asks questions and is not satisfied with the status quo
- Someone who has a vision: for themselves and for the profession

---

Winding-down: experiencing changes in the relationship as each individual evolves to a different point of development, has new goals, and seeks new opportunities

Moving-on: ending the formal relationship, though the mentor and protégé may remain colleagues or become professional friends

Caveats Regarding a Mentor Relationship

When considering entering a mentoring relationship, both individuals should consider the following caveats or "commandments" (Sandler, 1995):

- Be careful not to confuse a mentor relationship with a personal, emotional one.
- Many people can be mentors—you need not be at the top of your profession to be of assistance to novices.
- The protégé must take personal responsibility for learning.
- The mentor should not be expected to fulfill every need and meet every demand of the protégé.
- The confidences of the mentor must be respected.
- Expectations of both the mentor and protégé (e.g., time, type of assistance) need to be clarified early on in the relationship.
- Protégés should know if they are asking for too much, or too little, of the mentor.
- The feedback from the mentor to the protégé should take the form of praise and constructive criticism, with specific suggestions for improvement.
- The relationship should be used to open doors for future protégés.

- Mentors and protégés need not come from the same educational, ethnic, racial, religious, or any other type of background.
- Recognize that the relationship goes through stages (National Institute for Health and Care Research, 2022)—from dependence, uncertainty, and hesitancy to mutual give-and-take to termination or separation, at which point the protégé is more independent and identifies their separateness from the mentor.
- Be careful not to fall into mentoring because it's the thing to do or the "in" thing.

Benefits to the Protégé/Mentee

As described, mentoring is a special kind of relationship between two individuals that is intense, personalized, and long lasting and that has positive outcomes for both participants. Indeed, studies have documented several positive outcomes from engagement in a mentoring relationship.

In one of the first studies of "nurse influential," Vance (1977) found that 83% of the 71 individuals studied had mentors, and 93% of them were consciously aware of being mentors to others. A follow-up study (Kinsey, 1986) revealed similar findings—namely, that many of those nurses who were thought of as influentials in the profession had, themselves, been mentored by others and had served as mentors to novices.

A classic study of 1,250 top executives (Roche, 1979) revealed that almost two-thirds of those studied had mentors, and most mentoring relationships started when the protégé was in their 20s or 30s. Roche found that executives who had mentors moved into successful positions more quickly, earned more money at a younger age, were more likely to follow a personal career plan, were better educated, were more satisfied with their career progress, received greater pleasure from their work, and eventually sponsored protégés themselves.

In a more recent study of nurses transitioning to primary healthcare roles, junior members of the profession believed the mentor–mentee relationship was "invaluable," and development opportunities allowed for greater advancement and increased confidence (Cox et al., 2023). Additionally, mentors can help mentees navigate internal organizational structures and processes, research, and developing professional networks (Todoran, 2023). Thus, one can conclude that engaging in a mentoring relationship is beneficial to the protégé/mentee.

Benefits to the Mentor, Organization, and Profession

Although it may sound as if the only person who benefits from a mentor relationship is the protégé, nothing could be further from the truth. Indeed, mentoring is a mutually supportive, mutually beneficial relationship in which the mentor also gains a great deal. In their mixed method design, related to the mentor's perspective on the mentor–protégé relationship, Rossiter et al. (2024) concluded that in addition to guiding and challenging protégés to grow personally and professionally, mentors themselves experience positive impacts on their practice (e.g., reading more in the field), personal satisfaction, professional success, and a sense of contributing significantly to the organization and profession. Organizations can also benefit through cost savings from staff retention and satisfaction, along with improved clinical outcomes and patient satisfaction that result from a well-developed nursing staff (Anderson, 2024).

The strength of mentors comes from their own professional experience, self-worth, and autonomy. They must be capable of motivating neophytes to be creative and possess a good sense of their own creative selves. They also must be careful not to direct or control every facet of their protégé's life, and they must be open and willing to learn from the protégé.

As individuals engage in this evolving relationship, the protégé often pursues more sophisticated lines of investigation, develops skills the mentor may not possess, and establishes new networks. The mentor who is open to and willing to learn from a protégé will grow enormously from the relationship.

It is incredibly rewarding for mentors to see novice clinicians, educators, researchers, administrators, and leaders grow and evolve. In many cases, the accomplishments of the mentees far surpass those of the mentors, and mentors take great pride in seeing their protégés receive awards, make changes in practice, receive offers of significant positions, be elected to office in professional associations, receive competitive grants, receive major awards for their contributions, and publish articles or books that influence others.

Increasingly, scholars are recognizing that the mentoring relationship is mutually rewarding and results in growth in both the mentor and the protégé. In addition to the personal growth one experiences, both individuals expand their networks of professional colleagues and "influentials."

Summary

Because this relationship is mutually beneficial, those who are more junior in the field may need to take the initiative to seek out those in the field who have the expertise, experience, networks, and scholarly agendas that align with their own career goals. They can call or write to those whose published work they admire or whose research matches their own interests; approach such individuals at conferences; suggest such individuals as consultants at their place of employment or as speakers at conferences they are involved in planning—and then use those opportunities to connect with the more experienced individual to point out common interests, talk about their career goals, and explore the possibility of a mentor relationship. Likewise, those who are more senior in the field may need to seek out those more junior whose passions are aligned with their own professional work and who have the potential to make significant contributions to the organization or field, or to respond positively when more junior colleagues come forward (as noted earlier) and suggest a mentoring relationship. This kind of reaching out and responding to nurse colleagues is a hallmark of mentors and effective protégés.

In her book designed to guide nurses as they embark on the road to leadership, Huston (2018) asserts that the first leadership lesson individuals need to learn is "the importance of finding a mentor and positive role models to guide [them] on [their] professional journ[ies]" (p. 2). She shares personal experiences as a protégé and as a mentor, noting that "having a mentor is only valuable . . . if the relationship is honest and constructive" (p. 3). Thus, there continues to be evidence to support the value of mentoring, including the networking opportunities that are typically part of such a relationship.

NETWORKING

As noted, a mentoring relationship can help both participants develop contacts and expand their professional networks, networks they may call on throughout their careers for assistance, support of ideas, and guidance. Although some take offense at the idea of "using" people to one's benefit, the whole concept of networking is built on the assumption that who one knows is important and can be helpful.

Networks form for the purpose of providing access to contacts, referrals, information, support, feedback, understanding, and empathy. They also can serve to help nurses maintain a social and professional identity and provide a means of working toward organizational, professional, or societal reform.

Nurses might tap into their networks when they are looking for a guest speaker for a program, a consultant, someone to fill a key position in an organization, someone to nominate for appointment to a community board, or an expert in a clinical area. They might also use their networks to gather data about practices in other institutions that can help advance a proposal for a change in their own settings. Thus, networks serve a number of useful purposes, without the sustained, intense investment of a mentor relationship.

Does everyone need a mentor to make it and get ahead? No, but most people do need guides, support systems, sounding boards, and peer "pals" to help during certain times throughout their careers, and this is where one's network can be most effective.

Peer "pals" may help one another manage a particularly difficult community health problem or deal with an arrogant physician. *Guides* know easier ways to do something or have experienced a particular situation and share those insights with others. For example, nurses who are enrolled in a master's program may serve as guides to colleagues who are in the process of deciding whether they should pursue graduate education and, if so, what school to attend and what specialty to pursue. Nurses who have particularly good writing skills may review and critique an abstract before it is submitted in response to a call for presentation at a conference or a manuscript before it is submitted to a journal for review. *Sponsors* act on behalf of others, promote them, and advance them, much the same way a mentor does, but in more isolated instances, rather than over a lengthy period of time. For example, a faculty member may nominate a graduate for an award or suggest that graduate as a candidate for office in a professional association. All these are examples of a patron-type system in which nurses "use" their networks but do not necessarily enter into an extended, intense mentoring relationship.

Networks—both formal and informal (Broome & Marshall, 2021)—are most effective to enhance one's development as a leader. Nurses should be cautious not to fall into the trap of believing myths such as the following: networking is only for extroverts; networking is important only when you are looking for a new job; networking is something you do only outside your own organization and community;

networking is an idea that is no longer relevant in the age of social media and the Internet; and networking is relevant to managers and executives, but not to those who are not in such positions (Tandon, 2024). Instead, we need to broaden our web of professional contacts and use those contacts to help us face and manage difficult situations, grow professionally, and develop as leaders.

CONCLUSION

The development of leadership knowledge and skills throughout one's career requires (1) purposeful, goal-directed action; (2) honest, extensive self-assessment; (3) a willingness to ask for assistance or guidance; and (4) a willingness to accept help or guidance when it is offered. It is enhanced by the development and effective use of professional networks, as well as by engagement in mentoring relationships.

Regardless of their role, their level of education, or their scope of practice, nurses who are in positions of influence must take on the responsibility of coaching other promising nurses. Those seeking to be more influential and to become leaders must start early to seek experiences and colleagues—and possibly mentors—who will provide the professional and personal nourishment necessary for success. They must identify the people who are in a position to help, let them know they respect their ability, and seek their support. They also must convey to those who are in a position to help that they have something to gain by helping, guiding, and possibly mentoring them.

Each nurse must create a personal plan for leadership development throughout their career and then take responsibility for implementing that plan and documenting the results of various actions, perhaps through maintaining a professional portfolio. Such a plan may include advancing formal education or enrolling in courses or workshops that will help develop a better understanding of the phenomenon of leadership or enhance specific skills, such as assertiveness or public speaking. It may include looking for a work setting or professional association that is empowering or one in which strong role models exist. One's personal plan for leadership development may incorporate seeking a mentor, expanding professional networks, becoming more involved in the political process, running for office in one's specialty organization, submitting a manuscript for publication, or responding to a call for paper presentations at a regional or national conference.

Whatever the specific course of action, nurses will develop as leaders through a well-thought-out plan, and not through the waving of some magic wand. Taking responsibility is a large part of what leadership is all about, and such responsibility grows out of honest self-assessment about one's leadership abilities and potentials, as well as positive, focused action. Taking responsibility for one's own development as a leader is an excellent way to achieve professional goals, realize visions, and shape a preferred future for the nursing profession.

Leaders also are responsible for developing other leaders. Leadership in nursing is about creating future leaders. Nursing students and nursing leaders can work together to co-create a succession plan to engage innovative nursing leaders who can meet the challenges of the current healthcare climate to enhance the quality of patient care and advance the nursing profession (Parniawski et al., 2024).

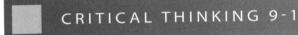

CRITICAL THINKING 9-1

1. Read at least three journal editorials. To what extent do these individuals express controversial ideas and convey a passion about their topic? Do you see any differences in the uniqueness of perspective, challenging nature of the ideas put forth, or passion expressed by those writing the editorials? What can you learn from this comparison about the nature of risk-taking that is inherent in a leadership role? If you were given the opportunity to write a controversial editorial for a prominent nursing journal, what would you write about? How would you express your ideas? Who would you ask to review your manuscript before you submitted it?

2. Complete the Leadership Environment Assessment Survey (see Box 9-2). To what extent does your organization provide an environment that promotes leadership? What can you do to make your environment more conducive to the development of leadership skills?

3. Review the discussion about what mentors look for in a protégé. How do you rate in each of the areas listed? What assets do you think you would bring to a mentoring relationship?

4. List the qualities you would like to see in your mentor. Whom do you know—in your immediate environment, from your educational program, in your specialty organization, in your local community, through your professional readings—who possesses all or most of those qualities? Consider making contact with that person to discuss the possibility of establishing a mentoring relationship.

5. The next time you attend a professional conference or convention or attend a meeting or event in your own organization, make it a point to meet at least three new colleagues. Talk to each one about their interests, areas of expertise, goals, current position, and so on. You also should be prepared to tell them about your goals, interests, and areas of expertise. Exchange contact information with each new colleague; note pertinent information about the individual, along with when and where you met the individual, and file it when you return home. This will help you build your professional network.

6. Reflect on the "results" of the assessments you completed earlier and any other tools you have found. What areas repeatedly emerge as strengths? How can you use those to develop as a leader throughout your career? In what areas do you need to develop? What will you do to overcome those limitations and enhance your leadership potential?

7. Write your personal career goals: What position would you like to hold 25 years from now? What types of offices would you like to hold? What awards would you like to have won or honors to have been bestowed on you? What types of books or articles would you like to have published? What would you like to be known for in the nursing profession? How influential would you like to be on the local, national, and international levels? Think big! Now, for each goal, list the types of actions you will need to take in order to achieve that goal and plot a timeline for each action. For example, if you would like to publish an article in the *Journal of Nursing Scholarship*, you may want

to take an intensive writing course and carefully read the articles published in that journal during the past 5 years to better understand the nature of what is published and its format. Take a paper you wrote for school or a difficult, challenging patient case study you presented at rounds and rewrite it to fit the guidelines of that journal; then submit it to a former faculty member or a trusted colleague at work for critique and comment. Talk to other nurses who have published in the *Journal of Nursing Scholarship* or other prestigious journals about their experience breaking into the publication arena and seek a mentor to assist you with writing for publication.

References

American Association of Colleges of Nursing. (2021). *The essentials: Core competencies for professional nursing education.* https://www.aacnnursing.org/Portals/0/PDFs/Publications/Essentials-2021.pdf

Anderson, S. (2024). A nurse anesthesiology mentorship program: An evidence-based project for implementation. *AANA Journal, 92*(1), 57–62. https://pubmed.ncbi.nlm.nih.gov/38289688/

Bernhardt, J. M., Sipe, M. H., Tagliareni, M. E., O'Brien, L. B., Donati, C., & Evans, L. A. (2023). Leadership in nursing education for advancing a school of nursing-led center for climate change, climate justice, and health. *Journal of Nursing Education, 62*(9), 528–531. https://doi.org/10.3928/01484834-20230509-10

Booher, L., Yates, E., Claus, S., Haight, K., & Burchill, C. N. (2021). Leadership self-perception of clinical nurses at the bedside: A qualitative descriptive study. *Journal of Clinical Nursing, 30*(11–12), 1573–1583. https://doi.org/10.1111/jocn.15705

Broome, M. E., & Marshall, E. S. (2021). *Transformational leadership in nursing: From expert clinician to influential leader* (3rd ed.). Springer.

Cantalupo, G. (2023, April 20). Top five myths about employee mentoring. *Forbes.* https://www.forbes.com/sites/forbescommunicationscouncil/2023/04/20/top-five-myths-about-employee-mentoring/?sh=553447595c02

Cox, R., Robinson, T., Rossiter, R., Collison, L., & Hills, D. (2023). Nurses transitioning to primary health care in Australia: A practice improvement initiative. *SAGE Open Nursing, 9.* doi:10.1177/23779608231165695

Dopelt, K., Shevach, I., Vardimon, O. E., Czabanowska, K., De Nooijer, J., Otok, R., Leighton, L., Bashkin, O., Duplaga, M., Levine, H., MacLeod, F., Malowany, M., Okenwa-Emegwa, L., Zelber-Sagi, S., Davidovitch, N., & Barach, P. (2023). Simulation as a key training method for inculcating public health leadership skills: A mixed methods study. *Frontiers in Public Health, 11*, 1202598. https://doi.org/10.3389/fpubh.2023.1202598

Egan, J. D. (2024). Why games for leadership? *Journal of Leadership Studies, 17*(4), 27–31.

Frilund, M., Fagerstrøm, L., & Vasset, F. (2023). The challenges of change processes for nurse leaders—A qualitative study of long-term leaders' experiences over 25 years. *Nursing Open, 10*(8), 5423–5432. https://doi.org/10.1002/nop2.1781

Houser, B. P., & Player, K. N. (2004). *Pivotal moments in nursing: Leaders who changed the path of a profession* (Vol. 1). Sigma Theta Tau International.

Houser, B. P., & Player, K. N. (2007). *Pivotal moments in nursing: Leaders who changed the path of a profession* (Vol. 2). Sigma Theta Tau International.

Huston, C. J. (2018). *The road to leadership.* Sigma Theta Tau International.

Institute of Medicine. (2021). *The future of nursing 2020–2030: Charting a path to achieve health equity.* The National Academies Press. https://doi.org/10.17226/25982

Kelley, R. (1992). *The power of followership: How to create leaders people want to follow and followers who lead themselves.* Doubleday Currency.

Kinsey, D. C. (1986). The new nurse influentials. *Nursing Outlook, 34*(5), 238–240.

Lasley, J. (2024), Role-playing games as a new adventure for leadership-as-practice: Forming a leadership framework around collective creativity and development. *Journal of Leadership Studies, 17*(4), 47–55. https://doi-org/10.1002/jls.21876

Leal, L. A., Silva, A. T., Ignácio, D. S., Soares, M. I., Ribeiro, N. M., & Henriques, S. H. (2022). Educational strategy to develop nursing students' management competencies in hospital practice. *Revista Brasileira de Enfermagem, 75*(6), e20210928. https://doi.org/10.1590/0034-7167-2021-0928

National Institute for Health and Care Research. (2022). *Maintaining momentum in the mentoring relationship.* https://www.nihr.ac.uk/documents/Maintaining-momentum-in-the-mentoring-relationship/32283#:~:text=Typically%2C%20mentoring%20relationships%20broadly%20transition,they%20can%20work%20productively%20together

Parniawski, P., Simonette, P., Green, C., Jacovino, E., Boyd, B., Antonino, K., & Ashman, A. (2024). The succession plan: Using competency-based curriculums to educate a new generation of nurse leaders. *Teaching and Learning in Nursing, 19*(1), 86–90. https://doi.org/10.1016/j.teln.2023.09.019

Rath, T. (2009). *Strengths based leadership: Great leaders, teams, and why people follow.* Gallup Press.

Raza, T., Ali, S. A., & Majeed, M. U. (2024). Transformational leadership and project success: The roles of social capital and self-efficacy. *International Journal of Management Studies, 31*(1), 335–371. https://doi.org/10.32890/ijms2024.31.1.12

Roche, G. R. (1979). *Much ado about mentors.* Harvard Business Review. https://hbr.org/1979/01/much-ado-about-mentors

Rossiter, R., Robinson, T., Cox, R., Collison, L., & Hills, D. (2024). Mentors supporting nurses transitioning to primary healthcare roles: A practice improvement initiative. *SAGE Open Nursing, 10,* 23779608241231174. https://doi.org/10.1177/23779608241231174

Rozimela, Y., Fatimah, S., & Fudhla, N. A. (2024). Contextualized reflective practice model: Responding to EFL teachers' needs. *Asia-Pacific Education Research.* https://doi.org/10.1007/s40299-024-00821-w

Ruben, B. D., De Lisi, R., & Gigliotti, R. A. (2023). *A guide for leaders in higher education: Concepts, competencies, and tools* (2nd ed.). Routledge

Saeed, I., Khan, J., Zada, M., & Zada, S. (2024). Employee sensemaking in organizational change via knowledge management: Leadership role as a moderator. *Current Psychology, 43,* 6657–6671. https://doi.org/10.1007/s12144-023-04849-x

Sandler, B. R. (1995). Women as mentors: Myths and commandments. *Educational Horizons, 73*(3), 105–107. https://www.jstor.org/stable/42925924

Tandon, R. (2024, March 11). Myth debunking 101—"Networking is only for extroverts." *The Economic Times.* https://economictimes.indiatimes.com/jobs/fresher/myth-debunking-101-networking-is-only-for-extroverts/articleshow/108383114.cms?from=mdr

Todoran, G. S. (2023). The contribution of formal and informal mentorship to faculty productivity: Views of faculty in public affairs programs. *Journal of Public Affairs Education, 29*(4), 404–420. https://doi.org/10.1080/15236803.2023.2220096

Vance, C. N. (1977). *A group profile of contemporary influentials in American nursing* [Unpublished doctoral dissertation]. Teachers College, Columbia University.

Vierra, K. D., Beltran, D. R., Denecker, L., & Robnett, R. D. (2024). "Research mentors should support students of color by taking an extra step." Undergraduates' reasoning about race and STEM research mentorship. *Education Sciences, 14*(2), 162. https://doi.org/10.3390/educsci14020162

Vuorivirta-Vuoti, E., Kuha, S., & Kanste, O. (2023). Nurse leaders' perceptions of future leadership in hospital settings in the post-pandemic era: A qualitative descriptive study. *Leadership in Health Services, 37*(5), 33–48. https://doi.org/10.1108/LHS-05-2023-0032

Yoon, H. J., Song, J. H., Donahue, W. E., & Woodley, K. K. (2010). Leadership Competency Inventory: A systematic process of developing and validating a leadership competency scale. *Journal of Leadership Studies, 4*(3), 39–50.

Zhao, X., Ren, Y., & Cheah, K. S. L. (2023). Leading virtual reality (VR) and augmented reality (AR) in education: Bibliometric and content analysis from the web of science (2018–2022). *Sage Open, 13*(3). https://doi.org/10.1177/21582440231190821

Zheng, G. G., Zhou, Y., & Wu, W. (2024). Followers matter: Understanding the emotional exhaustion of servant leadership. *Applied Psychology, 73*(1), 215–239. https://doi.org/10.1111/apps.12473

CHAPTER 10

Leadership, Excellence, and Professional Involvement
Essential Components to Creating the
Future for Nursing

LEARNING OBJECTIVES
• Analyze the concept of excellence.
• Discuss the responsibility for promoting excellence that rests with leaders who will create the future for nursing.
• Examine the interrelationships among leadership, excellence, and professional involvement.
• Propose strategies related to leadership, excellence, and professional involvement that influence the creation of the future for nursing.

INTRODUCTION

One of the responsibilities of those leaders who will create the future for nursing is to promote excellence. Every nursing professional is responsible for striving for excellence in their practice and delivering safe, quality healthcare to consumers. However, those professionals who take on the leadership responsibility to create the future for nursing—a future that acknowledges and takes full advantage of the myriad talents nurses bring to the healthcare arena—must have an even greater commitment and take deliberate action to promote excellence.

This chapter examines the concept of excellence in depth. Excellence is then related to leadership, and the role of leaders in advancing the notion of excellence

193

is explored. Finally, both concepts—excellence and leadership—are blended with professional involvement throughout one's career to promote nursing and create the future for our profession.

> *In all that you do, reflect the excellence that's in you.*
> —*Dr. Martin Luther King Jr.*

The case study presented in this chapter depicts an individual's nursing career. Referring back to the case study as the concept of excellence is discussed and as it is related to leadership and professional involvement should help the reader understand those ideas.

Case Study

ADRIENNE'S CAREER TRACK: STAFF NURSE TO NURSE MANAGER

Adrienne has been a staff nurse for 8 years at the local community hospital. She recently completed a baccalaureate program in nursing and now holds the position of nurse manager in a 30-bed telemetry unit in the area's medical center. As a nurse manager, Adrienne aims to lead the unit efficiently and provide optimal patient care. Adrienne believes that a cohesive and motivated team is vital to achieving the unit's goals. Despite her efforts, she notices that during mandatory management team meetings, several team members appear disengaged and are reluctant to contribute or share new ideas. This lack of engagement is concerning to Adrienne, especially as a new leader.

REFLECTION QUESTIONS

1. What initial steps should Adrienne take to understand the team members' disengagement during meetings?
2. What are some ways Adrienne may foster a more engaging environment for the team?
3. As a new leader, what are some resources Adrienne should consider to improve her overall leadership ability?

THE CONCEPT OF EXCELLENCE

Excellence is a common word in our personal and professional sectors.

- The American Nurses Association (ANA) promotes excellence in clinical practice and offers the Magnet designation to acknowledge excellence in nursing practice environments.
- The National League for Nursing (NLN) promotes excellence in nursing education and invites nursing schools to apply for a Center of Excellence in Nursing Education designation.
- Sigma Theta Tau International advances excellence in scholarship and presents biennial awards recognizing excellence in practice, research, education, technology, communications, and leadership/ professionalism.
- Most colleges and universities claim excellence regarding their program offerings, faculty complement, student accomplishments, and facilities.

However, just what is excellence? Moreover, what is meant by this often-used but little-examined concept?

Excellence means striving to be the best you can be in everything you do—not because some teacher, parent, or other authority figure pushes you to do it, but because you cannot imagine functioning in any other way. It means setting high standards for yourself and the groups in which you are involved, holding yourself to those standards despite challenges or pressures to reduce or lower them, and not being satisfied with anything less than the best.

This kind of perspective or approach applies to all spheres of life—providing care to elderly patients in a long-term care facility, teaching school-aged children about good nutrition or sexually transmitted infections, completing assignments for a course, preparing for a final examination, driving a vehicle, or working to secure more resources for underserved populations. Individuals committed to excellence do not—and will not—settle for mediocre performance or merely getting by.

When we allow ourselves and the systems in which we function to be minimally adequate, we sell ourselves short and do little to advance the profession of nursing and ensure the quality of care for patients, families, and communities. We fail to be challenged, grow, make change, and help others develop. Excellence means not allowing this state of affairs to exist!

Excellence also means being unwilling to accept the status quo. In a classic test, Wergin (2003) argued that the "most useful way to build and sustain a culture of excellence is to create a culture of critical reflection and continuous improvement" (p. xiii), sentiments that remain relevant today. Critical reflection, however, does not mean that all one does is criticize how things are being done and then walk away, hoping that someone else will correct what is wrong. Instead, individuals who strive for and expect excellence question and challenge the status quo; engage in critical conversations about current practices; examine the assumptions that underlie existing practices; and offer thoughtful, realistic, and evidence-based alternatives for how things could be done in other ways. More importantly, they are willing to invest time and energy to implement those alternatives, evaluate their effectiveness, and orchestrate change so the new approaches become integral to the system. A new, preferred future can be shaped.

Excellence means to excel, to surpass, and to be the best. Excellence is not an impossible dream. In fact, if we look at just what excellence is, we see it is not so foreign or so unattainable. Many people have written about excellence, but the description of that concept offered by Diers and Evans (1980) many years ago is still particularly helpful. These authors said that excellence involves several things:

- *Discipline:* drawing on our knowledge and experience to practice in a systematic way that is of the highest caliber
- *Choreography:* successfully balancing competing demands in our pursuit of goals
- *Responsibility:* acknowledging what we have done well or poorly and blaming no one

- *Caring:* consistently demonstrating a concern and a compassion for others (including our colleagues) and for ourselves
- *Skepticism:* keeping a proper distance from what is thought to be the truth and not accepting everything blindly; keeping our minds open to new ideas, new information, and new approaches
- *Perseverance:* continually striving to fulfill a goal or realize a vision
- *Passion:* the essence of excellence; being inflamed by our work

Diers and Evans (1980) said, "Excellent nurses are inflamed by nursing. . . . To be an excellent nurse is to be suffused with a deep and almost inexpressible passion for humankind" (p. 30).

The rapid development and distribution of the COVID-19 vaccine exhibited this passion for humankind. During the onset of the pandemic, the race to develop a vaccine against COVID-19 quickly began as the virus swept across the globe (Marcus et al., 2021). As nurses and healthcare leaders planned for the education about and distribution of the vaccine to local communities, particularly in rural and underserved areas, this led to a global effort to prevent the spread of the virus and save lives. These efforts saved countless lives and contributed to global vaccination campaigns and public education efforts.

Business guru W. Edwards Deming was inspired by Foster's quote and used it as a foundation to outline 14 key principles that, although directed toward managers who wished to transform business effectiveness, have relevance for our discussion and understanding of excellence. Among the points made by Deming (1986) almost 40 years ago but that still have relevance today (Deming, 2024) are the following:

- Create constancy of purpose toward improvement, with the aim to become competitive.
- Awaken to the challenge, learn responsibilities, and take on leadership for change.
- Cease dependence on inspection to achieve quality . . . build quality in from the start.
- Constantly and forever improve the system.
- Institute leadership . . . help people and systems do a better job.
- Remove barriers that rob individuals of their right to pride in workmanship.
- Institute a vigorous program of education and self-improvement.
- Create a climate where all participants collaborate to accomplish the transformation.

A commitment to pursuing excellence does not just happen; it does not just randomly occur. Doing whatever it is that must be done requires ongoing attention that is initiated and maintained by top management in an organization. In fact, Deming (1986, 2024) advocated that extensive training was needed to help everyone develop the courage that would be needed to break with tradition and to excel because pursuing excellence—just like taking on leadership responsibilities—is risky and requires courage.

Management recruits individuals committed to excellence and to consistently producing exceptional work. However, achieving excellence and a sense of accomplishment occurs only with individual investment. Executive leadership and the organization can do only so much. What each of us needs to remember is that every job is a self-portrait of the person who did it. Therefore, each of us needs to autograph *our* work with excellence. *Pursuing* excellence must be vigorously and relentlessly incorporated into everything we think, say, and do. The individual who autographs their work with excellence does not ignore or forget the little things, just as they do not forget the big things. Each of us who hopes to make a significant contribution to our organization, our profession, our community, or the world needs to make this commitment. The quality of our lives will be enhanced as a result.

As mentioned earlier, excellence needs to be a way of life, and for those who do make it a habit, it sets up a vicious cycle. In other words, excellence begets excellence—for ourselves and for those around us. Striving for excellence is highly contagious because peer pressure and collegial influence have powerful effects and they can usually do more than management ever could. Dr. Beverly Malone, president and chief executive officer (CEO) of the National League for Nursing, is one of the nation's leading healthcare executives and champions for pursuing excellence in nursing and beyond (National League for Nursing, 2024). Dr. Malone asserts that if you have colleagues who are co-creating with you, they will help give you a lift up, but you cannot do it all by yourself (Alonso, 2022).

In 2006, Peters and Waterman reflected on the eight attributes of excellence they outlined in their seminal 1982 book on the topic. They acknowledged all the work related to excellence that they and others had done and recognized that while others might outline a different set of attributes, the eight they presented initially are still relevant. The attributes are as follows: exhibit a bias for action, stay close to those you are serving in order to best understand their needs, articulate clear goals and allow those in the organization the autonomy to use their talents to meet them, treat everyone with respect, be clear about your values and use them to drive all you do, stay focused, minimize unnecessary complexity so that things can get done, and allow for flexibility (Peters & Waterman, 2024).

Excellence is relevant not only to the individual or a particular unit but also to an entire organization. In an article in which they propose institutional policies to foster civility, Clark and Ritter (2018) discuss the need to strive toward excellence in how all members treat and interact with one another. They acknowledge the following outcomes of workplace incivility, which include disrespectful behaviors exhibited by individuals as well as the failure of others in the system to address those behaviors: psychological or physiological distress, decrease in work effort and quality of work, decline in commitment to the organization, taking out frustrations on others, and high turnover rates. Thus, all those in an organization have the responsibility for creating and sustaining healthy work environments that strive for excellence, and it is essential, according to these authors, to have clear policies about how uncivil behavior is addressed and the consequences should it occur.

Clark (2022) states, "As nurses and leaders, we must courageously address the urgent need to foster civil, inclusive, healthy work and learning environments so that all members may prosper and thrive" (p. 1). The direct link between healthy work environments and nursing satisfaction and retention is undeniable. Employees are more likely to reciprocate respectful behaviors when the work environment demonstrates concern and commitment to them (Memon et al., 2021).

Finally, the Magnet Recognition Program of the American Nurses Credentialing Center needs to be acknowledged as an ongoing initiative designed to identify healthcare facilities that have a commitment to quality improvement, especially in terms of nursing care delivery. It reflects the following key principles, all of which can be thought of as describing excellence: transformational leadership, structural empowerment, exemplary professional practice, and new knowledge, innovations, and improvements. The impact of a work environment that expects excellence continues to be supported by Magnet recognition for healthcare facilities.

Excellence comes from within, and improves our personal investment. If staff tolerate mediocrity in what they do, practice will be mediocre. Management can create an environment that expects, fosters, and rewards excellence, but it is only when each individual in the organization can honestly say that they have done their very best that excellence will occur.

Unless we try to do something beyond what we have already mastered, we will never flourish. Excellence, therefore, involves knowing and challenging ourselves—accepting challenges that are offered to us (e.g., writing a grant proposal, pursuing advancement through our agency's clinical levels, facilitating a research project, or accepting an invitation to speak at a professional meeting or to the media). Excellence also involves seeking new experiences (e.g., asking to serve on a committee, agreeing to have our name placed on a ballot for election to a committee or office, assuming new responsibilities with cross-training, submitting an abstract in response to a call for papers, or revising the new edition of a textbook). Excellence is not allowing ourselves to get too comfortable or too complacent or so wrapped up in our own world that we lose this broader perspective. No one ever attains eminent success by simply doing what is required. It is the amount and excellence of what is done above and beyond that determines the greatness of ultimate distinction.

The organizations and professions that will make a difference—to the recipients of their services and to those providing the services—are the ones that prize the absolute best at every level. Such organizations need effective leaders, and in healthcare, nurses—as front-line care providers—are primed to take on this responsibility. It has been said that only those who dare to fail greatly can ever achieve greatly. In other words, it is only when we strive for excellence that we will achieve it. In that process, we may fail; therefore, taking risks is a critical component of achieving excellence.

LEADERSHIP AND EXCELLENCE

Just as excellence is a complex phenomenon, so too is leadership. As noted, Burns (1978, p. 2), in a classic work on the topic, asserted, "Leadership is one of the most observed and least understood phenomena on earth." This assertion was reiterated by Richardson (2000), who noted that "leadership has often escaped precise definition, yet we respect its power to transform and are quickly able to sense its absence" (p. v). Despite a lack of full understanding, however, many elements of leadership are universal, elements that have already been addressed but that bear reviewing.

First, there is agreement that, unlike management, *leadership is not necessarily tied to a position of authority in an organization.* In other words, there is a need for and opportunities to function as a leader at every level of every organization, society, and institution. One can be a leader as a staff nurse or as a student, just as well as if one is a nurse manager, the vice president for nursing, a faculty member, a dean, or the president of a professional association. In fact, it may be easier to be a leader if one is not in a position of authority because then one is not expected to promote any given agenda, and it may be easier for the person to raise difficult questions, articulate a bold vision, and work toward changing the system.

Second, *leadership is a relationship of influence* more than a relationship of authority. People follow leaders by choice, not because they are required to do so.

Perhaps one of the most essential characteristics of leaders is that *leaders have a vision;* they see new possibilities, new horizons, and different options. They have some notion of circumstances being able to be better than they are now, regardless of how good they are now. In addition, this vision is their cause or purpose in life, and they are willing to invest enormous amounts of energy to see it realized. Think again about Dr. Martin Luther King Jr., who worked all his life for racial equality and the peaceful resolution of differences. Mother Teresa devoted her life to helping people experiencing poverty and disenfranchisement. Many others have envisioned a better world and worked to see it materialize. We must ask if we are leaders—if we have a vision of a better world.

In accord with this drive toward realizing a vision, *leaders are change agents.* They are innovators who continually challenge the status quo, make new initiatives known, and take the risk of being rejected. They strive to keep people and organizations inspired and moving forward. Again, each of us must ask ourselves if we are leaders—if we work toward positive change. If leaders are going to be agents of change, they also must be *comfortable with conflict.* Leaders must be able and willing to navigate conflict, introduce it if necessary, and use it to achieve the group's goals. They do not always want to minimize or eliminate conflict because they know that conflict is healthy and promotes growth in individuals and organizations. Ask yourself if you are a leader—if you can manage the conflict we face in our daily and professional lives.

Leaders are *willing to use intuition* in making decisions, they are *comfortable with ambiguity and uncertainty,* and they are *creative.* They want to see new forms take shape and do not need to rely on predictability or rationality. They *see the big picture,* are *effective communicators,* and *want to collaborate* with others to achieve goals rather than having a narrow, limited, self-centered interest or focus. Each of us needs to ask ourselves if we are leaders, if we are creative, if we can tolerate uncertainty, and if we can look beyond our needs.

Finally, leaders are *characterized by excellence,* and they work to promote excellence in themselves and others. Driven by their vision, they strive to be the best they can be, and they inspire others to do the same. Dissatisfied with the status quo, they take risks, try innovative approaches, call on their creativity, and work to co-create change. Energized by a desire to continue to grow and learn, they seek new opportunities, take on challenges, and know how to manage conflict. Appreciative of the diverse and complex world in which we live, they do not allow themselves to become too highly specialized or too narrowly focused.

PROFESSIONAL INVOLVEMENT

When one thinks about the history of Sigma Theta Tau International, the Honor Society of Nursing, or the interdisciplinary Honor Society of Phi Kappa Phi, one is inspired by what could be characterized as authentic leadership and actual excellence. Sigma Theta Tau was started in 1922 by six nursing students who wanted to create some way to recognize and acknowledge nursing scholarship. Phi Kappa Phi was started in 1897 by one young individual who dreamed of scholars from all disciplines being recognized on college campuses to the same extent that athletes were recognized. Those six nursing students and that one young individual each had a vision; they banded together and enlisted the support of others; they took action and worked tirelessly, and they formed two of the most prestigious honor societies in our country.

Today, these organizations have hundreds of chapters and thousands of members. They are dedicated to scholarship and leadership (in the case of Sigma Theta Tau) and to promoting academic excellence (in the case of Phi Kappa Phi). They are proactive and forward-looking. Sigma Theta Tau is international in scope and purpose. Each organization is clear about its purpose, focused in its efforts; and highly regarded, well respected, and emulated. All of this from a handful of students who saw a need, had a vision, believed in excellence, and exercised leadership.

Members of Sigma Theta Tau are among the most influential innovators in our field. A historical context demonstrates this influence: Dorothy Brooten's research on the effects of nursing care on low-birth-weight infants who have been discharged early from the neonatal intensive care unit to home has received accolades from the nursing and medical professions. Lois Evans and Neville Strumpf's extensive work on restraint-free care of older adults has humanized that care in countless ways. Imogene King's contributions in theory development have been significant in advancing the science of nursing. Melanie Dreher's commitment to advancing the concept of clinical scholarship has been influential in helping nurses in practice develop more significant insights into their practice and be creative in where and how they deliver quality care. Mary Naylor's pioneering work in the design, evaluation, and spread of healthcare innovations has significantly improved the outcomes of chronically ill older adults and their family caregivers, while reducing healthcare costs. Dan Pesut's writings about the future have opened the minds of many. And the late Virginia Henderson helped us crystallize the professional nursing role in a way few others have.

By being involved in organizations like this—or in many other professional organizations—each of us has the opportunity to interact with and learn from outstanding individuals. We have the opportunity to see leaders in action, connect with and seek possible mentors, be involved in activities that promote excellence, and learn more about ourselves as potential leaders. Individuals such as these have an intense passion for the profession and their area of work, and they do not hesitate to reach out to, guide, and help others in the field. They share a commitment to advancing the profession in whatever way they can, and they want to invest in others.

Professional involvement also means participating in organizational, community, and political activities to advance our vision and make it a reality. Nurses who serve on committees where they work, on the board of the local community health center, on school boards, as mayors, or as U.S. senators all are in positions of influence and have many opportunities to promote excellence, exercise leadership, and create a preferred future for nursing.

Nurses who publish or give presentations by sharing ideas and advancements put forth a high standard of practice, and this helps to create nursing's preferred future. The same is true for nurses who conduct special projects (funded or not), conduct research and disseminate the findings, mentor others, and engage in collaborative practice with other nurses and with members of other healthcare disciplines. The opportunities to promote excellence and function as a leader are limitless, and each time a nurse engages in activities that advance nursing or demonstrate leadership to realize a vision, they are contributing to creating a preferred future for the profession.

Case Study, continued

ADRIENNE'S CAREER TRACK: STRIVING FOR EXCELLENCE AND BEING A LEADER

Adrienne sought out a former nurse manager as a mentor, and regularly communicates with the mentor about nursing practice issues, career advancement, and other professional matters. Adrienne seeks out opportunities to attend conferences and workshops as a way to learn more and expand professional networks, and participates actively in professional organizations at the state level, often with support from the institution. She now initiates regular team meetings focused on brainstorming and discussion unit challenges, encouraging collective problem-solving. In addition, Adrienne schedules quarterly feedback sessions to allow the team an opportunity to share their thoughts on the unit's progress and suggest improvements.

REFLECTION QUESTIONS

4. How might Adrienne measure the effectiveness of the changes she has implemented?
5. What lessons can be drawn from Adrienne's experience that are applicable to new nurse leaders?

CONCLUSION

As we develop as leaders, each of us should take advantage of the opportunities presented to become involved professionally. Each of us is responsible for participating and trying to make a difference. Through networking, role-modeling, mentoring relationships, thoughtful self-reflection, and the continued study of leadership and excellence, practice will be enhanced, and we will grow enormously. The outcomes will be excellence in our spheres of influence and in the future of nursing. Indeed, "leadership holds the key to transforming our institutions . . . and our society" (Richardson, 2000, p. v).

Nursing would do well to systematically study the phenomena of leadership and followership in our field to understand better how we can best prepare, support, and nurture our leaders and influential followers. A few research questions are offered to stimulate our thinking about these concepts:

- How do graduates of programs that feature learning experiences designed to help pre-licensure students view themselves as evolving leaders contribute to creating practice environments that embrace excellence?
- What are the most influential experiences in a transition-to-practice program for new graduates that contribute to those nurses' sense of empowerment and willingness to advocate for changes in practice?
- What work environment characteristics are most effective in encouraging nurses to function as leaders and influential followers?

Although there are many more questions that could be, and perhaps need to be, pursued through research, it is hoped that those noted here stimulate thinking about the many dimensions that influence how we prepare and nurture our leaders and followers. In conclusion, a contemporary piece of advice seems to capture the essence of leadership, excellence, and professional involvement:

Excellence can be attained if you:

CARE more than others think is wise,
RISK more than others think is safe,
DREAM more than others think is practical, and
EXPECT more than others think is possible.

We hope each student and nurse who reads this book will take on the challenges of excellence and leadership. You are the future of our marvelous profession. We have every confidence that you will take up this challenge with all seriousness and will succeed in creating a preferred future for nursing.

CRITICAL THINKING 10-1

1. Ask several nurses how they define excellence or what goes into something being called excellent. Pose this same question to individuals in other professional roles (e.g., teacher, physician, social worker). What common themes emerge in the responses you receive? Are there any differences in how various groups talk about the concept? What conclusions can you draw about why the commonalities and differences exist?

2. Identify a nurse who recently received an award that acknowledges excellence—in clinical practice, education, research, contributions to the profession, care for a particular population (e.g., people experiencing homelessness), and so on. The award can be local, regional, national, or international. Interview the award recipient about their recognition. Talk about the individual's background, philosophy, accomplishments, contributions, and ideas about excellence and leadership. What have you learned from this interview that you can use to promote excellence and exert leadership in your arena of practice? Outline specific strategies that could lead you to receive such an award.

References

Alonso, M. (2022). Together, we are better. *AAACN Viewpoint, 44*(4), 16–17. https://ezproxy.gardner-webb.edu/login?url=https://www.proquest.com/scholarly-journals/together-we-are-better/docview/2878102523/se-2

Burns, J. M. (1978). *Leadership*. Harper Torchbooks.

Clark, C. (2022). *Core competencies of civility in nursing & healthcare*. Sigma Theta Tau.

Clark, C. M., & and Ritter, K. (2018). Policy to foster civility and support a healthy academic work environment. *Journal of Nursing Education, 57*(6), 325–331.

Deming, W. E. (1986). *Out of the crisis*. MIT Press.

Deming, W. E. (2024). *Enriching society through the Deming philosophy*. W. Edwards Deming Institute.

Diers, D., & Evans, D. L. (1980). Excellence in nursing [Editorial]. *Image, 12*(2), 27–30.

Marcus, B., Danielson, L., & Frenkel, T. (2021). Vaccination during the COVID-19 pandemic: What nurses need to know. *Online Journal of Issues in Nursing, 26*(2), 1–16.

Memon, K. R., Zada, M., Ghani, B., Ullah, R., Azim, M. T., Mubarik, M. S., Vega-Muñoz, A., & Castillo, D. (2021). Linking corporate social responsibility to workplace deviant behaviors: Mediating role of job satisfaction. *Frontiers in Psychology, 12*, Article 803481.

National League for Nursing. (2024). *Beverly Malone, PhD, RN, FAAN: President & CEO*.

Peters, T. J., & Waterman, R. H. (2006). *In search of excellence: Lessons from America's best-run companies*. HarperCollins.

Richardson, W. C. (2000). Foreword. In A. W. Astin & H. S. Astin, *Leadership reconsidered: Engaging higher education in social change* (pp. iv–vi). W. K. Kellogg Foundation.

Wergin, J. F. (2003). *Departments that work: Building and sustaining cultures of excellence in academic programs*. Anker.

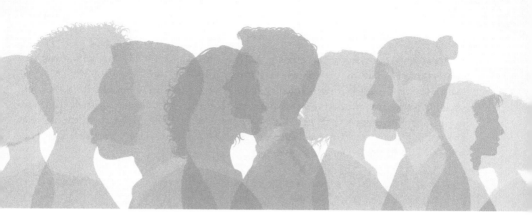

Annotated Bibliography

Adams, R. (1972). *Watership down*. Avon Books.

Watership Down is a book about the adventures of a group of rabbits that leave their comfortable warren in search of a better, safer place to live. Originally thought of as a children's story, this book is an excellent portrayal of leadership styles, leader–follower interactions, and the qualities of effective leaders and followers.

The group of rabbits that serves as the focal point of the story travels extensively to create a new life for themselves, and they encounter several different warrens along the way. They experience warrens that are leaderless, those that are headed by a totalitarian despot, and those where the "leader" provides direction and the basic needs of rabbits in the warren are met, but there is an aloofness between the leader and followers, and high-order needs are not met.

The Watership Down warren rabbits come to form a democratic, participating group where the talents of each rabbit are known and called upon as needed, where followers assume the role of leader when circumstances require a particular type of leadership, and where there is a constant exchange of ideas and support. In essence, this group of rabbits exhibits all that is good about leaders and followers.

This book exposes the reader to various types of leadership and leader–follower relationships. One sees risk taking, acting in uncertainty, clarity of vision, clear communication, and many other behaviors of leaders . . . all within the context of a beautiful story that captures the imagination and holds one's attention.

Andersen, E. (2012). *Leading so people will follow*. Jossey-Bass.

The author describes human beings as having a "deeply wired-in need for leaders who will guide us well and safely; who care more about the success of the enterprise than about their own comfort; who call out the best and take full advantage of who we are" (p. 1). She then reports on findings from research she conducted to identify the key components of the leadership archetype. Those key components—farsightedness, passion, courage, wisdom, generosity, and trustworthiness—are then explored in depth, giving the reader great insight into what effective leadership looks like in our current society and what is needed if individuals are to entice others to follow their lead. This is an informative book that includes many examples and is uplifting and can serve as an excellent source to stimulate personal reflection about the extent to which each of us measures up to the leadership archetype.

Arussy, L. (2018). *Next is now: 5 steps for embracing change—Building a business that thrives into the future.* Simon & Schuster.
This book talks about "cataclysmic" change and how new knowledge and technology will prepare us for today and for the future. The author emphasizes the importance of dynamic change and not treating change as a one-time incident. Additionally, he points out that every single person must acquire skills of adaptability so people can "reinvent" themselves. He describes three forces involved with any change: (1) how you adjust to the change, (2) the competition to the change, and (3) what happens if you do nothing.

With the *Harvard Business Review*, the author's company, Strativity, conducted a landmark study (*n* > 400 executives of Fortune 500 companies) about change. Results, including poor communication (62% of the time) and not understanding the reason for the change (50% of the time), are discussed with recommendations for adapting to constant change. He developed five steps to follow to develop change resilience: (1) identify the trends and facts, (2) analyze all the data, (3) reinvent it, (4) help the process to grow, and (5) own what evolves. This book is exhilarating to read and gives guidance regarding adapting to change and reinforces the importance of dynamic change in one's life.

Babcock, L., & Laschever, S. (2003). *Women don't ask: Negotiation and the gender divide.* Princeton University Press.
When Linda Babcock asked why so many male graduate students were teaching their own courses and most female students were assigned as assistants, her dean said, "More men ask. The women just don't ask." It turns out that whether they want higher salaries or more help at home, women often find it hard to ask. Sometimes they don't know that change is possible—they don't know that they can ask. Sometimes they fear that asking may damage a relationship, and sometimes they don't ask because they've learned that society can react badly to women asserting their own needs and desires.

By looking at the barriers holding women back and the social forces constraining them, *Women Don't Ask* shows women how to reframe their interactions and more accurately evaluate their opportunities. It teaches them how to ask for what they want in ways that feel comfortable and possible, taking into account the impact of asking on their relationships. And it teaches all of us how to recognize the ways in which our institutions, childrearing practices, and unspoken assumptions perpetuate inequalities . . . inequalities that are not only fundamentally unfair but also inefficient and economically unsound.

With women's progress toward full economic and social equality stalled, women's lives becoming increasingly complex, and the structures of businesses changing, the ability to negotiate is no longer a luxury but a necessity. Drawing on research in psychology, sociology, economics, and organizational behavior as well as dozens of interviews with men and women from all walks of life, *Women Don't Ask* is the first book to identify the dramatic difference between men and women in their propensity to negotiate for what they want. It tells women how to ask and why they should.

Bass, B. (1985). *Leadership and performance beyond expectations*. The Free Press.
Written in 1985, this outstanding book describes leadership in terms of transformational and transactional components and still has relevance. The author says transformational leadership is found in varying amounts in everyone and needs to be tapped. He offers traditional leaders (e.g., Moses, Buddha, Jesus Christ, and Mohammed) as well as more recent leaders (e.g., Theodore Roosevelt, John F. Kennedy, and Gandhi) as examples for study. He also cites how each of these individuals exemplified charisma, individualized consideration, and intellectual stimulation. Bass gives behavioral examples of transactional leadership and defines the principles of management-by-exception and contingent rewards.

Perhaps the most interesting aspect of this book is the description of the data collected from the author's classic study of 104 military officers who completed the author-developed Leadership Questionnaire. This instrument asked the officers about their perceptions of their immediate supervisor's leadership skills, and the findings regarding what these individuals believe make someone an effective leader are extremely interesting. The results of this study also point out how an effective leader can influence the followers in a group. (A copy of the Leadership Questionnaire and parameters for scoring are included in the book.)

Bass, B. M. (2008). *The Bass handbook of leadership: Theory, research, and managerial applications* (4th ed.). The Free Press.
This is a classic volume that provides a historical perspective on leadership, an analysis of the meaning of leadership, descriptions of various categories or typologies of leadership, and an examination of leadership theories and models (including Great Man, trait, situational, psychoanalytic, and other theories). Beyond this introductory material, the major emphasis of this 1,000-plus-page book is research that has been completed about leaders and leadership.

The research reported focuses on leadership traits, tasks of leaders, leadership styles, women and leadership, leader–follower interactions, and the significance of values to leaders. Concepts such as charisma, inspirational leadership, power, and conflict also are addressed.

This handbook is an excellent resource for any serious student of leadership. Sadly, however, although the author notes that leadership and management are different phenomena, most of the studies reported use managers as subjects, thereby suggesting that one needs to be in a position of authority to be considered a leader. Despite these limitations, *The Bass Handbook of Leadership* is a classic that should be read and used as a reference source.

Beatty, J. (1998). *The world according to Peter Drucker*. The Free Press.
This book chronicles the life of Peter Drucker and delineates how he constantly pushed himself to become a stronger and more successful person by thinking about what

people *can* do, not only what they *cannot* do. Drucker is a firm believer in frequent self-evaluation, which he calls "keeping score on self" (p. 14), and this theme is inherent in all his work.

Drucker is perhaps best known for his philosophy of "management by objectives," which emphasizes the significance of planning, goals, and evaluating results against preestablished expectations. All this clearly is management, but it is a crucial part of being an effective leader . . . namely, having a vision and evaluating, on a regular basis, the progress being made toward realizing the vision.

This book is easy to read and gives the reader a feeling that anyone can be whatever one wants to be. It also stresses the importance of making a difference in people's lives and not being remembered merely for writing a book or developing a theory. This book is good for helping individuals develop their leadership abilities.

Bennis, W. (1993). *An invented life: Reflections on leadership and change.*
    Addison-Wesley.
This is a retrospective look by Bennis about his own life and work. He candidly explains leadership through his lens as a social scientist and business administrator and offers thoughts on comparing leaders with managers: "I decided that the kind of university president I wanted to be was one who led, not managed. That's an important difference. Many an institution is well managed yet very poorly led. It excels in the ability to handle all daily routine inputs yet never asks whether the routine should be done in the first place" (p. 31).

Bennis speaks of a democratic leadership style as what is most promoted in U.S. industry and defines it as including: "1) full and free communication, regardless of rank and power; 2) a reliance on consensus rather than on coercion or compromise to manage conflict; 3) the idea that influence is based on technical competence and knowledge rather than on the vagaries of personal whims or prerogatives of power; 4) an atmosphere that permits and even encourages emotional expression as well as task-oriented behavior; and 5) a basically human notion, one that accepts the inevitability of conflict between the organization and the individual but is willing to cope with and mediate this conflict on rational grounds." He ends with the importance of leaders of all organizations, small and large, to partner with others and collaborate in order to best set the stage for change.

Bennis, W. (2009). *On becoming a leader: Leadership classic—Updated and expanded*
    (4th ed.). Perseus Books.
Written by one of the foremost authorities on leadership, this book is a classic in the field. Beginning with the conviction that everyone can potentially be a leader, this book is a reflective exploration of the nature of this elusive phenomenon and the qualities and characteristics of those who serve as leaders. Bennis asserts there are few people answering our nation's call for leaders, and he worries about the impact of this lack of leadership because our "quality of life depends on leaders." He gives many examples of where leadership is lacking in our world, including U.S. business and the Roman Catholic Church. Bennis says leaders tend not to seek a leadership position but rather wish to express themselves.

Although leadership can be provided by almost anyone, leaders are not ordinary people, according to Bennis. They work everywhere, they serve as guides, they take risks, and they fail. Leaders always learn from those failures; they engage in continuous learning and self-development, and they know themselves.

By using many examples—from Norman Lear to Gloria Steinem to the executive director of the American Association of University Women to the chairperson and CEO of Johnson & Johnson—Bennis helps the reader understand how leaders need to master the contexts in which they find themselves, create new contexts, use their instincts and intuition, and be innovators who help others move through chaos, among other things. These examples also are used to illustrate the differences between leadership and management.

Serious students of leadership will want this classic reference in their collection. It is insightful and offers many practical suggestions for developing as a leader.

Bennis, W., & Biederman, P. (1998). *Organizing genius: The secrets of creative collaboration.* Addison-Wesley.

This book starts out reminding us that "none of us is as smart as all of us" (p. 1). Charles Handy says in the foreword that "Warren Bennis's great gift is the ability to find meaning and messages where the rest of us see only happenings" (p. xi). This is accurate because as one reads through this book, it is the observations seen on a daily basis that Bennis and Biederman have used to convey their ideas of great leadership being made up of great followers and leaders who have the freedom to do their very best every step of the way and then to enjoy the "personal transformation" that such accomplishments bring. This book provides strategies for success by collecting a group of great people, led by a leader who facilitates each and every individual to perform their absolute best, in order to accomplish excellent results.

Bennis, W., & Nanus, B. (2003). *Leaders: Strategies for taking charge* (3rd ed.). Harper & Row.

This is the third edition of the seminal work in which Bennis first claimed that managers are those who do things right and leaders are those who do the right things. The authors speak to the dramatic changes taking place in our world and acknowledge the dire need for competent leadership and for more flexibility and awareness on the part of leaders and followers alike.

Based on the results of a 2-year study of individuals who were thought to be leaders, Bennis and Nanus identified four major themes/areas of competency/"human handling skills" that emerged: attention through vision (i.e., creating a focus or having an agenda, particularly one that draws others in); meaning through communication (i.e., expressing ideas powerfully so that others understand and want to support them); trust through positioning (i.e., making one's position known, being reliable, and being persistent with relentless dedication); and the deployment of self (i.e., having a positive self-regard, knowing one's strengths and weaknesses, and setting high goals). Each of these strategies is discussed thoroughly, and many ideas are offered as to how one can implement each.

The authors conclude by recommending that we must increase the search for new leadership to a national priority. They urge the purposeful and continuous development of leaders because without effective leaders, the best our society can do is maintain the status quo; at worst, our society could disintegrate. (There is a 2007 paperback version of this.)

Bennis, W., & Thomas, W. (2002). *Geeks and geezers: How eras, values, and defining moments shape leaders.* Harvard Business School Press.
This book is a compilation of ideas on leadership development and the generational differences between the geeks (people under 30 years old) and the geezers (people over 70 years old). It focuses on the young and the old more so than on the people between 30 and 70 years of age. The leadership development model described in this book can help readers develop the four areas that these authors define as leadership: voice, integrity, adaptive capacity, and ability to engage others by creating a vision. A great emphasis is on what the authors call "crucible moments," which are life-changing experiences that people have throughout their lives and that call for leadership. This book is easy to read, worthwhile, and helpful in improving self-confidence and general self-concept regarding one's ability to achieve dreams and personal visions.

Bolman, L. G., & Deal, T. E. (2011). *Leading with soul: An uncommon journey of spirit* (3rd ed.). Jossey-Bass.
Using the story of Steve, a dispirited leader in search of something more meaningful in his life than the bottom line, these authors help the reader see and appreciate the spiritual dimensions of leadership and how work and spirit can and, in their opinion, need to be connected. They discuss the interrelationship of leaders and followers, the "gifts" of leadership (love, power, and significance), and the legacy of leadership. This book challenges the reader to look deep inside oneself and reflect on one's true self and values. Finally, the dialogue between the authors and an interviewer that concludes the book provides insights into why they examined the concept of the soul of leadership and how this work has affected individuals in various positions in diverse organizations.

Book, E. W. (2001). *Why the best man for the job is a woman: The unique female qualities of leadership.* HarperBusiness.
This book reports on intensive studies the author conducted with 14 women who have exhibited leadership, primarily in the corporate world. Among the strengths that were common to all women were "a gravity-defying level of self-confidence . . . a preternatural sense of exactly what their [followers] want . . . [and a tendency to] foster a more collegial environment" (p. xiii). The author claims that "evidence is mounting that the style of leadership women offer is beneficial not only to employees but also to the bottom line, [perhaps because] women are better at communicating, empowering people and being positive" (p. xv).

The author provides extensive descriptions of the key characteristics of what she calls "new paradigm leadership": selling one's vision, reinventing the rules, having a laser focus to achieve, maximizing high touch in an era of high tech, turning challenge into opportunity, and having courage under fire. She contrasts these with features of the old paradigm—masculine, hierarchical, command-and-control oriented, opposed to change, focused on individual efforts, and limited communication—and describes the advantages of new paradigm leadership.

In conclusion, Book offers a number of tips on becoming a new paradigm leader and encourages women to assume such roles with enthusiasm. As such, this book provides a thoughtful analysis of women's leadership styles and serves as a helpful guide to those wishing to integrate such styles into their own repertoire.

Brown, B. (2018). *Dare to lead. Brave work, tough conversations, whole hearts.* Random House.

Using interview data collected over a 20-year period, her own and others' published research, and years of experience in numerous organizations, Brown discusses the courage one needs to be a leader. She notes that anyone can be a leader, as this responsibility is not tied to a title or a position or a certain level or status, and asserts that to be a leader means to recognize the potential in people and ideas and exhibit the courage to develop that potential. Being a leader involves being vulnerable, but that is not necessarily a bad thing; and Brown offers many strategies to confront and accept one's vulnerability. This book is of particular value to those who fear taking risks or being open to challenge and criticism, and it is quite reader friendly.

Burns, J. M. (1978). *Leadership.* Harper Torchbooks.

This book is truly a classic! It was Burns who first acknowledged that "leadership is one of the most observed and least understood phenomena on earth" (p. 2) and then proceeded to help us understand this complex concept.

He noted how little we knew at the time about leadership and how to develop it—despite the hundreds of definitions of the term!—and how little attention was given to the significance of followers and the "interwoven texture of leadership and followership" (pp. 4–5). He also analyzed the nature of power and the role of power in leadership and explored the ways in which leaders help release the potentials of others.

In his attempt to clarify the meaning of leadership, Burns offered distinctions between *transactional* and *transformational* leadership and introduced the notion of *moral* leadership. In recent years, many authors have carried the banner of transformation leadership, but Burns was the first to name it and describe it exquisitely.

As a result of Burns's seminal work on leadership, our understanding of this complicated concept has progressed enormously. This is a book that must be read as a foundation to subsequent works about leadership.

Burns, J. M. (2003). *Transforming leadership: A new pursuit of happiness.* Atlantic Monthly Press.

In this book, Burns expands on his notion of transformational leadership. He asserts that "to transform something . . . is to cause a metamorphosis in form or structure, a change in the very condition or nature of a thing" (p. 24) . . . a change of breadth and depth.

The primary focus of this book is an examination of how a number of leaders in the past, including the American Founding Fathers, embraced and lived the three standards or norms that Burns claims constitute a good leader: virtue, ethics, and transforming values. He then conducts an extensive analysis of how these standards shaped the

Declaration of Independence's emphasis on life, liberty, and the pursuit of happiness, with particular emphasis on the latter (hence, the book's subtitle).

Although Burns offers many insightful comments about leaders, leadership, followers, empowerment, and other topics relevant to a study of leadership, they often are difficult to cull from the discussions of the pursuit of happiness. Leadership scholars will want to study this book carefully, but novices to leadership studies are likely to benefit more from other resources. (There is a 2004 paperback version.)

Cain, S. (2013). *Quiet: The power of introverts in a world that can't stop talking.*
   Broadway Books.
Cain's thoughtful analysis serves to bring a sigh of relief and a sense of hope to those who think of themselves as introverts, individuals who, according to the author, make up one-third to one-half of the U.S. population. She acknowledges the common negative perceptions of and biases against introverts, then proceeds to challenge those ideas, noting that being an introvert does not mean one is necessarily shy and withdrawn but that one prefers to work more slowly and deliberately, to connect with fewer individuals and have deeper conversations with them rather than be a social butterfly who has superficial exchanges with everyone in the room, to focus on character more than on personality, to listen carefully to others, and to prefer contemplative activities to constantly busy ones. She notes that we tend to think of talkers as smarter and as leaders but defuses that myth by noting the lack of correlation between outgoingness and GPA, SAT scores, intelligence test scores, insight, and leadership.

Although this book does not focus on leadership, Cain notes people may overestimate the importance of being an outgoing leader, acknowledges the impact quiet leaders can have, and encourages those who see themselves as introverts to take on the challenge of leadership with confidence.

Chaleff, I. (2009). *The courageous follower: Standing up to and for our leaders*
   (3rd ed.). Berrett-Koehler.
This book gets to the heart of what leadership truly is and how it grows from followership. The author describes followership in a very positive way and avoids the negative connotations often associated with being a follower.

Chaleff speaks to being an *effective* follower and how such individuals are critical to generating effective leaders. He offers many fundamental, common-sense, helpful ideas that could be most useful to the person interested in empowering herself or himself and others, creating a vision, making a change, and preparing for a leadership role.

The author makes a point of explaining the significance of being a follower, supporting the leader's vision, and participating actively in change processes. A major point made by Chaleff is that followers do not do things simply at the bidding of leaders, nor do they hide behind leaders. Instead, followers do things because they think those things are best for themselves and for the organization. Followers, according to Chaleff, are not weak or passive. They are dynamic and passionate about many issues.

This book is a must read for understanding the relationship between leaders and followers and for appreciating the significance of followers in making change and realizing visions.

Chapman, G., & White, P. (2019). *The 5 languages of appreciation in the workplace: Empowering organizations by encouraging people* (2nd ed.). Northfield.
Chapman and White suggest several tangible ideas to assist in empowering organizations by supporting and appreciating people at the workplace. Their main theme is that all levels of employees, from CEO to maintenance staff, seek appreciation for a job well done. This edition speaks to the need for appreciating all employees along with special ideas for communicating to those who work remotely and also specifics for dealing with individuals from various generations. They developed the Motivating by Appreciation Inventory tool to measure employees' feeling of appreciation from both supervisors and coworkers. They identified five appreciation languages for people to use when communicating appreciations effectively to team members and supervisors: words of affirmation, quality time, acts of service, tangible gifts, and physical touch. The authors do an excellent job of describing what kind of people react best to these five appreciation languages with specific strategies for communicating appreciation.

Clampitt, P., & DeKoch, R. (2001). *Embracing uncertainty: The essence of leadership.* M. E. Sharpe.
The authors make the case that embracing uncertainty is more effective and rewarding than trying to eliminate it. They advocate that leaders recognize that they will never have all the right answers and that "not knowing" is quite legitimate. Leaders should never feel bad about not knowing but should attempt to foster this belief in their followers so that increased creativity and increased morale are the outcome. The *Working Climate Survey* developed by these authors to measure one's tendency to embrace uncertainty provides fascinating insight into one's comfort with uncertainty and ambiguity. This tool is included in this book, along with directions for interpreting results.

Coles, R. (2001). *Lives of moral leadership: Men and women who have made a difference.* Random House.
This book powerfully conveys the meaning of moral leadership using well-known and influential, as well as ordinary, people as examples. The lives and work of individuals like Robert Kennedy, Gandhi, and Albert Jones (a Boston bus driver) are used to illustrate the bond that develops between true leaders and their followers and how "moral energy" helps our society respond to crises and challenges. Coles asserts that "we need heroes, people who can inspire us, help shape us morally, spur us on to purposeful action" (p. xi), and he acknowledges that "from time to time we are called on to *be* those heroes, leaders for others, either in a small, day-to-day way, or on the world's larger stage" (p. xi). Reading this book helps one appreciate what moral leadership is and how it is achieved. As such, it is a most significant resource in today's environment.

Conger, J. (1992). *Learning to lead: The art of transforming managers into leaders.* Jossey-Bass.
Conger firmly believes that leadership can be broken down into specific behaviors and that those behaviors can be taught and learned. In fact, this book is an account of the author's own experiences in learning to be a leader, specifically through his participation in the following innovative leadership development programs: Kouzes and

Posner's Leadership Challenge, the Center for Creative Leadership's Leadership Development Program, the Experiential Pecos River Learning Center Program, and the Vision Quest Program.

The author explains the significance of leaders having a vision so that they can provide some type of direction and meaning, being inspirational, demonstrating charisma, being empowered, and acting as a transformational change agent. He asserts that one can learn these skills.

Work experiences, taking advantage of opportunities that present themselves, educational advancement, mentors, and experiencing hardship all are variables identified by Conger as fostering leadership. He explains the historical development of leadership training and points out the importance of having such programs focus on providing feedback to participants regarding their conceptual development, skill building, and personal growth.

Conger also explores some of the more "common" theories about leadership. He explains how situational leadership and the "task-versus-relationship" contingency model of the 1980s lack the strategic envisioning, inspirational speaking, and management of change that he feels is absolutely essential for an effective leader in today's environments. He believes that all aspiring leaders need to participate in the kind of personal growth programs that he discusses in this book.

Covey, S. (1992). *Principle-centered leadership*. Summit Books.
This book is grounded in the idea that having principles to guide one's life, like a compass guides one's journey, makes for a more productive, fulfilling life. Covey presents his ideas regarding the principles of vision, leadership, and human relationships as the way to make decisions in one's personal, interpersonal, managerial, and organizational lives. He offers suggestions on how to cultivate eight characteristics that facilitate the making of what he calls a "principle-centered leader."

This excellent book on self-leadership can be used as a rich resource to assist others in their development as leaders, particularly principle-centered leaders. Covey's ideas center around the importance of a leader being a pathfinder—someone who can align an organization's or an individual's structure with an individual's behavior, *not* the organization's behavior—and a facilitator or empowerer of others. By *pathfinder*, Covey means being able to move an individual or group down a path or to realize a vision. The pathfinder is an individual who, by using leadership, moves individuals or organizations in new directions, an approach that is vastly different from making changes merely in response to revised organization policies and expectations.

Covey, S. (2004). *The 8th habit: From effectiveness to greatness*. Running Book Press.
This book is an excellent sequel to *The 7 Habits of Highly Effective People*. The author has added the idea of "finding your voice and encouraging others to find theirs" as the eighth habit. He describes how all individuals can discover the voices that evolve from three gifts at birth: freedom to choose, natural laws, and the four intelligences (mental, physical, spiritual, and emotional). He gives multiple examples of how people can use these ideas to improve themselves and become more holistic people and leaders.

Covey discusses how leadership roles have changed and gives examples of how individuals can maximize their leadership skills with new roles. He also describes what he sees as new roles for leaders: modeling, pathfinding, aligning, and empowering. He discusses the value of vision, discipline, passion, and conscience in leaders and gives many real-life examples for using the new roles of leadership. The book also offers advice on how a person can change from being a "want to" person to a "can do" person, and the Frequently Asked Questions section regarding his ideas of leadership is helpful. There is a paperback version.

Covey, S. (2013). *The 7 habits of highly effective people: Powerful lessons in personal change*. Rosetta Books.
The author, Stephen Covey, celebrates the 25th anniversary of this wildly successful book in this edition. He highlights how one must take responsibility and be accountable for one's life. He offers multiple quotes from leaders from around the world who answered his question, "How did the earlier edition of this book impact your life?" Reading through these quotes is especially good for self-reflection of one's life, both professionally and personally. Covey also shares how he lived his life with a carpe diem (seize the day) attitude and "sucked the marrow out of life." It is very motivating and may be able to assist an individual or group to really make a change and get out of a status quo situation. Covey offers excellent ideas on how to make a positive and constructive culture rather than seeing things so negatively. He suggests that for each problem one identifies, one needs to recommend some suggestions to solve the problem and that one should dwell more on implementing the solution than "whining" about the problem. Another major idea this book offers is that leaders must be effective communicators and be successful in empowering others to be confident leaders.

Csikszenthihalyi, M. (2013). *Creativity: Flow and the psychology of discovery and invention*. Harper Perennial.
The major purpose of this book is to remind the reader that creativity is a process that unfolds over a lifetime. It is "based on histories of contemporary people who know about [creativity] firsthand" (p. 1) because they have experienced the challenges, disappointments, and joy in promoting creative ideas or approaches. As an outcome of scholarly, in-depth interviews with selected individuals known for their creative endeavors, the author offers several conclusions: Creative ideas arise from the synergy of many sources and not from the mind of a single individual; it is easier to enhance creativity by changing conditions in the environment than by trying to make people think more creatively; and a genuinely creative accomplishment is almost never the result of a sudden insight but comes after years of hard work.

Reading about creativity in the young, middle-aged, and elderly is inspiring and informative, and anyone wishing to better understand this phenomenon that is "a central source of meaning in our lives" (p. 1) is encouraged to explore this book. The author recommends everyone try to increase their creativity because it will allow them to live more fully.

Dempsey, M., & Brafman, O. (2017). *Radical inclusion: What the post-9/11 world should have taught us about leadership*. Missionday Publishers.
The authors are extremely persuasive in their views regarding the need for stronger leadership with the ability to obtain followers who can trust the leaders. They give examples of this use of inclusion leadership in the military, academia, government, and business. They point out that leaders must be committed and able to protect people from drowning in "digital echoes" or social media that is allowing people to become more "isolated, more suspicious, less positive, and less optimistic" (p. 169). They say this suspicion that is cast over the world now is "affecting the way we interact with one another" (p. 169) in all aspects of life—both professionally and personally. Their premise is that to be successful, leaders must be radically inclusive of their followers, be transparent so they can be trusted, show they are not leading for autocratic power and control, be dynamic, and constantly collect data and new networks. The authors share real-life stories that are both entertaining and very informative.

Denhardt, R., & Denhardt, J. (2006). *The dance of leadership: The art of leading in business, government, and society*. M. E. Sharpe.
This book emphasizes the need for each individual to lead, no matter what their role. The authors assert that each person should use their leadership ability to improve the work setting, home situation, or other circumstance. They offer a view of leadership that originates from the arts, noting that "artists see the world in a way quite different from others . . . they see the world in terms of an especially intense and textured interplay of space, time, and energy" (p. 6). Denhardt and Denhardt tell an interesting story about how one cannot really have a single operational definition of leadership, and they assert that "the only thing that really counts in leadership is that which you can't explain" (p. 10).

This book is interesting, entertaining, and challenges the reader to think seriously about the emotional aspects of leadership and the importance of the leader's audience (i.e., followers). The authors explore various concepts such as rhythms of human interaction, communication, spontaneity, and creativity, and they share their rendition of the difference between leadership and management. These authors make a strong argument that leadership originates from art, not science.

DePree, M. (2004). *Leadership is an art* (2nd ed.). Doubleday Currency.
Leadership Is an Art is about how the art of leadership frees people to do what is required of them in the most effective way possible. As an art, leadership is something one learns over time. The foreword to this second edition stresses the importance of having a mentor in one's life to assist in developing one's leadership ability.

One of the most significant aspects of leadership, according to DePree, is a genuine concern for and about others. Leaders understand the diversity of the talents, gifts, and skills others possess and find ways to allow each individual to contribute to a cause or purpose in her or his own way.

The author asserts that leaders serve others. They are responsible for identifying, developing, and nurturing future leaders, and they bind people together to accomplish great things. They provide and help to maintain the momentum of a group, and they keep the group focused on the values and visions that guide them. DePree describes the three most important themes of the book: integrity, ability to build and nurture relationships, and community building. He relates all these components of leadership to knowing who we intend to be in the future, which, he says, will help us to generate exactly what we will end up doing with our lives.

This easy-to-read book includes many insightful points about leaders and leadership that stimulate one's thinking in new ways. The conceptualization of leadership as an art, but an art that can be learned, is a useful one for the would-be leader.

DePree, M. (2008). *Leadership jazz: The essential elements of a great leader* (2nd ed.). Doubleday.
This is the second edition of a classic book on leadership that was described by Sam Walton as "one of the best books I have ever read in my life on the subject of leadership and business management philosophy." The basis for this book is an assertion that without followers, leaders can do nothing but play solo. The book tells how leaders can facilitate leadership in others because, as DePree asserts, it is more important to develop leaders than to direct them. He expands on four questions that he believes assist one in gaining insight about leaders and leadership: (1) How can I know what's in the hearts of my followers? (2) What gifts of leadership have I come to treasure most? (3) What questions do I now wish I had been asked? and (4) What questions would I ask you? DePree believes these four questions underlie one's future in becoming a global citizen prepared to take advantage of multiple opportunities.

Dreher, D. (1996). *The Tao of personal leadership*. Harper Business.
This book is a rich blend of the principle of centering and balancing one's life and the Taoist philosophy of engaging in compassion while remaining detached. It emphasizes the importance of realizing the power of living systems that generate energy all around us, and it reinforces the appreciation of all people potentially becoming leaders, regardless of their station in life.

Communication, team building, having an appetite for constant change, credibility, risk taking, and the ability to facilitate others in accomplishing goals/vision are necessary assets of a strong leader, according to Dreher. The author describes the Tao leader as being a pioneer, a pathfinder, a person who guides with intuition, someone who constantly faces the unknown with excitement, and someone who turns conflict into opportunities for stronger relationships, greater knowledge, and better solutions. The author has written an exhilarating account of how one can develop one's leadership capacity in exponential fashion.

Gardner, J. W. (1990). *On leadership*. The Free Press.
John Gardner is one of the experts on the topic of leadership, and he reports, in this book, insights gained from a 5-year study of the phenomenon. He distinguishes leadership from management and expresses the great need we have for true leaders, individuals "who are exemplary, who inspire, who stand for something, [and] who help us set and achieve goals" (p. xi).

One of the most significant contributions Gardner makes through this book is helping the reader understand what he calls "the tasks of leadership." Included in those tasks are the following:

> Envisioning goals: pointing us in the right direction or asserting a vision
> Affirming values: reminding the group of the norms and expectations they share
> Motivating: stimulating and encouraging others to act
> Managing: planning, setting priorities, and making decisions
> Achieving a workable unity: managing conflict and promoting unity within the group
> Explaining: teaching followers and helping them understand why they are being asked to do certain things
> > Serving as a symbol: acting in ways that convey the values of the group and its goals
> > Representing the group: speaking on behalf of the group
> > Renewing: bringing members of the group to new levels

In fulfilling these tasks, leaders must work collaboratively with followers, whom Gardner refers to as *constituents*. He acknowledges that "followers often perform leader-like acts" (p. 23) and recognizes the significant role that followers play in accomplishing change and realizing a vision.

Finally, Gardner draws on the work of many researchers to identify several attributes of leaders, including the following: physical vitality and stamina (i.e., a high energy level); intelligence and judgment-in-action (i.e., ability to identify and solve problems, set priorities, etc.); willingness to accept responsibilities (i.e., exercise initiative, bear the burden of making a decision, and step forward when no one else will); task competence (i.e., knowing the task at hand and the system); understanding followers/constituents and their needs; skill in dealing with people; a need to achieve; the capacity to motivate others; and courage. He also discusses how leaders need to use power and how they need to be morally responsible.

Gladwell, M. (2005). *Blink: The power of thinking without thinking*. Little, Brown.
Although this book is not about leadership per se, it nevertheless offers valuable insights for anyone who strives to fulfill the role of leader. It is a book about how we think without thinking and how this process can be very valuable or have disastrous consequences.

Gladwell notes that "our world requires that decisions be sourced and footnoted" (p. 52). He then challenges that approach and labels it a mistake, asserting that "if we are to learn to improve the quality of the decisions we make, we need to accept the mysterious nature of our snap judgments. We need to respect the fact that it is possible to know without knowing why we know" (p. 52).

While somewhat unorthodox, Gladwell's perspective is congruent with much of the leadership literature, which notes that leaders often rely on their intuition and do what they believe—in their hearts—is right. As such, readers interested in developing themselves as a leader could benefit from these ideas that help one see the world in a different way.

Gladwell, M. (2008). *Outliers: The story of success.* Little, Brown.
As noted by the author, this book is about outliers, men and women who do things that are out of the ordinary—those who have been given opportunities and had the strength and presence of mind to seize them. He asserts that in studying those who have been successful, we must consider their upbringing and the life events that have shaped them because all that comes together to make them outliers. Additionally, while there is such a thing as innate talent and it does have a role to play in success, achievement is talent plus preparation, and it is preparation that seems to play a much larger role. Thus, those who aspire to greatness or who accept the responsibility of leadership must work hard, be deliberate, invest a great deal of energy, accept help from others, reflect on how their life experiences have shaped them, and use those experiences to advance new ideas and facilitate change. In fact, he says, hard work is "a way to find meaning in the midst of great uncertainty," (p. 239) and "if you work hard enough and assert yourself, and use your mind and imagination, you can shape the world to your desires" (p. 151)—ideas that are congruent with the idea of persistence, which is a noted characteristic of leaders.

Goleman, D. (2018). *Emotional intelligence: Improve your emotional quotient for business and relationships/unleash the empathy in you—Practical ways to improve your people skills.* Millenia Publishing.
Goleman's research indicates that emotional intelligence is nearly twice as significant as IQ in becoming a leader. People are born with certain cognitive abilities, or IQ, and that is not likely to change dramatically throughout one's life; emotional intelligence, on the other hand, is something one can acquire and use to improve one's professional behavior. This book has advice on how to increase your empathic skills, become more socially aware, and be successful in networking and making relationships. Goleman shares many interesting stories, such as how managers are more apt to hire and promote individuals with high emotional intelligence versus high intelligence, and then delves deeper to teach the reader how to gain more emotional intelligence.
    It is essential for nurses to realize the power they have in making positive change on their units, in their agencies, and in the health policy arena, and this book can be a good guide to help nurses change the status quo.

Goleman, D., Boyatzis, R., & McKee, A. (2013). *Primal leadership: Realizing the power of emotional intelligence* (2nd ed.). Harvard Business School Press.
This book speaks to the concept of resonance, which is defined as "a reservoir of positivity that frees the best in people" (p. ix). The authors expand on this concept as they explain that at its root, the primal job of leadership is emotional. Being intelligent about emotions is extremely significant to leaders being successful, and the authors discuss how maximizing the power one derives from being emotionally intelligent improves performance. The relationship between neurotransmitters and mood is exciting to read about because it illustrates how leaders' moods affect their behavior and the behavior of those they lead.
    Examples of how emotionally intelligent leaders are successful in guiding organizations during chaotic times are excellent and well worth reading. The leadership competencies of emotional intelligence—self-awareness, self-management, social awareness,

and relationship management—are clearly explained, and the idea that "most people are leaders so there is not just one leader" pervades the book.

Greene, R. (1998). *The 48 laws of power*. Viking.
This author claims that "all of us hunger for power, and almost all of our actions are aimed at gaining it" (p. xix), and he asserts that "if the game of power is inescapable, better to be an artist than a denier or a bungler" (p. xix). Given these perspectives, Greene then goes on to thoroughly describe 48 laws that, he claims, will help one attain and retain power. Among those laws are the following: conceal your intentions, learn to keep people dependent on you, keep others in suspended terror, play all the way to the end, and preach the need for change, but never reform too much at once.

It is obvious that these laws reflect a Machiavellian perspective on power, and the author fails to discuss more positive sources or uses of power. For those who find themselves in cutthroat environments where one must do anything to survive, these laws may be helpful. For those who aspire to provide leadership in the way it has been discussed in *The New Leadership Challenge: Creating the Future of Nursing* and proposed by most authorities on the subject, such actions will not empower followers, create a sense of unity, or renew leaders or followers. Perhaps reading this book serves as a good lesson in what *not* to do as a leader.

Hagemann, B., Vetter, S., & Maketa, J. (2017). *Leading a vision: The Leader's Blueprint for creating a compelling vision and engaging the workforce*. Nicholas Brealey.
With the majority of workers now being Generation Y (75% of all workers will be Generation Y by 2025), it is now more important than ever for leaders to be aware of the needs of the multigenerational employees. The authors are all dynamic and frequently sought-after speakers to lead audiences about vision development. They recommend that employees be very involved in this development. They describe how leaders need to be courageous, very clear in their communications, network with each and every employee, and continuously be shaping the organization's work culture.

The authors collected data from leaders of greater than 400 successful companies, such as OluKai, Bumble Bee, Coresystems, Jimbo's, and Bunge, to name a few. From this research, they used the results to develop a blueprint with step-by-step actions for leaders to successfully develop an organization's vision.

Hames, R. D. (2007). *The five literacies of global leadership: What authentic leaders know and you need to find out*. Jossey-Bass.
As noted in the foreword to this book, "The future is shaped by the quality of leadership" (p. xvii). With this in mind, Hames examines the current state of leadership throughout the world and creates "a manifesto of a group of remarkable people who are intent on creating better futures" (p. xxi). The remarkable people highlighted in this book are well-known politicians, scientists, and "the man next door," but whether they reside in rich, powerful nations or very poor ones, the author claims they have five things in common: they are passionately optimistic, their curiosity and craving for wisdom drives them to continually explore new possibilities, they acknowledge the

power of collective action, they embrace uncertainty and system-wide change, and they are compassionate.

Through the narratives and stories provided, this book helps the reader appreciate what individuals can do to mobilize and collaborate with others to create a preferred future. It is inspiring and reinforces the commonalities among us.

Hansen-Tarton, T., Sherman, S., & Ferguson, V. (2007). *Conversations with leaders: Frank talk from nurses (and others) on the front lines of leadership.* Sigma Theta Tau International.

Although this book was written more than 10 years ago, it continues to offer insights about leadership and stories of the leadership journey of many key figures in the nursing profession. The themes about leadership identified by the authors based on the narratives provided by and/or interviews with various individuals are that leadership is inspiring, challenging, collaborative, intentional, transformative, and visionary. For those new to the field, as well as those who have been in nursing for some time and wish to know more about those who have provided leadership within our profession, this book offers a moving collection of stories that will inspire and, hopefully, ignite action.

Harvard Business School Press. (1998). *Harvard Business Review on leadership.* Harvard Business School Press.

This collection of eight articles reflects some of the foremost thinkers in the area of leadership, including Mintzberg, Kotter, and Zaleznik. Many of the articles are accompanied by an executive summary, and most are followed by a retrospective commentary by the author. Mintzberg, for example, even offers some self-study questions after his chapter.

Clearly, these writings are significant in that they raise key questions such as the following: Are managers and leaders different? What do leaders really do? How do chief executives really lead? Why is providing leadership difficult?

At the end of the text is a short paragraph describing all the contributing authors and their accomplishments since their seminal pieces were originally published. This book is definitely a must read for those wishing to develop a comprehensive understanding of the complex phenomenon of leadership.

There are additional books of compilations of *Harvard Business Review* articles that relate to leadership that may be of use to readers. Examples of subtitles are *Leadership in a Changed World, Breakthrough Leadership,* and *Leadership at the Top.*

Heifetz, R. A., Grashow, A., & Linsky, M. (2009). *The practice of adaptive leadership: Tools and tactics for changing your organization and the world.* Harvard Business Review Press.

This book by authorities on organizational leadership discusses the concept of adaptive challenges and how leaders can help groups be effective when faced with those transformative types of situations. The authors distinguish between leadership and authority and provide numerous examples of how leaders and followers need to collaborate to thrive in a constantly changing world that calls for both adaptation and the need to upend the status quo, regardless of its tenacity. The book is filled with stories and examples from business and public life, offers many practical tools and realistic tactics, and is designed to help readers better understand the systems in which they operate, put ideas into action, understand themselves, connect with their leadership purpose and those who are critical in realizing it, and continually grow and be renewed.

Helgesen, S. (1990). *The female advantage: Women's ways of leadership.* Doubleday Currency.
In this book, one of the few and one of the earliest texts dealing specifically with women as leaders, Helgesen describes ways in which women lead differently than men. Based on a study of women leaders in the workplace, she found patterns of behavior and approaches to making decisions and setting priorities that were quite different from what had been reported in studies of male leaders.

Women in Helgesen's study were very concerned about being involved in the work of the organization, keeping relationships healthy and productive, making time for activities that were not directly related to their work (e.g., parenting responsibilities), and maintaining a "big picture" orientation. They also viewed their jobs as only one element of who they were, not as *the* factor that defined who they were, and they preferred to see themselves at the center of or in the midst of things, rather than at the top.

As a result of these values, perspectives, and preferences, women tended to create operational structures that were more weblike rather than hierarchical. Such structures provide for more interaction among members of the group, allow for more participation of all players in goal setting and decision making, and result in greater inclusion.

Helgesen views these differences in the ways women lead as great strengths, strengths that are having and will continue to have dramatic effects on the nature of our organizations. The book provides a provocative analysis of women leaders and the way they can use their different perspectives and values to change organizations.

Hennessy, J. (2018). *Leading matters: Lessons from my journey.* Stanford University Press.
Some lessons about leadership shared by John Hennessy, previously president of Stanford University and sometimes referred to as the "godfather of Silicon Valley," seem helpful and merit review by nurses at every level. He shares 10 very attainable and learnable qualities that could assist individuals in improving leadership skills: (1) humility, (2) authenticity and trust, (3) leadership of service, (4) empathy, (5) courage, (6) collaboration and teamwork, (7) innovation, (8) intellectual curiosity, (9) storytelling, and (10) legacy. Each of these skills would benefit a nurse, or anyone for that matter, but one way to begin improving these skills is to read this book and see how Hennessy shares how he gained them through various real-life situations. Stories about his experiences as both a professor and entrepreneur are most entertaining and will be helpful to anyone learning how to lead. The book is a fast read and very informative, and it even has a list of books that Hennessy recommends reading.

Houser, B. P., & Player, K. N. (2007). *Pivotal moments in nursing: Leaders who changed the path of a profession* (Vol. 2). Sigma Theta Tau International.
This book spotlights 11 nurses who moved the discipline ahead in significant ways. Included among those studied are Mary Elizabeth Carnegie, Imogene King, Ruth Watson

Lubic, and Margaret McClure. Each nurse was interviewed and her history analyzed; from these analyses, the authors then drew conclusions about leaders. Their work helps the reader appreciate how leaders meet and overcome barriers and challenges to the ideas they propose that are out of the mainstream, how they use their high energy level and passion to keep moving forward, how they are willing to always go the extra mile for their colleagues and for the profession, and how they become politically astute to deal with influential people in their environments.

It is clear from the study of these nurse leaders that they viewed themselves as rebels and were comfortable with that role. In addition, each of the individuals spotlighted had a vision and was able to see a bigger picture than others were able to see. The book, therefore, helps define what leadership is and offers insights into how one develops as a leader.

NOTE: The first volume of this book was published in 2004. It followed a similar format but presented 12 different nurse leaders, including Joyce Clifford, Luther Christman, Vernice Ferguson, Rheba de Tornyay, and Claire Fagin, among others.

Hurwitz, M., & Hurwitz, S. (2015). *Leadership is half the story: A fresh look at followership, leadership, and collaboration.* University of Toronto Press.
In this engaging and down-to-earth book, the authors challenge the notion of followership being referred to as "the F-word" and speak to the essential role followers play in any group, organization, or profession. They provide evidence of how followership is linked to substantial improvements on many "performance metrics" and assert, therefore, that emotional intelligence on the part of followers is ever more important to a team and to goal accomplishment than is the emotional intelligence of the leader.

Hurwitz and Hurwitz offer several principles related to partnerships and collaboration: leaders and followers both are needed, and both are equal and dynamic and contribute different strengths; leaders set the frame (or articulate the vision), but followers are the ones who create within that frame or vision; both leaders and followers need to invest in significant ways (i.e., have passion and commitment) to build connections and realize a vision; focusing and building on the positive is most effective; and leaders and followers must hold shared goals. They assert that our current environment calls for new perspectives in which leadership is exercised by any number of individuals in a group, and followership is a role that needs to be nurtured, encouraged, and rewarded. Those aspiring to leadership would do well to reflect on the principles offered in this book and imagine how new leader and follower roles can be maximized.

Huston, C. J. (2018). *The road to leadership.* Sigma Theta Tau International.
In this short, engaging book, Huston shares leadership lessons, personal stories, and numerous quotes that challenge the reader to reflect seriously on the nature of leadership and how to help oneself and others become a leader. She reflects on things that will facilitate the leadership journey—mentors, self-awareness and authenticity, humility, vision, personal power, effective communication, appreciating and empowering followers, "choosing your battles carefully," and enjoying the journey. She also offers ideas that serve to inspire the reader and strengthen one's resolve to accept and effectively implement the role of leader, regardless of the scope of one's impact, one's educational preparation, or the setting in which one works.

Jaworski, J. (2011). *Synchronicity: The inner path of leadership* (2nd ed.). Berrett-Koehler.
This author calls on Jung's classic definition of *synchronicity*—"a meaningful coincidence of two or more events, where something other than the probability of chance is involved"—to discuss what he refers to as "the most subtle territory of leadership, creating the conditions for 'predictable miracles'" (p. ix). Thus begins this fascinating book that focuses on how leaders shape the future instead of simply responding to the present.

Jaworski notes that most contemporary institutions are leaderless and bemoans this state of affairs in light of his expressed belief that there is leadership potential in everyone. Using his own personal journey, he describes how "we can shape our future in ways that we rarely realize" (p. 9) and "participate in the unfolding process of the universe" (p. 44), not merely accepting what comes our way. By facing and overcoming personal challenges (i.e., being afraid to step outside one's own narrow circle, being afraid to take the risk of stepping into the unknown, fearing that one cannot make a difference anyway), Jaworski responded to the "call to redefine what is possible, to see a vision of a new world and . . . undertake, step-by-step, what [was] necessary . . . to achieve that vision" (p. 58).

The personal journey described in this book helps the reader appreciate the risk taking inherent in a leadership role, as well as the rewards of serving in such a role.

Johnson, S. M. (2014). *How we got to now: Six innovations that made the modern world*. Penguin Group.
This book is about how innovative individuals in North America and Europe (the author emphasizes that the innovation process in other cultures would be a different journey) came up with ideas and developed light bulbs, sound recordings, air-conditioning, clean tap water, a wristwatch, and a glass lens. They describe how they received assistance from others, sometimes serendipitously and other times after reaching out for help, and revised and improved their original projects. The author discusses the multiple connections between various individuals who impacted the success or demise of the innovations. The process of lesson learning with these innovations is easily compared with the phenomenon of leadership and followership and how the interrelationships that occur simultaneously in multiple networks lead a project to its fulfillment. For readers interested in gaining skills in improving their ability to be innovative, it may be prudent to also watch the Public Broadcasting Service (PBS) series *How We Got to Now*, which illustrates how the modern world evolved through various collaborative networks.

Of course, with the great advantages innovation generally brings come some adverse events that would never have been imaginable. It is wise to think of innovation like any other change and realize that we are in constant flux; hence, growth, no matter good or bad, will occur. Johnson explains the evolution of the hummingbird in gaining the ability to float as it extracts nectar from plants and how this natural process can be paralleled to leaders who step up to solving problems and developing solutions that previously would have been thought impossible. The author suggests we need to appreciate how innovation affects society and how to predict the "hummingbird effects" that will influence us after an innovation transpires. According to Johnson, "most innovation happens in the present tense of the adjacent possible, working with the tools and concepts that are available in that time" (p. 252). The author notes that innovative leaders are able to see past their own setting or discipline and work "at the margins of their official fields, or at the intersection point between very different disciplines" (p. 252). The book also includes a comprehensive bibliography.

Kahnweiler, J. B. (2013). *The introverted leader: Building on your quiet strengths* (2nd ed.). Berrett-Kohler.

As noted by the author, "most people think of leaders as being outgoing, very visible, and charismatic people," but this is a perspective she finds to be quite narrow. If the "key challenge for leaders today is to get beyond the surface and unlock the full potential of all their colleagues," as Kahnweiler asserts, introverts are well equipped for this role because they are characterized by traits that help them meet this challenge: listening, preparation, and calmness. In fact, she notes that "often it is the quietest people who have the loudest minds" and can be, therefore, quite effective as leaders who have vision and see the big picture. Introverts draw energy from within themselves, tap into their reflective side, and have quiet strengths that they harness, all of which contribute to their being effective leaders. The author compares introverts and extroverts along several dimensions, and offers ways to deal with the six key challenges faced by introverted leaders. For those who think of themselves as leaders who cannot possibly be leaders, this book challenges, inspires, and assists in building your quiet strengths.

Kellerman, B. (2008). *Followership: How followers are creating change and changing leaders.* Harvard Business Press.

Recognizing that the preparation of leaders has become an industry while attention to followers has been virtually nonexistent, Kellerman sets out to help the reader appreciate how "people without obvious sources of power, authority, and influence are far more consequential than we generally assume" (p. xxi). She is clear in asserting that good followership matters and acknowledges that we are now more willing than ever before to recognize that followers are integral to the leadership process.

Through a careful analysis of Germany during the Nazi regime and other real-life situations, the author guides us to think about five different kinds of followers: isolates (who are completely detached and alienated), bystanders (who observe but make a conscious decision not to participate), participants (who invest some of what they have [e.g., time] to try to have an impact), activists (who are fully engaged and energetic, either in support of or against the leader), and diehards (who are prepared to "put everything on the line" for the cause). She points out the value and concerns about each type of follower, acknowledges clearly that all of us are followers at some point, and suggests that self-reflection regarding the type of follower one is in various situations is in order.

Kellerman, B. (2015). *Hard times: Leadership in America.* Stanford University Press.

This book explains how to "think like a leader and not necessarily how to be a leader" by using a dynamic framework of the leader, followers, and context. Kellerman suggests we view the term *context* as a "series of concentric circles" in whatever setting the leading is supposed to be present. She emphasizes the importance of every leader and follower developing "contextual expertise." Another significant point she makes is that leading may be different in various places in America, but will be more so outside of the country. The time factor is also unique. So this book focuses only on leading in the United States in 2015.

Kellerman offers a flexible checklist to assist us in thinking like a leader and developing our contextual expertise with the following categories: history and ideology, media and money, class and culture, risks and trends, leaders and followers, to name a few.

She gives realistic examples of how leaders and followers exist successfully in several corporate work settings, professional organizations, health-care environments, and academia in America. The idea of how leading has become more difficult in the 21st century in all settings is a strong theme and supports the title of the book, *Hard Times: Leadership in America.*

The book has seven themes—technology, money, America in decline, a divisive America, pressure on the leaders, relentless sense of danger, and leaders are disappointments—that the reader will want to explore with regard to their own situation while using the checklist framework to increase contextual expertise.

Kelley, R. E. (1992). *The power of followership: How to create leaders people want to follow and followers who lead themselves.* Doubleday Currency.
Robert Kelley presented one of the first and best discussions of followership available in the literature. His goal in writing this book was to "shift the spotlight toward followership as *the* important phenomenon to study if we are to understand why organizations succeed or fail" (p. 5), and he achieved that goal extremely well.

This author talks about the increasing emphasis on teams and collaboration and the kind of power that followers can and do have in groups and organizations. He notes that "followers determine not only if someone will be accepted as a leader but also if that leader will be effective" (p. 13), and he asserts that effective followers are critical for success.

The term *effective follower* is not used lightly in this book. Indeed, Kelley describes five different followership styles: passive, conformist, pragmatist, alienated, and exemplary/effective. He offers ways to help the reader identify her or his followership style, argues for the importance of developing one's followership skills, and offers very convincing arguments why individuals should become followers.

This book, therefore, is unique in its attention to a critical but frequently ignored role in the leadership process. It is one that must be read to gain a better appreciation of the concept of followership.

Keohane, N. O. (2010). *Thinking about leadership.* Princeton University Press.
Written by a former president of Wellesley College and Duke University, where she was the first woman to hold that position, Keohane offers a perspective on leadership "from the inside." This book is a masterful combination of theory and practical points that incorporates political theories, literature, biographies, and other sources to examine the leader–follower dialectic, the need for balance in leaders, the importance of vision, and whether gender makes a difference in leadership. This is a thoughtful, scholarly, informative book about leadership that challenges leaders to consider the ethics of their behaviors, how power can be easily abused, and the uniqueness of providing leadership in a democratic society that values equality, involvement of its citizens, and expertise.

Kethledge, R., & Erwin, M. (2018). *Lead yourself first: Inspiring leadership through solitude.* Bloomsbury.
The authors share the importance of using solitude as a leader and give excellent examples with Martin Luther King Jr., Jane Goodall, Dwight Eisenhower, and others to explain how and why this works. They say it is more difficult to use solitude with the constant bombarding of social media 24/7, but it is imperative that leaders try to use solitude in order to increase creativity, emotional balance, clarity on issues, and moral courage. They share information obtained from interviews they conducted with multiple leaders and challenging experiences to help leaders and also strategies to find solitude in their busy schedule. Most importantly, they reinforce the fact that one must be able to lead oneself before leading others.

Knowles, B. (2017). *The quiet rise of introverts: 8 practices for living and loving in a noisy world.* MJF Books.
The intention of this book, the author notes, is not to turn introverts into extroverts; instead, it is to teach introverts how to have a grasp of themselves and listen to their internal voice while also being comfortable and effective with relationships and inter-dependence. Like Cain (*Quiet;* see earlier), Knowles discusses society's seeming prefer-ence for extroverts and myths or unfounded assumptions often made about introverts. Although the book is not directed specifically at helping introverts be successful as lead-ers, the advice offered in this book has relevance for those in leadership roles and, in fact, highlights many qualities discussed in the leadership literature. Among those qual-ities are self-awareness, caring for oneself, having confidence in oneself, learning from conflict, being attentive and responsive to others, promoting unity and collaboration, and—perhaps most importantly—being oneself.

Koestenbaum, P. (2002). *Leadership: The inner side of greatness* (2nd ed.). Jossey-Bass.
This book is a philosophical analysis of individuals and what it takes for successful leaders to achieve specific goals. It is not a synthesis of stories about people who have been successful but rather a compilation of how to create environments and socie-ties that will facilitate the achievement of goals. Koestenbaum describes his Leadership Diamond Model, which revolves around the concepts of time, democracy, motivation, teamwork, and salesmanship.
   This is a good book to read if one wishes to analyze one's leadership ability and/or develop one's leadership skills. There are some excellent cases, such as the Enron scandal, that examine marketing morale and history, and the exercises and checklists to assist the reader in leadership development are helpful.

Komives, S. R., Wagner, W., & Associates. (2009). *Leadership for a better world: Understanding the social change model of leadership development.* Jossey-Bass.
This book is unique in that it shares the voices of students who are engaged in activities designed to help them develop as leaders who can influence social change. It provides a set of principles about how knowing oneself, engaging in meaningful ways with others, and adopting a systems perspective can promote the socially responsible leadership many argue is so desperately needed in today's world.

Through case studies, thought-provoking questions and scenarios, pointed content, and a clear commitment to social change being at the heart of the leadership experience, this book is an excellent resource for educators who are in search of learning activities related to leadership development, service learning directors looking for meaningful ways to engage students in the life of their communities, or individuals desiring to make a difference in the world.

Kotter, J. (2008). *A sense of urgency*. Harvard Business Press.
This book—a sequel to Kotter's previous books on change such as *Leading Change, The Heart of Change*, and *Our Iceberg Is Melting*—points out the absolute necessity for leaders to help others appreciate the urgency for change. In fact, Kotter believes the biggest error that people make in implementing a change is not being able to create a sense of urgency for a specific change. He points out how most successful people become complacent and do not want to "rock the boat" by instituting a change but soon find themselves not being successful because they actually did miss out by not implementing change. He further points out that some embark on change not because they feel the urgency but because they are motivated by anxiety, anger, or frustration; as a result, they create a frantic culture that does not allow a clear focus on the needed change. Kotter offers several strategies to assist in acquiring the skills to lead change. This skill is especially important today when change seems to be continuous and not episodic in occurrence.

Kotter, J. P. (2012). *Leading change*. Harvard Business Review Press.
This book speaks to the rapid pace of just about everything and how important it is to be aware of the social and technological trends occurring. Kotter says a winning organization has to have constant change 24/7 to keep winning. We will not be able to become complacent nor will we be able to just experience short hectic periods of change like we did in the 20th century. Kotter says those days are long gone. He emphasizes the importance of rapid data dissemination that is accurate and not designed just to make the system "look good." The focus has shifted from management development to leadership development that he says must occur for global success. He believes we can develop more leaders to lead the world's population of approximately 5.7 billion people and that successful organizations must become incubators of leadership (p. 174). The book gives multiple examples for leaders to discuss best practices of change processes by supporting cultures that are adaptive to change, encourage teamwork at the top, and demand less bureaucracy.

Kouzes, J., & Posner, B. (2003). *Encouraging the heart: A leader's guide to rewarding and recognizing others*. Jossey-Bass.
The main theme in this book is that people who are recognized for their good work and encouraged are more likely to achieve higher levels of success. The authors recommend how leaders can support the human need to be appreciated for what we do and who we are. They describe the process of "encouraging the heart" with four ideas: leaders must follow general principles that reward people for work well done, leaders will not be perceived as being "soft" for encouraging the heart, leaders have multiple methods they

use to encourage the heart, and all leaders must be aware of the soul and spirit involved in any organization. This book gives the reader ideas on how to keep hope alive and explains how ordinary people can actually be effective leaders by being encouraging to others. This is a good book for all to read, especially when the organizations in which we function appear to be losing their edge and failing to be responsive to all those involved in the work of the organization, and there is still a need to get extraordinary things done.

Kouzes, J., & Posner, B. (2017). *The leadership challenge: How to make extraordinary things happen in organizations* (6th ed.). Jossey-Bass.
This sixth edition of this excellent book reflects the authors' observations of what leaders do to encourage extraordinary accomplishments when they are leading, not managing. This edition includes interviews with some of the most significant leaders around the globe and shares a new and more global perspective of leadership. There are many examples of international leaders. Kouzes and Posner's classic "five sets of behavioral practices" and "ten behavioral commitments" are described fully, and the importance of leaders having perseverance, having direction, empowering others, being role models, and recognizing others' contributions are all discussed thoroughly. Each of the five behavioral practices are correlated with two of the behavioral commitments and discussed with reality-based examples.

The book describes leadership as a skill that can be developed by coaching and through experiential learning. In fact, this sixth edition gives excellent examples of how to apply coaching skills in assisting others to gain leadership ability. There are specific examples of this with business issues. The necessity of purposefully developing one's leadership is advanced, as is the notion that leadership is now more important today than ever before if we are to achieve success in the future. Ideas on how to be more effective as a great, and not just good, leader are described. The authors remind us that leadership is everyone's business and, therefore, that everyone should accept the leadership "challenge" on a daily basis and offer creative strategies to tackle the complex problems of today.

Kouzes, J. M., & Posner, B. (2011). *Credibility: How leaders gain and lose it . . . Why people demand it* (2nd ed.). Jossey-Bass.
The purpose of the second edition of this book is to explore, in depth, the quality of a leader whom constituents (i.e., followers) would want to follow: credibility. Based on extensive research, the authors conclude that people have very high expectations of their leaders, wanting them to "hold to an ethic of service, [be] genuinely respectful of the intelligence and contributions of their constituents, [and] put principles ahead of politics and other people before self-interests" (p. xvii). This new edition offers updates to the research and also emphasizes the book's major theme of credibility, which they explain as saying what you mean and always meaning what you said.

Kouzes and Posner view leadership as a relationship and a service, with credibility clearly at its foundation. This book examines leadership as a relationship, talks about the benefits of credibility, and discusses the behaviors that convey and establish credibility. Among those behaviors are the following: knowing yourself and your values, appreciating the strengths and talents of followers, reinforcing shared values, developing others to reach their fullest potential, making meaning out of the work or tasks to be done, and sustaining hope in the followers. Strategies for how leaders develop and gain and can even lose credibility also are discussed.

This analysis stimulates the reader to thoughtfully reflect on her or his own actions and how they establish or undermine credibility. Although other writers imply the significance of credibility in the leader–follower relationship, Kouzes and Posner make a most valuable contribution to our understanding of how leaders can be most effective by their careful study of the concept. Any discussion of leadership would be incomplete without a discussion of credibility; this book, therefore, is an excellent resource for enhancing such understanding. Additionally, in this new edition, Kouzes and Posner share some cases studies from around the world that are helpful as the world becomes more globally integrated.

Krzyzewski, M. (2000). *Leading with the heart: Coach K's successful strategies for basketball, business, and life.* Warner Business Books.

"Coach K," as the author is known, is the winningest men's basketball coach in NCAA history. He has been head coach at Duke University since 1980 and coached the gold-medal-winning 2008 U.S. Olympic men's basketball team. In this book, Coach K shares tips for being a successful leader, one whose players say they learned lessons like the following from him: "setting the bar high so that you can strive to be the best you can be; the value and rewards of a hard-work ethic; building close relationships based on trust; setting shared goals; sacrificing; giving of yourself; winning with humility; losing with dignity; turning a negative into a positive; being a part of something bigger than yourself; [and] enjoying the journey" (pp. x–xi).

Among the guiding principles offered by Coach K are those that have implications for individuals aspiring to provide leadership: know your team, help the entire team think in terms of "we" rather than "I," build on the strengths of team members and expect everyone to help one another achieve their full potential, be clear about shared goals and expectations, be honest, be passionate about what you do, strive to do your best 100% of the time, and have fun. By following such principles, leaders will constantly be energized, team members will grow, and great things can be accomplished.

Leadership in Nursing. (1994). *Holistic Nursing Practice, 9*(1) [Entire issue].

This journal issue offers a thoughtful collection of articles about the nature of leadership, particularly as it relates to nursing. It is a useful resource because each article can be read independently of the others. The articles focus on many significant areas, all of which facilitate an understanding of the complex nature of leadership. Included among those areas are the following: the nature of leadership and ways to conceptualize it that make sense for 21st-century practice; the holistic nature of leadership; transformational leadership, particularly as it relates to women leaders; the significance of followers; ethical aspects of leadership; the preparation of leaders; an exploration of the leadership that is needed to shape a preferred future for nursing; and an analysis of 10 years of nursing leadership research.

All the articles in this issue are intended to "provide new insights and to explore important issues related to leadership" (p. vi). They accomplish that goal in a stimulating way that has relevance for our profession.

Loue, S. (2011). *Mentoring health science professionals*. Springer.
This is an interesting book that provides examples of mentoring faculty, students, and junior professionals in health fields. It provides an overview of the concept of mentoring, highlights and critiques various formal mentoring programs, and shares the journey of a mentor and protégé as they collaborate to help the protégé develop a successful career trajectory as a faculty member in an academic medical setting. Although the foundations of mentoring presented in this book are similar to those offered in other works, the fact that the examples provided reflect the uniqueness of health fields and health settings may be particularly useful to those in nursing.

Broome, M. E., & Marshall, E. S. (Eds.). (2021). *Transformational leadership in nursing: From expert clinician to influential leader* (3rd ed.). Springer.
This book provides a helpful overview of major leadership theories, then focuses in depth on transformational leadership. The authors acknowledge the need to be aware of the context, situation, or culture in which the leadership role is enacted; they examine the importance of collaboration, networks, and communication for leaders; and they offer strategies to help one develop as a leader.
    Building on these foundations, Broome and Marshall seem to bring an administrative or management perspective to the discussion as they talk about challenges in complex health-care organizations, new practice models, and shaping the organizational environment and culture to support practice excellence. While such topics certainly are relevant to the leader who also holds a position of authority, they may not be as relevant for the individual providing leadership on a smaller scale.

Maxwell, J. C. (2019). *Leadershift: The 11 essential changes every leader must embrace*. HarperCollins.
In this book that clearly acknowledges our fast-paced, constantly changing world, Maxwell offers an analysis of ways in which individuals need to change if they are, indeed, to provide leadership in such environments. Among those changes are the following: moving from maintaining systems to creating them; doing less directing and more connecting; appreciating and capitalizing on the diversity of the team rather than seeking uniformity; and viewing one's work as a calling, not merely a career. For those who seek to or are called upon to provide leadership in the 21st century, the following quote serves to summarize the focus of this book: "You cannot be the same, think the same, and act the same if you hope to be successful in a world that does not remain the same" (p. 7). Maxwell's book is a compelling read that captivates the reader's attention until the very end.

McBride, A. B. (2010). *The growth and development of nurse leaders*. Springer.
This is an interesting book focused on leadership, not management. McBride divides the book into three parts—personal leadership, leadership as it pertains to organizational goals, and transformational leadership—and offers multiple examples that illustrate various aspects of leadership development both personally and professionally. Each chapter ends with a list of "Take-Away Points," which further serve to assist the reader in gaining insight into one's own leadership style. The book is written with the

idea that one will want to reflect on one's own lived experiences regarding leadership and how best to augment one's success with leading and inspiring others to also lead. This book will give readers many ideas to use to transform their own leadership style and ultimately help them to lead in a more productive fashion.

McCall, M. W. (1998). *High flyers: Developing the next generation of leaders*. Harvard
    Business School Press.
The major emphasis in this book is on corporate executives who have a bent toward management more so than leadership. Despite this emphasis, however, McCall presents many interesting ideas about leaders and what needs to be done to prepare individuals to be effective in leadership roles.

The author asserts that "organizations not only overlook people with the potential to develop but also frequently and unintentionally derail the talented people they have identified as high flyers by rewarding them for their flaws, teaching them to behave in ineffective ways, reinforcing narrow perspectives and skills, and inflating their egos" (p. xi). He notes that we often keep people from developing their full potential as leaders, and as a result, neither they nor their organizations progress as much as they otherwise could.

McCall firmly believes that leadership can be learned and points out that "the development of leaders is itself a leadership responsibility" (p. xii). Learning leadership, he says, is a "lifelong journey, with its lessons taught by the journey itself" (p. 17). He challenges each of us—as aspiring leaders who must take responsibility for our own growth, and as practicing leaders who must take responsibility for the leadership development of others—to attend to the conscious development of ourselves and others as leaders.

Nickerson, J. (2014). *Leading change from the middle: A practical guide to building
    extraordinary capabilities*. Brookings Institution Press.
Nickerson was challenged with renovating the Brookings Executive Education (BEE), a subunit of the Brookings Institution. Not only was BEE located in Washington, D.C., and Nickerson was a professor at Washington University Olin Business School in St. Louis, but he also knew no one at the BEE. The book is an excellent account of how to make a change from the middle of the organization and provides examples of successful changes in the public, private, and nonprofit sectors. Leaders can be successful if they follow the Leading at the Crossroads of Change framework that has three components: (1) stakeholder categories; (2) communications, strategies, tactics, and the sequencing of actions (CoSTS) that are specific to each category; and (3) general CoSTS to use to manage emotions (disrespect, envy, anger, and fear) that (many times) stop the change.

The author provides ideas for helpful reflection exercises that, if followed regularly, should also positively influence one's leadership abilities. Exact methods of dealing with change are detailed with interesting explanations of subtle differences the leader should use given specific situations, stakeholders, and unaccounted variance that could occur. The author actually states his purpose for writing the book is to provide "a road map for midlevel leaders who are attempting to build extraordinary capabilities" (p. 123).

Orr, M. (2019). *Lean out: The truth about women, power, and the workplace.* HarperCollins.

A former employee at Google and then Facebook, where she connected with Sheryl Sandberg (author of *Lean In* [see later]), Orr realized that the ideas put forth by that author were "completely antithetical to . . . and ran counter to" (p. xxi) everything she believed. She did not believe that women needed to change to be more like men (e.g., more assertive, ambitious, and demanding), as was implied by Sandberg; instead, she believed that women would be more influential in workplaces if those institutions themselves changed in ways that acknowledged and valued the strengths women possess and their ways of leading. She admits to a bit of "corporate rebelliousness" (p. xxi) as she offers critical analyses of organizational changes that are needed to benefit from the strengths of all members, men and women alike. Women need not be victims, according to Orr.

Palacios-Huerta, I. (Ed.). (2013). *In 100 years: Leading economists predict the future.* MIT Press.

This book is composed of 10 economists' (including Daron Acemoglu, Robert Shiller, Alvin Roth, and Robert Solow) predictions for the world of the 22nd century. Trends such as the improving economy in China and India, climate change, political extremism, technology, and the continuing increase of inequality throughout the world are all greatly impacting us. Each author writes about their perception of this impact—for example, will the weapons of mass destruction from improved technology ultimately destroy Earth as we know it? Will the varying natural disasters, greenhouse gas emissions, and rising sea levels—possibly caused by extreme climate change—cause such catastrophic damage to the environment that Earth's inhabitants will all die? Or will there be a political change so huge that will eliminate personal freedom and current property ownership? Some warn that the more dangerous risks the world faces will be a result of biological or social origin such as with health problems and conflicts or wars. Others have a more positive spin for 2113 (100 years from the publication of Palacios-Huerta's book) and predict health longevity, material prosperity, and an increasing population but also believe geoengineering will be necessary to manage the climate change.

The book has been compared with John Maynard Keyne's 1930 *Economic Possibilities for Our Grandchildren*, which offered predictions for what he felt would be happening in the 21st century, that the standard of life in progressive countries in 2030 would be between four and eight times as high as it was in 1930—that has already transpired for some, but certainly there is no global economic prosperity. The contributors speak to the need for standard accreditation of products, programs, and specific workers. Competency, authority, and credibility will not just be believed from someone's say-so but will be granted only if standards are met. The editor also provides a succinct biosketch of each contributor.

Quibell, D., Selig, J., & Slattery, D. (2019). *Deep creativity: Seven ways to spark up creative spirit.* Shambhala Publishers.

The authors are most innovative and assist the reader in gaining creativity in many different ways. The reflective exercises are very helpful and are offered as pathways for anyone to use in their organization to achieve the creative, reflective organizational culture they are striving for. They use seven unique pathways—love, nature, the muse, suffering, practice, the sacred, and art—to assist the reader in finding their creativity and also offer 15 principles of how to find creativity from yourself and others.

Quibell, Selig, and Slattery describe deep creativity as the ability to spark up the creative spirit and, consequently, the morale of a group. The book shares stories on how groups have come together and expanded their production and improved outcomes just by being more creative in all aspects of the work. This book is a must-read, especially for health-care professionals who are involved in more and more intraprofessional teamwork and networking.

Rath, T., & Conchie, B. (2008). *Strengths-based leadership: Great leaders, teams, and why people follow.* Gallup Press.

This book challenges the reader to think about and assess her or his own leadership. Based on the assumption that each of us will have many opportunities to lead during our lifetime, the authors want us to be able to seize those opportunities and be effective as leaders. They analyzed decades of Gallup data (in-depth interviews with more than 20,000 senior leaders, Gallup polls about most admired leaders, and studies of more than 1 million work teams) and combined that information with the findings of their own study of more than 10,000 followers to summarize three key findings about the most effective leaders: (1) they always invest in strengths, (2) they surround themselves with the best people and then maximize their team, and (3) they understand the needs of the followers.

Given that "the path to great leadership starts with a deep understanding of the strengths [one] bring[s] to the table" (p. 3), the authors provide the StrengthsFinder (2.0) Assessment for readers to use to identify their strengths as a leader. Once that personalized report is received, the book provides an explanation of each of the three key findings and how one's own strengths can be used to meet followers' needs, to lead others who themselves are strong in various areas, and to continually grow as a leader. The assessment is easy to complete, the customized report is informative, and the self-reflection prompted by this analysis is revealing. Anyone who works collaboratively with others could benefit from learning about their own strengths and how to use them most effectively.

Robinson-Walker, C. (1999). *Women and leadership in health care: The journey to authenticity and power.* Jossey-Bass.

This book reports on intensive dialogue with nearly 100 women and men responsible for managing a significant portion of America's health care. It is clear that "women are simply not present in the numbers we would expect, nor do they ascend at the rate we would expect to the most senior leadership roles in health care" (p. ix). Given this reality, the author—who co-created the national Center for Nursing Leadership in the late 1990s—examines the significance of gender in the 21st century; stumbling blocks faced by women in reaching the top; and relationships among gender, values, and leadership.

The author asserts that the characteristics most commonly exhibited by women, particularly women interviewed for this book, are precisely the qualities needed by those providing leadership in health care: an ability to tolerate ambiguity, a collaborative style, dispersed power, consensus building, integrity, "doing the right thing—even when the price is high" (p. 185), and others. She then offers a number of "antidotes" to help women be more effective leaders: defusing gender's role in conflict, negotiations, and power; using communication as a bridge; renewing our careers; nurturing ourselves; and mentoring others.

Although this book—one of the first to study the relationship between gender and leadership—acknowledges the difficulties women often have with taking on the leader role, it also is positive and offers specific strategies to overcome those difficulties. As such, it is an excellent resource on gender issues related to leadership.

Rosenbach, W. E., Taylor, R. L., & Youndt, M. A. (Eds.). (2012). *Contemporary issues in leadership* (7th ed.). Westview Press.
This book is one of the best collections of readings about leadership, as are all previous editions of it. None of the articles—many of which have been published originally elsewhere, and several of which are classics in the field—has focused specifically on nursing (to date), but each offers many rich ideas that could easily be applied to a nursing context. The seventh edition reemphasizes followership as an integral component of leadership, discusses the importance of leaders as mentors, helps navigate the hazards of leadership, and presents a renewed framework for understanding leaders and leadership from a contemporary perspective. The book, therefore, continues to be a most valuable one for students and teachers of nursing.

This book draws on experts in various areas and includes original articles as well as those previously published in the *Harvard Business Review, Leader to Leader, World Futures*, the *Wall Street Journal*, and *Compass: A Journal of Leadership*. It is, therefore, exciting and inclusive of diverse perspectives. Although several of the articles are from management journals, they clearly are focused on leadership, and this is one of the things that makes this collection of readings so valuable—it does not confuse management and leadership.

NOTE: All previous editions of this book also are quite valuable and include collections of different readings. The first edition was published in 1984, the second in 1989, the third in 1993, the fourth in 1998, the fifth in 2001, and the sixth in 2006.

Sandberg, S. (2013). *Lean in: Women, work, and the will to lead.* Knopf Doubleday.
Sandberg was chief operating officer at Facebook and had been vice president of Global Online Sales and Operations at Google, as well as chief of staff at the U.S. Treasury Department. This book focuses on women as leaders, partly in response to her observations that "when it comes to making the decisions that most affect our world, women's voices are not heard equally" (p. 6).

She notes that women who aspire to leadership face many external barriers erected by society, but they also are hindered by barriers that exist within themselves. She asserts that women hold themselves back by lacking self-confidence, not raising their hands, pulling back when they should be leaning in, internalizing the negative messages they get throughout their lives, and lowering their own expectations of what they can achieve.

In response to such circumstances, Sandberg "makes the case for leaning in, for being ambitious in any pursuit" (p. 10), and she offers advice on how to do just that, including believing in and having confidence in oneself, continually learning, seeking out leadership roles, accepting leadership opportunities when they present themselves, accepting and embracing uncertainty, and disrupting the status quo. In essence, the advice she offers is for women to understand the qualities of leaders and learn to enact such qualities.

Sashota, N., & Ashley, M. (2019). *Own the artificial intelligence revolution: Unlock your artificial intelligence strategies to disrupt your competition.* McGraw-Hill.
Artificial intelligence (AI) is an exciting phenomenon already occurring in our world today. The authors describe the complex impact that AI is having and will continue to have on our lives. It is a concept most people understand but only in basic terms. This book discusses the huge innovations and changes that AI brings to many formats.

Readers can gain enormous amounts of knowledge to help them plan their future personal and professional lives. Many helpful strategies (including legal, technological, ethical, and scientific) for leaders to use are illustrated with facts as well as case studies and interviews with AI thought experts. Most readers will be fascinated by the discussions of how AI is the "fourth Industrial Revolution," its use with analyzing big data and connecting various people, and how it will impact our everyday life now through the 2030s.

Schiff, K. G. (2005). *Lighting the way: Nine women who changed modern America.* Hyperion.
Written by the daughter of former vice president Al Gore, this book chronicles how nine extraordinary women worked behind the scenes and against the odds in the major political movements of the last century. It tells powerful stories of women who influenced women's suffrage, the decision to enter World War II, the struggle for civil rights, environmental health, the AIDS crisis, and other significant issues of the past 100 years.

In telling these stories, Schiff points out that women have always been consequential, if often unrecognized, political leaders and have been responsible for many of the most creative ideas that helped shape history. This book is uplifting and powerful and is an excellent resource for the study of women as leaders.

Schulze, H. (2019). *Excellence wins. A no-nonsense guide to becoming the best in a world of compromise.* Zondervan.
Although this book, written by the co-founder and former president of the Ritz-Carlton Hotel Company, focuses on businesses and management—perhaps more than on leadership—it is still a valuable read, primarily because of its focus on achieving excellence and not settling for merely getting by. Schulze acknowledges that leading is an acquired skill, something that one can learn and continue to develop over time, and effective leaders exhibit the following qualities: they strive to inspire others with their vision and engage them in achieving it; they never settle for less than the very best; they ensure that the crystal-clear vision guides everything; and they are always looking to improve. For

those who want to be challenged and guided by a spirit of excellence, this book could be quite helpful.

Senge, P. (2006). *The fifth discipline: The art and practice of the learning organization* (2nd ed.). Doubleday Currency.
This newer edition of Senge's seminal work, *The Fifth Discipline*, describes how many of his ideas regarding leadership and management have been operationalized in organizations since its original 1990 publication. He shares the outcomes of his interviews with people from companies such as Intel, Ford, BP, and HP, as well as organizations such as the World Bank, Roca, and Oxfam. Some new and particularly interesting chapters in this edition are *"Impetus,"* which describes how to build learning-oriented cultures instead of staying in one's comfort zone, "Leaders' New Work," and "Frontiers for the Future."

Through this book, Senge teaches the reader how to see things differently (e.g., seeing the forest *and* the trees), how to deal with the constant struggle of being tugged by personal *and* work issues, and how to maximize one's creativity. This is perhaps a more management-focused book, but because being a good manager serves to strengthen one's leadership ability, it is a valuable resource.

Sinek, S. (2017). *Leaders eat last: Why some teams pull together and others don't* (2nd ed.). Penguin Random House.
This is a great book to read to gain insight on how to lead for the good of others and not oneself. Sinek shares the importance of caring for one's teams and gives real-life examples of this caring, or what he refers to as the "Circle of Safety," which allows for a trusting culture in the team or organization where people will do just about anything for one another. It is, according to Sinek, due to the leader's belief that leaders must always think of the followers before themselves that makes for a trusting and happy work culture. Hence, the title of the book refers to "leaders eat last," and the followers should always go first unless it is a dangerous situation, and then the leader should forge ahead first with the followers following. This author is known as the speaker of the third most frequently watched TED Talk, *How Great Leaders Inspire Action*, and describes how to maintain optimism and think positively in the chaotic world we know today.

Soder, R. (2001). *The language of leadership.* Jossey-Bass.
The author suggests that management is a larger, more encompassing concept than leadership; however, he goes on to say, "This book deals with elements of leadership as applied to those in elected and other public offices . . . and those in the private sector" (p. xv), meaning, largely, that the focus is on individuals in management positions.

The author asserts that persuasion is "a critical aspect of leadership" (p. 3) and focuses most of the book on an analysis of the concept of persuasion and how leaders can use it to get others to do what they want. In addition, the author makes leadership seem like little more than political maneuvering (p. 28), almost as if one needs to be quite Machiavellian (e.g., use devious means to get information) to be successful as a leader. These perspectives are contradictory to most other literature on leadership.

In addition, the author seems to want to impress the reader with his knowledge of a wide range of literature by inserting quotes and snippets from various philosophers, historical figures, and so on. A few such quotes and examples are helpful to illustrate a point, but after a while, it seemed that the author was inserting such items simply to impress the reader. Instead of accomplishing this goal, however, this style may obfuscate the real point of the book.

Spears. L. C. (Ed.). (1995). *Reflections on leadership: How Robert K. Greenleaf's theory of servant-leadership influenced today's top management thinkers.* John Wiley & Sons.
This collection of 27 essays—written by some of the leading thinkers and practitioners of servant leadership—brings together into one volume some of the most significant ideas about the concept and the growing influence of Robert K. Greenleaf's legacy. It begins with several chapters by Greenleaf himself, describing the evolution of his thinking and the development of his theory.
This book is an excellent source of information about servant-leadership and how a variety of people have interpreted and lived the concept. It is inspiring and uplifting, and helps one think about leadership in a different way.

Spears, L. (Ed.). (1998). *The power of servant leadership: Essays by Robert Greenleaf.* Berrett-Koehler.
This book captures the vision and writings of the late Robert K. Greenleaf, who was the first to use the term *servant leadership.* According to Greenleaf, "servant leadership" is a way of leading that puts serving others (e.g., customers, patients, employees, students) first. This collection includes the following eight essays written by Greenleaf throughout his career: "Servant-Leadership: Retrospect and Prospect, Education and Maturity"; "The Leadership Crisis: Have You a Dream Deferred?"; "The Servant as Religious Leader"; "Seminary as Servant"; "My Debt to E. B. White"; and "Old Age: The Ultimate Test of Spirit."
All the essays in this collection reflect Greenleaf's ideas about spirit, commitment to vision, and wholeness. Given this focus, this is a most reflective book that leaves the reader with a feeling of "wanting to do things right."

Tabrizi, B., & Terrell, M. (2013). *The inside-out effect: A practical guide to transformational leadership.* Evolve Publishing.
This book is extremely helpful for all nurses who want to improve their leadership ability and general performance, identify and maximize their best strengths for personal fulfillment, and evolve and transform to their fullest potential. As indicated in the book's title, the focus is on realigning one's inner–outer balance in all aspects of one's life. The authors describe stories of all kinds of people who are successful in transforming themselves—some with major changes and others with minor tweaks. Theories from multiple disciplines such as psychology, leadership development, human potential research, and the newest findings in neuroscience are integrated into the book. They apply Bronnie Ware's philosophy of making one's life everything one chooses instead of trying to live one's life according to others' expectations. Their mantra is Know-Be-Lead and includes these three issues: (1) Who am I at my very core? (2) Who am I actually? (3) Am I authentically leading? They offer solutions to increasing one's self-awareness and personal/professional alignment through real cases. It is easy to identify with many

of the case examples and obtain the courage one needs to make the changes that are so necessary to accomplish one's core goals.

Tye, J. (2014). *The Florence prescription: From accountability to ownership. Manifesto for a positive healthcare culture* (2nd ed.). http://www.TheFlorenceChallenge.com
In the foreword to this engaging book, Charles S. Lauer asserts the following: This book "reminds us of the importance of healthcare heroes—as sources of intelligence and inspiration, and as the conscience for everything we say, do, and feel" (p. xxvii) and that the barriers we encounter in facing today's challenges are as much internal ones as they are external ones. It is a work of fiction about an imagined medical center populated by individuals who, like Florence Nightingale, are committed to transformation of the system to best meet patient care needs.

The author continually asks, "What would Florence do or tell us to do?" and he repeatedly concludes with advice that is relevant for every nurse who takes on the challenge of leadership. "What Florence would advise" is what Tye calls the eight essential characteristics of a culture of ownership: commitment, engagement, passion, initiative, stewardship, belonging, fellowship, and pride. All of these—with the exception of pride—are qualities of effective leaders discussed throughout the analysis of the phenomenon of leadership offered in *The New Leadership Challenge: Creating the Future of Nursing*; thus, this book is an excellent resource for those who are or strive to be leaders in nursing, particularly because it focuses on the health-care arena and spotlights the founder of our profession.

Walsh, M. (2018). *The algorithmic leader: How to be smart when machines are smarter than you.* You Two Publishers.
Mike Walsh, a futurist and CEO of Tomorrow, interviewed the world's top business leaders and AI experts and developed 10 core principles to assist people with understanding AI. He says we must reinvent ourselves and stay ahead of the machines. He offers guiding points to help us with our transformation for the future. He calls them his 10 principles to try to achieve success in an algorithmic world: (1) Imagine the future and work backward not forward toward the future; (2) maximize growth in every sector continuously; (3) strategize like a computer; (4) try to be less wrong but definitely do not strive to always be right; (5) be human; (6) engage all and insist on their input for decisions; (7) foster reinvention of everyone—you cannot always get the best results; (8) always look beyond the answer and think about what else it could be; (9) obtain fresh ideas and opinions; and (10) attempt to accomplish the purpose with the profit being less of a priority. It seems these recommendations would correlate well with helping nurses or other professionals in multiple situations. This book was not only informative but also entertaining, since the stories and case studies provide realistic examples that most readers can totally relate to in their work and life.

Wheatley, M. (2006). *Leadership and the new science: Discovering order in a chaotic world* (3rd ed.). Berrett-Koehler.
This third edition of Wheatley's seminal work on the New Science reinforces ideas presented initially in 1992 and offers many new ideas to challenge our thinking. Contrary to the scientific or Newtonian model of step-by-step planning, the New Science

emphasizes the importance of exploring and accepting things the way they occur, as viewed from the perspectives of quantum physics, chaos theory, and biology.

Wheatley speaks to how leaders and those responsible for running organizations can benefit from application of the New Science. She asserts that by moving toward holism and appreciating the intricate relationships that exist between and among all things, one can develop and effectively use methods to change how people act, how they work, and how they view life. As a result of this interconnectedness between every single thing in the world (actually everything *plus* the world, according to Wheatley), every moment of one's day is dynamic and unpredictable. She emphasizes the importance of relationships, even at the subatomic level. Also, the idea that change and chaos are the most significant ways to transform positively is integrated throughout the book.

This edition offers examples of how self-organizing networks can flourish in our new world, and it presents information on how best to respond to disasters and stop terrorism. The author concludes that the fundamental work of our time centers around all of us discovering new ways of working and being together.

Wheatley explains how order and chaos can be seen as identical images and how these two seemingly opposite forces actually drive each other. Using natural phenomena (e.g., the evolution of the Grand Canyon, a babbling brook, and stormy weather), Wheatley creates complexity from simplicity and excites the reader with ideas of how the future will evolve from the whole rather than from the parts. This is an essential book for anyone interested in learning more about chaos theory and the New Science.

Wheatley suggests people organize their own "Leadership & the New Science" discussion groups by going to www.bkconnection.com or joining the listserv group.

Wheatley, M. (2017). *Who do we choose to be? Facing reality, claiming leadership and restoring sanity.* Berrett-Koehler.
Wheatley describes how leaders need to come forward in this most chaotic and tumultuous time. She shares ideas of how to bring back humaneness, strength, grace, and sanity. Wheatley discusses the celebrity culture we are currently living in and how superficial it is. Guidelines to use in being more reflective, suggestions for use of less social media and more one-to-one communication via talking, and the idea that it is right to care and give back to community are discussed. It is certainly a book worth reading for anyone, and the knowledge readers will gain from this book will assist them in helping others become less fearful and vulnerable. Wheatley shares her ideas on what is real and of value and serves as a source of helping us gain back our true feelings.

Wheatley, M., & Kellner-Rogers, M. (1996). *A simpler way.* Berrett-Koehler.
This book offers a way of thinking about life in a dynamic and totally different way, and it is critical reading for those who wish to better understand the New Science of Leadership. The authors share a magnificent collection of photographs of life, poems that convey the importance of being oneself, and narratives about simpler ways of viewing what most people define as a stress-filled, unenjoyable life.

This is a remarkable book about how to view life within the vastness of the universe. The authors speak to how life "self-organizes" without our planning every minute of every day and how this organization creates our identities. The advantages of seeing the world self-organize without human manipulation are challenged, and ways to foster more creativity, freedom, and real meaning in life are generated. In addition, the notions of play, organization, self, emergence, and coherence are explored.

Yudkowsky, M. (2005). *The pebble and the avalanche: How taking things apart creates revolutions.* Berrett-Kohler.
The basic premise in this book is that revolutions—in how we think, how we do business, how we use technology, and so on—can be relatively easy to create by taking things apart, a process the author calls *disaggregation.* Disaggregation and innovation, the author asserts, have positive results, such as heightened creativity in organizations, healthy competition, cost reduction, greater simplicity, and synergy, all of which "sweep aside old infrastructures" (p. 22).

The notions of taking things apart and questioning basic premises or assumptions are valuable ways to stimulate change, and they can be helpful to leaders. In addition, the idea that a small change can trigger a huge avalanche of change has merit to the leader who attempts to influence complex, tradition-laden systems. This book, however, suggests that revolutionary change is relatively easy to achieve, which is a conclusion that must be questioned.

Yukl, G. (2013). *Leadership in organizations* (8th ed.). Prentice Hall.
Much like the classic reference by Bass (2008) noted earlier, this book continues to be an excellent resource about leadership. It summarizes research related to key leadership concepts—followership, power, transformation, change, gender considerations, developing leadership skills, and others—and provides the reader with a rich and comprehensive overview of the field. Although much of the book focuses on management, rather than leadership, it still serves as a worthwhile, scholarly book on the latter and would be a useful addition to any library on leadership.

Zaleznik, A. (1977). Managers and leaders: Are they different? *Harvard Business Review, 55*(3), 67–78.
This article is indispensable reading. It is one of the earliest works in which leadership is clearly distinguished from management, and as such, it is a classic in the field.

Zaleznik talks about the differences between managers and leaders in terms of how they relate to other people, to the organization, and to goals. He explores the different conceptions of work, different perspectives on solitary activity, and different views about conflict and status quo held by leaders and managers. For purposes of illustration, the author talks about leaders and managers in the extreme, but he does acknowledge that managers can also be leaders, and leaders also can be managers.

This article is clearly written and is extremely helpful in clarifying the distinctions between these two related phenomena. It is an essential reading in one's quest to understand leadership.

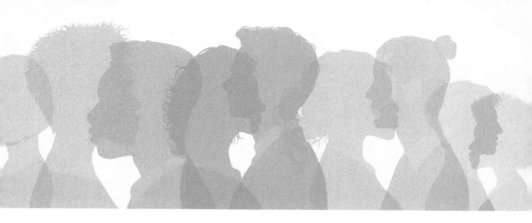

INDEX

Note: Page numbers with "f" refer to figures; those with "t" refer to tables.